W9-AOA-067

THE ECONOMICS

OF HEALTH

RECONSIDERED

Second Edition

THE ECONOMICS

OF HEALTH

RECONSIDERED

Second Edition

Thomas Rice

Health Administration Press, Chicago, Illinois
AcademyHealth, Washington, D.C.

Your board, staff, or clients may also benefit from this book's insight. For more information on quantity discounts, contact the Health Administration Press Marketing Manager at (312) 424-9470.

Library of Congress Cataloging-in-Publication Data

Rice, Thomas H.
    The economics of health reconsidered / Thomas Rice.—2nd ed.
      p. cm.
    Includes bibliographical references and index.
    ISBN 1-56793-193-6 (alk. paper)
      1. Medical economics—Mathematical models.   2. Medical care—Cost effectiveness.
    3. Medical economics—United States—Mathematical models.   I. Title.
    RA410.R53   2002
    338.4'33621—dc21   2002027615

The paper used in this publication meets the minimum requirements of American National Standard for Information Sciences—Permanence of Paper for Printed Library Materials, ANSI Z39.48-1984. ⊚™

Acquisitions manager: Audrey Kaufman; Project manager: Helen-Joy Bechtle; Book design: Matt Avery; Cover design: Anne LoCascio.

Health Administration Press
A division of the Foundation
of the American College of
Healthcare Executives
One North Franklin Street
Suite 1700
Chicago, IL 60606
(312) 424-2800

AcademyHealth
1801 K. Street, NW
Suite 701-L
Washington, DC 20006
(202) 292-6700

To Clara, Danny, and Kate, and to my parents,
Dorothy and Jim Rice

Contents

Foreword

OUR ENDLESS NATIONAL "conversation" about health policy has always revolved around what social role health services should play in the nation. Should health services be viewed merely as one of several basic, private consumption goods—such as food, clothing and shelter—of which society might be willing to make a basic quantity and quality available to those who cannot afford it on their own, but otherwise let the individual's care experience vary with that person's ability to pay for health services? Or should health services be viewed as a special social good that should be financed collectively, with contributions based on the individual's ability to pay, and distributed by criteria other than the individual's ability to pay?

It is appropriate to revisit and debate these value-laden questions regularly, and one could respectably favor one or the other of the two visions for health services. Alas, for some reason the participants in this debate rarely ever discuss these questions openly. Instead, participants conduct the debate with judiciously composed imagery or resort to the seemingly value-free but often quite treacherous jargon of economics—using words such as "efficiency," "rationing," and "cost effective." The result has been considerable confusion in our debate on health policy. Suspicion has also been cast on economists in their role as social scientists, when the ethical precepts hidden in their normative policy recommendations clash with the divergent ethical precepts held by decision makers in the public sector.

In an ideal world, one should never be able to infer the ideology of economists from their policy analyses. However, in the real world economists routinely are engaged by public decision makers on the basis, first, of the economist's political allegiance and, second, on their analytic prowess. Such is not a healthy state of affairs for a discipline that aspires to the label of "science."

Tom Rice's *The Economics of Health Reconsidered,* now in its second edition, addresses this troublesome facet of health policy analysis. The author carefully instructs readers on the crucial distinction between the purely *normative* and the purely *positive* facets of policy analysis, and how not to confuse the two with one another in *normative* policy analysis. Rice does so by laying bare the ethical premises that may be deeply buried in what may seem to the laity to be objectively scientific economic analysis. In principle, policy analysts should push their analysis to the point where moral trade-offs come into play and then allow those trade-offs to be made by those whose task it is to make them. Alternatively, economists should begin with a clearly stated social goal that is itself the product or a moral trade-off made by others, and then seek for methods to reach that goal with the least necessary sacrifice of real resources—that is, efficiently.

Rice also reminds readers of the many conditions that would have to be fulfilled before the market for health services could be said to approximate the standard textbook model of freely competitive markets. These conditions are much more stringent than seems widely supposed in the debate on health policy. Since Ronald Reagan's presidency 20 years ago, for example, health-policy circles have talked about a health services retail market in which savvy "consumers" (formerly "patients") could shop around freely for cost-effective care. It was taken for granted at the time that the requisite information infrastructure for such a market soon would emerge on the back of private entrepreneurship. So far, however, the American market for health services continues to resemble a haberdashery in which shirts are stored in white boxes, each labeled "shirt," but without showing on the outside of the box any information on the shirt's size or material, let alone price. Several months after freely choosing one of these boxes, the customer is sent an incomprehensible bill whose only understandable text is a red-framed box containing the statement "Pay this amount: $69.99." That, in a nutshell, remains the real-world model of the American health services market.

The air is full of promises once again that "soon" the information infrastructure for a flourishing retail market in health services will emerge, but the word "soon" might well mean another two decades. Much of that infrastructure would be a public good; however, private markets will not produce public goods in efficient quantities, and the public sector in this country will not likely step up to the task of financing the information infrastructure. In addition, the politically powerful supply side of the health market has little to gain from the greater transparency required by an adequate information infrastructure and will do everything in its power to retard the development of such a market.

That circumstance raises a question of professional ethics for economists, namely: can one fairly and responsibly advocate health policies that would thrust individual patients into a "consumer-driven" albeit opaque health services retail market that functions like the haberdashery described earlier? Should not the establishment of an adequate information infrastructure come first? Precisely how would that be done? For example, how would one convey to consumers (patients) in a given market area information on the fees charged by individual physicians in that market, when the CPT-4 code maintained by the American Medical Association and used by the federal Medicare program contains over 7,000 distinct items, each of which must be priced? Even if that information were available on a website, how would one convey to consumers information about the individual physician's practice style—that is, the resource-intensity of the physician's treatments and hence their cost? Finally, precisely how would one convey to consumers reliable information on the quality of a physician's services?

It is one thing for economists to repair the frictionless, virtual worlds they construct from axioms, theorems, and assumptions, and there to conduct the clever *Gedankenexperiments* that lead to tenure and possible renown. It is quite another, much more serious matter when economists use their analytic prowess to rearrange the real world, which may not sufficiently reflect the axioms, theorems, and assumptions made in modeling exercises, especially when that rearrangement may vastly redistribute economic privilege among members of society. One can certainly recommend such changes in the role of a citizen-advocate. One should not do so in the guise of objective science, with appeal to seemingly scientific methods that may embed hidden value judgments and with professional jargon that is apt to confuse the non-initiated. As Nobel Laureate Kenneth Arrow remarked on this point in his seminal article "Uncertainty and the Welfare Economics of Medical Care"[1]:

---

1. Arrow, K. J. 1963. "Uncertainty and the Welfare Economics of Medical Care." *American Economic Review* 78 (Dec.): 942–73.

A definition is just a definition, but when the *definiendum* is a word already in common use with highly favorable connotation, it is clear we [economists] are really trying to be persuasive; we are implicitly recommending the achievement of optimal states. (p. 942)

The much-used terms "efficiency" and "rationing" are examples of such words. To lay persons, "more efficient" typically means "better." As is well-known to students of economics, however, and as Tom Rice explains in this book, the word has no such connotation in the economist's dictionary. Similarly, lay persons are apt to think that a health system that rations care is worse than one that does not. Once again, economists may conclude quite the opposite.

The graph shown below exhibits so-called marginal-value curves for a baby's visit with a pediatrician. The curves represent two families, the high-income Chen family (the solid curve) and the low-income Smith family (the dashed curve). A new baby has just arrived in each family; Baby Chen is in perfect health, while Baby Smith was born with a number of health problems., Assume that neither family has health insurance coverage for routine baby care or, alternatively, that each family has a catastrophic insurance policy with a $5,000 deductible and is a long way from attaining that deductible with its health spending.

A family's marginal value curve indicates the maximum price it would bid for the nth annual visit, in addition to the previous $(n-1)$ visits. Presumably, that maximum bid price would be the monetary measure of the subjective *value* the family would attach to the nth visit. Another descriptive name for the curves therefore would be *willingness to pay curves*, where willingness to pay reflects in part the family's economic circumstance. In textbooks, the curves would be called simply *individual families' demand curves for pediatric visits*. These marginal value curves have great significance in economic analysis, because they are taken as indicators of the value that the decision makers they represent attach to the goods or services underlying the curves. Careless analysts might even call them indicators of "social value," although no presumption can be made that the value an individual family may attach to the nth pediatric visit for a baby will also be the value that society as a whole attaches to that visit.

The shapes and positions of the two families' marginal value curves would be determined in part by the families attitude toward this type of care—their "taste" for care, as economists would put it. The families would also be driven, however, by their willingness to pay for visits to

Figure: Individual Demand for Physician Visits

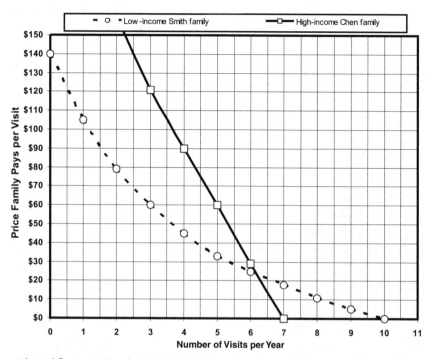

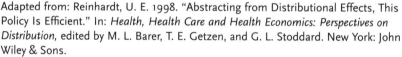

Adapted from: Reinhardt, U. E. 1998. "Abstracting from Distributional Effects, This Policy Is Efficient." In: *Health, Health Care and Health Economics: Perspectives on Distribution*, edited by M. L. Barer, T. E. Getzen, and G. L. Stoddard. New York: John Wiley & Sons.

the pediatrician, which, as noted, reflects also their ability to pay for that care. In many discussions on health policy the pretense is made that these curves are driven primarily by differences in "consumers' tastes" for health services. The role of ability to pay is given shorter shrift, if it is mentioned at all. Here it seems reasonable to suppose that, whatever the two families' tastes for pediatric visits might be, the shape and position of the curves are strongly dominated by the families' ability to pay for care. In other words, ability to pay, and not a difference in tastes for pediatric visits, leads the high-income Chen family to attach a value of $120 to the third annual visit, while the low-income Smith family would value that visit at only $60.

Efficiency

If, in the example illustrated above, the market for pediatric visits approximated the requirements of a competitive market in the two families' town, and if such visits could be procured at the going market price of $60 per visit, then, under the insurance regime assumed above (and already reflected in the families' demand curves) the sickly Baby Smith would have three visits per year to the pediatrician and the healthy Baby Chen, five visits per year. Because at these relative "consumption" rates each family would have paid for the last visit it purchased an amount equal to the marginal monetary value the family attaches to that visit, this resource allocation would be judged "efficient" by economists. Another way to put it is that it would not be possible to reallocate visits between the two families in a way that would make one family feel better off and the other not feel worse off.

Now suppose that, initially, a government-run health insurance program made pediatric visits free at point of service to all families, but rationed the total capacity available in the system in a way that would allocate five visits to sickly Baby Smith and only three visits to healthy Baby Chen. Suppose next that this system were replaced by the more market-based, catastrophic insurance regime assumed earlier, which means that as part of the adjustment to the new regime two pediatric visits per year would be reallocated from sickly Baby Smith to healthy Baby Chen. Would that transfer increase the "efficiency" of the health system and enhance "social welfare"?

Some economists would say so, on the following logic. Even under the government-run insurance system, the marginal value curves of the two families would have been latently in existence. Now that the market flushes them into the open, after the abolition of the government-run system, we can infer that the Smith family had associated a marginal value of $45 with the fourth visit that was transferred to health Baby Chen, and only $33 with the fifth visit, which also was transferred to healthy Baby Chen. In sum, the Smith family attached a value of only $78 to the two visits that were transferred from their baby to the Chen's baby. The Chen family, on the other hand, attached a monetary value of as much as $150 to the two extra visits Baby Chen now receives ($90 to the fourth and $60 to the fifth visit). Thus it might be said that the total net social value created by this transfer in the short run would be $72. Economists beholden to this form of "welfare analysis" might take this amount as the monetary measure of the net social-welfare gain achieved by switching from the assumed government-run health insurance system to the market-driven system with catastrophic health insurance. To phrase it slightly differently, economic welfare was increased by transferring two pediatric visits from a family that evidently values them relatively less to another that evidently values them relatively more.

Admittedly, the preceding example has been carefully constructed to highlight the precarious nature of words such as "efficiency" and "social welfare" in normative economic analysis of health policy. As Tom Rice illustrates in this volume, with his discussion of the concept of Pareto optimality, and as should be well-known by any properly trained economist, a resource allocation that would be said by economists to be more "efficient" than another is not necessarily "better" than the other. Under the efficient allocation, some people might live in gluttony while others are starving. In the less efficient allocation, no one might be starving. Unfortunately, among the laity the phrase "a more efficient resource allocation" is naturally thought to mean a "better resource allocation." It is sufficient reason for conscientious economists to use the term "efficiency" sparingly, and only in a manner that cannot possibly be misunderstood.

It could also be objected that the preceding example abstracted impermissibly from the possibility of "positive externalities" in the consumption of health services. Positive externalities would exist if someone other than the Smith and Chen families derived satisfaction from knowing that their babies received all medically necessary care. All economists recognize and acknowledge that, in the face of externalities, the demand curves representing individual consumers or families are not reliable measures of the social value of goods and services. Because the preceding example does not incorporate the possible presence of externalities, it might be said to be unfairly rigged to make a point.

The accusation would be valid. The example did abstract from externalities; but it did so to explore the oft-made proposition that third-party payment is the major source of inefficiency in our health system, and that greater efficiency could be attained by switching the health system to the market-driven, catastrophic health insurance system incorporated into the illustration. That proposition has been put by none other than the distinguished Nobel Laureate Milton Friedman, who offered it first during the health-reform debate of the early 1990s[2] and recently updated and

2. Friedman, M. 1991. "Gammons Law Points to Health Care Solution," *The Wall Street Journal* November 12: A21.

expanded it in an article entitled "How to Cure Health Care" published in the prominent policy journal *The Public Interest*.[3]

In his earlier commentary, in which he acknowledged the contribution of a fellow Nobel Laureate, economist Gary S. Becker of the University of Chicago, Friedman wrote that

> [T]he *inefficiency*, high cost and inequitable character of our medical system can be fundamentally remedied in only one way: by moving in the other direction, toward re-privatizing medical care. . . . The [proposed] reform has two major steps: (1) End both Medicare and Medicaid and replace them with a requirement that every U.S. family unit have a major medical insurance policy with a high deductible, say $20,000 a year or 30% of the unit's income during the prior two years, whichever is lower. (2) End the tax exemption of employer provided medical care. . . . Each individual or family would, of course, be free to buy supplementary insurance, if it so desired. (Emphasis added)

To put Friedman's policy recommendation in perspective, it may be noted that in 1990, at about the time Friedman formulated his recommendation, median pretax income in the United States was $29,943 for all households and $35,353 for "families," that is, for households with two or more members.[4] If we generously assume that Friedman meant to base the recommended deductible not on the sum of the family's income during the past two years but only the average annual family income over the prior two years, then that deductible in 1990 would have been $10,500 per year for a family with median pretax income of $35,353. The outlays on health services of a relatively healthy family probably would not have reached that deductible. A family stricken with serious illness almost surely would have had to pay that much out of pocket before insurance coverage would set in. In addition, of course, each family would have to pay the premium for the catastrophic insurance policy.

Evidently, in his commentary, Friedman the economist suggested to a lay readership that the replacement of an "inefficient" government-run health insurance system, such as Medicaid, with the market-driven, catastrophic insurance scheme he proposed would be more "efficient," which

---

3. Friedman, M. 2001. "How to Cure Healthcare." *The Public Interest* 142 (Winter).
4. Stockman, A. 1996. *Introduction to Microeconomics.* New York: The Dryden Press.

lay persons were bound to interpret as "better." As Kenneth Arrow would put it, with appeal to the issue of efficiency, Friedman sought to persuade readers to his own political preference. For, surely, neither Milton Friedman nor anyone else would assume for a moment that the distribution of health services in the United States, the distribution of the financial burden of illness, and the sociodemographic profile of health status would be the same under his proposal—including as it would the complete abolition of Medicare and Medicaid—as they would be in the presence of these programs or under yet other health-reform proposals. As every properly trained economist knows, or should know, two alternative public policies cannot be meaningfully compared in terms of their relative economic efficiency if they aim at different social goals—here, at different distributions of economic privilege among members of society. Thus, the call between the two policies in this illustration cannot objectively be made on the basis of relative economic efficiency. It is an inherently political call that economists are not entitled to make in their role as scientists—although they certainly could make it as a political argument in their role as citizen-advocates.

Rationing

In the stylized example used earlier, we had started with an initial position in which a government-run health system rationed care between the two babies on what appeared to be clinical criteria. We then assumed that this regime was replaced with a market-based, catastrophic insurance system. At the new, allegedly more "efficient" market-driven equilibrium, healthy Baby Chen had two more pediatric visits per year and sickly Baby Smith two less. A fundamental question that frequently comes up in debates on health policy is this: *did the switch from a government-run regime to a market-driven regime eliminate the rationing of care?* During the health reform debate of the mid 1990s, for example, the opponents of government-run universal health insurance often argued that such systems inevitably lead to the rationing of health services, which could be avoided under the market-driven systems. Is that proposition really valid?

Remarkably, economists are stuck in the semantic mud on this seemingly simple question.

In their well-known textbook *Microeconomics*, Michael Katz and Harvey Rosen flatly assert that "prices ration scarce resources."[5] Similarly,

---

5. Katz, M. L., and H. S. Rosen. 1997. *Microeconomics*, p. 15. Homewood, IL: Irwin.

in his textbook *Principles of Microeconomics,* James Kearl instructs students that "prices ration commodities on the basis of willingness to pay."[6] According to that interpretation of the word "rationing," which I fully share and which I inherited from my teachers at Yale University, the switch from a government-run to a market-driven health system would not avoid the rationing of health services. The switch would merely replace one form of rationing (non-price rationing) with another (price rationing), and would result in rather different distributional consequences.

Not all economists agree with this interpretation of the word "rationing." In his commentary on a presentation by economist Mark Pauly at a recent health services conference, for example, Brookings Institution economist Henry Aaron (2002)[7] argued that

> Eliminating care that is worth less than it costs is a precise definition of rational rationing. Rationing occurs when administrative rules prevent people who have money enough to buy from buying. (As an aside, the term "price rationing" should be an oxymoron for economists. To label as rationing a situation when people cannot afford to buy something because it is too expensive—as some do when they say that health care has always been rationed because the poor cannot afford as much of it as the rest of us—is equivalent to saying that people who lack money to buy everything they want are experiencing rationing. . . . Calling non-satiety "rationing" would drain the term of any meaning). (p. 5)

One can agree with Aaron that, as a matter of analytic convenience, economists might as well confine the term "rationing" to situations in which scarce resources are allocated by algorithms other than price and ability to pay, if only to avoid having to write "non-price rationing" and "price-rationing" every times the occasion arises. Economists would know that, with this particular definition of the word "rationing," a health system that rations care among citizens might be widely preferred

---

6. Kearl, J. R. 1993. *Principles of Economics,* p. 288. Lexington, MA: D.C. Heath & Co.

7. Aaron, H. J. 2002. "Should Public Policy Seek to Control the Growth of Health Care Spending?" (Mimeographed). Remarks prepared for the *Ninth Annual Princeton Conference,* sponsored by the Robert Wood Johnson Foundation and organized by the Council on Health Care Economics and Policy, Brandeis University, Waltham, MA.

by the citizenry to one that does not. Indeed, in his commentary Aaron goes on to argue, "the *only* way that a *civilized* society can rein in moral hazard [in health services] is through the imposition of effective budget limits in a way that constrains the supply of the health system" (p. 8, italics added). One gains the impression from that sentence that Aaron considers artificially limiting the capacity of the health system and then the rationing of this artificially scarce capacity by administrative or clinical algorithms a more "civilized" method of reining in moral hazard in health services than a market-driven system that seeks to limit the system through high deductibles and coinsurance—that is, by price and ability to pay.

Unfortunately, non-economists would be unlikely to grasp these semantic fine points. If, in a public debate on health policy, a lay audience were told by economists that policy A would lead to the rationing of health services while policy B would not, the majority in the audience would be likely to think of B as the superior health policy. Carefully and explicitly distinguishing in policy analysis between price and non-price rationing could help eliminate this dissonance.

Every economist and policy analyst always is both a social scientist and a political creature with his or her own ideology. Even the most conscientious economists face a challenge to keep analyses completely free from ideology. The questions raised, the analytic framework chosen, the assumptions made in analysis, and the data selected to support it all are conduits through which ideology can seep, wittingly or unwittingly, into the analysis,.

Given this perennial challenge to health policy analysts, it is a delight that colleague Tom Rice has gone to the trouble of returning the spotlight to intra-professional debates that had been decisively settled decades ago—by the then giants of our profession[8]—but whose outcome seems to have been all but forgotten or deliberately suppressed by subsequent generations of economists. If nothing else, the book should trigger the revival of a philosophical debate that should be had anew by every generation of economists and policy analysts.

A welcome addition to the second edition of the book is a lengthy chapter on the role of government in a nation's health system. The

---

8. See, for example, Bator, F. M. 1958. "The Simple Economics of Welfare Economics." *American Economic Review* 72 (Aug.): 351–79 and especially Baumol, W. J. 1969. *Welfare Economics and the Theory of the State.* Cambridge, MA: Harvard University Press.

author's extensive survey of rival theories on the role of government in the economy reminds readers that every nation must continuously choose between market failure and government failures, and that there is no obvious, ideal choice between the two. After a cross-national survey of health systems, accompanied by a wealth of statistical material, Rice boldly sets forth the ten lessons he draws from that survey, fully aware no doubt that not all serious students of the subject matter would concur. Whatever individual readers may conclude, however, it is surely helpful to be forced to think once more beyond the increasingly popular theory that has been distilled into a famous axiom by Congressman Dick Armey, formerly an economics professor and currently Majority Leader of the U.S. House of Representatives: "The market is rational and the government is dumb."[9] Perhaps the Congressman would sleep more soundly if our government's functions were taken over by the genius and the mores of the folks who run Wall Street, the telecommunications industry, or the energy industry. Millions of his constituents might not.

The sundry critiques of the market offered in this valuable book, and other critiques of the literature advocating the "market" for health services,[10] should not be read as aimed at any proposal to engage the market approach in health services, for the critique is not intended as such. In many instances market forces can, indeed, be constructively engaged in health to achieve explicitly stated social goals. Rather, the book and other such critiques should be read as pleas that social goals not be posited inadvertently or surreptitiously in policy analysis, either carelessly through normative economic analysis or through deliberately mischievous use. It is difficult enough at times for economists to see through such tactics; it is well-nigh impossible for even highly educated lay persons—let alone for the general public—to see through these tactics.

Uwe E. Reinhardt, Ph.D.
James Madison Professor of Political Economy, Professor of Economics
    and Public Affairs
Princeton University

9. Armey, D. 2002. [Online source.] http://armey.house.gov/axioms.htm

10. Barer, M. L., T. E. Getzen, and G. L. Stoddard. 1998. *Health, Health Care and Health Economics: Perspectives on Distribution* New York: John Wiley & Sons.

Acknowledgments

MUCH OF THE research contained in this book was conducted while I was on two sabbaticals from the University of California at Los Angeles. I would like to express my deep appreciation to a number of people for providing comments on the research itself or on the individual chapters. Material in the first edition was read and commented on by Henry Aaron, Ronald Andersen, William Comanor, Katherine Desmond, Robert Evans, Rashi Fein, Paul Feldstein, Susan Haber, Diana Hilberman, Donald Light, Harold Luft, David Mechanic, Glenn Melnick, Gavin Mooney, Joseph Newhouse, Mark Peterson, Uwe Reinhardt, John Roemer, Sally Stearns, Greg Stoddart, Deborah Stone, Pete Welch, and Joseph White. Chapter 6, which is new to this edition, was reviewed by Gerard Anderson, Miriam Laugesen, Gavin Mooney, Joseph White, and Miriam Wiley. Reviewers of the materials on the individual countries in the Appendix include John Creighton Campbell, Finn Diderichsen, Eddy Van Doorslaer, Susan Giaimo, Jeremiah Hurley, Gavin Mooney, Kieke Okma, Valérie Paris, Kristina Bränd Persson, Lise Rochaix-Ranson, Erik Schut, Björn Smedby, Clive H. Smee, Paul Talcott, and Peter Zweifel. My thanks also go to Charles Doran and Karen Gorostieta for preparing the figures included in the book. Finally, I would also like to express my appreciation to Miriam Laugesen for preparing most of the material in the Appendix on the health services systems of various countries. It goes without saying that all conclusions, and any errors, are entirely my own and are not the responsibility of any of the reviewers.

Acknowledgments

Preface to the Second Edition

IT HAS BEEN nearly five years since the first edition of *The Economics of Health Reconsidered* was published. That expanse of time alone is probably sufficient to justify an updated version, given the growth and rapid progress in health economics and health services research. Indeed, I have made efforts to update the text and references, and have added two new health applications on topics that have received much attention recently: how the distribution of income affects health (Chapter 2) and defined contribution insurance products, Medicare premium support proposals, and medical savings accounts (Chapter 3).

The primary reason for coming out with a new edition, however, stems from some criticisms of the previous material. It was claimed— I think, quite correctly—that while I was critical of markets in the health services area, I did not provide a parallel critique of government involvement (Dowd 1999; Pauly 1997). As a result, this new edition adds another chapter, entitled "The Role of Government" (Chapter 6). It begins by discussing government failure so as to parallel earlier material on market failure. But because policy conclusions tend to be based more on experiences rather than theory, the remainder of this chapter focuses on the ways in which countries actually organize their health sectors. The chapter categorizes the different choices that countries must make in tailoring their own health systems, provides evidence on health costs, access, and quality in ten selected developed countries, and concludes with ten "lessons" drawn from the preceding material. Although this new chapter in general, and the lessons in particular, are based on my own views, it is my hope that they will stimulate more thought on the appropriate roles of markets and government for achieving better organization, financing, and delivery of health services.

Chapter 1

Introduction

1.1 WHY SHOULD THE ECONOMICS OF HEALTH BE RECONSIDERED?

Recent years have seen a surge of interest in reforming the organization and delivery of health systems by replacing government regulation with a reliance on market forces. Although much of the impetus has come from the United States, the phenomenon is worldwide. Spurred by ever-increasing costs, coupled with the financial problems facing numerous countries' governments, many analysts and policymakers have embraced the competitive market as the means of choice for reforming medical care systems. To a great extent, this belief stems from economic theory, which purports to show the superiority of markets over heavy government involvement.

During the latter part of the 1990s, increased competition in the U.S. health services sector did help control the rate of increase in costs. The main manifestation of this competition was the increase in managed care enrollment, and concomitant decline in fee-for-service. Between 1993 and 2001, for example, the percentage of workers covered by conventional fee-for-service insurance declined from 49 percent to just 7 percent (Jensen et al. 1997; Gabel et al. 2001). The second half of the 1990s also showed much lower inflation in health costs than had been the case in the previous decades. Average per capita health expenditures rose only 5 percent annually, approximately the same amount as the economy as a whole, and far less than in previous years (U.S. DHHS 2001). In addition, various studies have shown that the geographic areas in which managed care penetration is highest have experienced the smallest increases in health costs (Zwanziger and Melnick 1996; Bamezai et al. 1999).

Whether this indicates that the health services market in the United States is indeed operating in a more efficient manner than it used to be is less clear, however, as improved efficiency depends not only on costs, but also on what we are getting for the money.[1] More Americans are uninsured than previously, most likely in part because of additional competition among health insurers.[2] In addition, although the empirical evidence is still ambiguous, much concern now exists about how increased competition among providers and insurers has affected the quality of care provided.

The onset of the new millennium also brings the signs of changes. Health-related costs in the United States are beginning to rise again. Premiums increased by 11 percent in the employer-sponsored market during 2001 (Gabel et al. 2001), and various factors point to continued double-digit rates—most notably, an explosion in pharmaceutical costs. Other factors include consumer dissatisfaction with "heavy-handed" managed care techniques; insurer and provider responses to the prospects of "consumer bills of rights"; and increasing consolidation of market power as more insurers and providers merge. Thus, whether markets will be able to repeat their cost-containment successes of the previous decade is in doubt.

Nevertheless, the perceived success of this increasingly competitive marketplace in health services is perhaps emblematic of a larger trend in the United States, in which markets are viewed as "efficient" and government is viewed as "inefficient." As Robert Kuttner (1997) has written, "America . . . is in one of its cyclical romances with a utopian view

---

1. Alain Enthoven (1988) makes this point nicely, writing, "An efficient allocation of health care resources to and within the health care sector is one that minimizes the social cost of illness, including its treatment. This is achieved when the marginal dollar spent on health care produces the same value to society as the marginal dollar spent on education, defense, personal consumption, and other uses. Relevant costs include the suffering and inconvenience of patients, as well as the resources used in producing health care. This goal should not be confused with minimizing or containing health care expenditures. Policy makers focus much attention on the total amount of spending on health care services, often as a share of gross national product (GNP). But, a lower percentage of GNP spent on health care does not necessarily mean greater efficiency. If the reduced share of GNP is achieved by denial or postponement of services that consumers would value at more than their marginal cost, then efficiency is not achieved or enhanced by the cut in spending" (p. 11).

2. In the four-year period between 1994 and 1998, the percentage of nonelderly Americans under age 65 who were uninsured rose from 14.3 to 16.5 percent (U.S. DHHS 2001).

of laissez-faire" (p. 4). This does not imply, either in the health services sector or in the economy as a whole, that policymakers have eschewed government involvement. My concern, however, is that the trend is going in this direction, and that economic theory is used—inappropriately, it will be argued—in support of further market-based health policies.

Indeed, all health economists—even those favoring a more competitive marketplace—recognize that government needs to play a significant role in the health system. Much of the work in this area is based on the writings of Alain Enthoven (1978a, 1978b, 1988; and Enthoven and Kronick 1989a, 1989b), who has over the past quarter century advocated reliance on consumer choice and markets to improve the efficiency of health markets, with government playing two key roles: ensuring that competition is based on price rather than the selection of the healthiest patients, and providing subsidies to low-income persons.[3]

The corollary to this viewpoint is that government *should* confine itself to only these two roles. Stated another way, competition should form the basis of policy in the health services area, with government playing a subsidiary role of ensuring that markets operate fairly and that disadvantaged people are helped out. This conclusion, however, does not fall out of a careful review of economic theory as applied to health.

This book contends that one of the main reasons for the belief that market-based systems are superior stems from a misunderstanding of economic theory as it applies to health. As will be shown, such conclusions are based on a large set of assumptions that are not met and cannot be met in the health services sector. This is not to say that competitive approaches in this sector of the economy are inappropriate; rather, their efficacy depends on the particular circumstances of the policy being considered and the environment in which it is to be implemented. There is, however, no a priori reason to believe that such a system will operate more efficiently, or provide a higher level of social welfare, than alternative systems that are based instead on governmental financing and regulation. This argument is further bolstered by the fact that so many other developed countries have chosen to deviate from market-based health systems.

---

3. Enthoven's earliest work in this area was published in *The New England Journal of Medicine* (Enthoven 1978a and 1978b), followed up by a book (Enthoven 1980). A significant revision of the proposal appears in Enthoven (1988) and Enthoven and Kronick (1989a and 1989b), in which "sponsors" such as large employers or consortia of small employers would serve as brokers for consumers who purchase health insurance.

Although economists are aware that claims about the superiority of competitive approaches are based on fulfillment of a number of assumptions, a reading of the health literature contains little mention of either the large number of such assumptions, or of their importance. One should not put undue blame on health economists, however, because this problem pervades the entire economic discipline. In this regard, Lester Thurow (1983) has written that "every economist knows the dozens of restrictive assumptions . . . that are necessary to 'prove' that a free market is the best possible economic game, but they tend to be forgotten in the play of events" (p. 22).

Although the conclusion that competition will result in optimal economic outcomes is based on many assumptions, no list has been generally agreed upon, and various economists have come up with different lists. The list presented below was drawn from several writers: Graaff (1971), Henderson and Quandt (1980), Mishan (1969a, 1969b), Nath (1969), Ng (1979), Rowley and Peacock (1975), and Sen (1982).

The book thus centers around a description, analysis, and application of these assumptions—and in particular, what happens if they are not met in markets for health services. The specific assumptions examined, along with the chapters in which they are analyzed, are shown in Table 1.1. (Some of these will not be self-explanatory to the noneconomist reader; they will be clarified in the specified chapters.) It is noteworthy that this is only a *partial* list of the assumptions on which the superiority of the competitive model is based. Other assumptions are not mentioned here either because they are essentially the same as those noted above, or because, in the author's opinion, the health economics profession has dealt with them adequately.[4]

---

4. One exception is the *theory of the second best.* Suppose that two or more of the assumptions in Table 1.1 are not met. It might seem reasonable to suppose that public policy should focus on trying to improve one of these particular market imperfections. This, however, is not necessarily the case. This theory states that if multiple factors cause a market to deviate from the assumptions of market competition, then it is not necessarily appropriate to try to make the market more competitive in selected areas (Lipsey and Lancaster 1956–1957).

A hypothetical example in the health field might help clarify this. Suppose that two of the assumptions on which economic competition is based do not hold: there are few firms, which results in monopoly power; and consumer information is poor. The theory shows that more competition in one of these areas will not necessarily bring us any closer to an optimal state and, in fact, may have the opposite effect. If there are a limited number of firms, then

1.2 PURPOSE OF THE BOOK

As the title suggests, the purpose of this book is to reconsider the economics of health. It does so by examining the assumptions on which the superiority of competitive approaches are based, and how, if they are not met, this affects health policy choices.

Although each chapter provides numerous applications, the book is also about theory—both its use and its misuse. The book will attempt to show that *economic theory* provides no support for the belief that competition in the health services sector will lead to superior social outcomes.

If one accepts the viewpoint that economic theory does not demonstrate the superiority of market forces in health, the obvious corollary is that all important questions must be answered empirically. And, to a large extent, that is exactly what most health economists and health services researchers are trying to do. The author has few reservations about the kinds of research studies that are being conducted; rather, the concern is that the work will suffer if researchers approach it with preconceived notions of what the results ought to be.

Economists often take the viewpoint that the way to test a theory—such as the purported advantages of market competition—is to see how well it predicts. This may work well when we are evaluating *positive* (i.e.,

---

better information about price might allow firms to set prices as in a cartel (Fielding and Rice 1993). Or if information were limited, then as the number of physicians in an area rose, it would become increasingly difficult for consumers to keep track of prices and reputation in the market. As a result, consumers might have to pay higher physician prices than they might otherwise (Satterthwaite 1979; Pauly and Satterthwaite 1981). Thus, even within the economic model, increased competition may not always be desirable.

Because so many assumptions of the competitive marketplace are not met in the health services area, second-best considerations are pervasive. The most important one, perhaps, is the existence of health insurance itself. When consumers have health insurance, the price they pay out-of-pocket for services is less than the cost of providing the services. (In a competitive marketplace, prices and costs are equivalent in the long run.) The theory of the second best therefore tells us that *other* competitive policies are not necessarily optimal in the presence of health insurance.

One problem with using second-best considerations to critique competitive economic policies in the health area is that, realistically, none can pass a second-best test. As indicated, nearly always, several aspects of a market do not conform to the assumptions of competition. None of the arguments made in this book rely on second-best considerations. Readers wishing to pursue this topic should examine Robert Kuttner's (1997) book, *Everything for Sale: The Virtue and Limits of Markets*, for a detailed analysis of applying the theory of the second best to the health services sector and to several other markets.

Table 1.1: Assumptions of Market Competition and their Further Treatment in the Remaining Chapters

Chapter 2: Market Competition
  1. There are no negative externalities of consumption.
  2. There are no positive externalities of consumption.
  3. Consumer tastes are predetermined.

Chapter 3: Demand Theory
  4. A person is the best judge of his or her own welfare.
  5. Consumers have sufficient information to make good choices.
  6. Consumers know, with certainty, the results of their consumption decisions.
  7. Individuals are rational.
  8. Individuals reveal their preferences through their actions.
  9. Social welfare is based solely on individual utilities, which in turn are based solely on the goods and services consumed.

Chapter 4: Supply Theory
  10. Supply and demand are independently determined.
  11. Firms do not have any monopoly power.
  12. Firms maximize profits.
  13. There are not increasing returns to scale.
  14. Production is independent of the distribution of wealth.

Chapter 5: Equity and Redistribution
  9. Social welfare is based solely on individual utilities, which in turn are based solely on the goods and services consumed.
  15. The distribution of wealth is approved of by society.

factual) issues—say, the effect of a change in patient copayments on service utilization. It is less helpful in evaluating *normative* issues—those that involve the word "should."

The field of *welfare economics* deals in the latter kinds of issues—for example, *should* we rely on competitive policies in the health services sector? In such instances, assessing how well the theory predicts does little good, because different analysts will disagree about which alternative state of the world is at a higher level of welfare. For example, if the United States were to adopt a Canadian-style "single-payer" system, there would likely be little agreement among health economists about whether the population was better off under the new system or the old one.

In this regard, Jan de V. Graaff (1971) has written,

> [W]elfare . . . is not an observable quantity like a market price or an item of personal consumption [so] it is exceedingly difficult to test a welfare proposition. . . . The consequence is that, whereas the normal way of testing a theory in positive economics is to test its conclusions, *the normal way of testing a welfare proposition is to test its assumptions.* . . . The result is that our assumptions must be scrutinized with care and thoroughness. Each must stand on its own two feet. We cannot afford to simplify much. (pp. 2–3, emphasis added)

Thus, it is vitally important that we get our theory right when applying economics to health—and the key to this is understanding the validity of the assumptions. If we do not, then we will blind ourselves to policy options that might actually be best at enhancing social welfare, many of which simply cannot be derived from the conventional economic model. One of the primary purposes of this book is to understand the implications that arise when many important assumptions that underlie the advantages of competition are not met in health services.

It is important also to set out what the book does *not* do. Some readers will be disappointed to see that, although the book critiques the competitive model, it does not explicitly offer a theoretical alternative in its place. It does however compare the health systems of countries that use different amounts of government versus markets. Unfortunately, the cross-national empirical data that can be used to draw conclusions about the success of alternative systems are still somewhat scanty. Ultimately, readers must draw their own conclusions about the most desirable sort of system using both theory and the extant empirical literature.

This leads to a second limitation. Unlike some other health economics texts, this one does not attempt to summarize the empirical work in the field. As such, it is not designed to serve as a stand-alone textbook for courses in health economics or health policy. Rather, the book can be used as a supplementary textbook, in addition to one of the more traditional health economics texts, or along with a reader of classic or current economics journal articles.

This book is intended to serve several audiences, not just students. One of its primary audiences is health economics professionals in universities, research firms, management, and government. Although the book contains economic background that is hardly necessary for such an audience, the main theme is intended to strike a nerve, making readers realize that the case for relying on competitive markets in health does not arise from a careful reading of economic theory.

Finally, the book is also addressed to noneconomics professions. Because practitioners in these disciplines obviously tend to be less schooled in the details of economic analysis, they often have to take health economists at their word when the latter speak about the policy implications of economic analysis. (In this regard, Joan Robinson has been quoted as advising, "Study economics to avoid being deceived by economists" [Kuttner 1984, p. 1].) It is hoped that this book will help put those in other disciplines on a more level playing field when it comes to discussions of health policy.

1.3 OUTLINE OF THE BOOK

The book is divided into seven chapters. Chapters 2 through 4 deal with the three central themes of microeconomic theory: market competition, demand theory, and supply theory. The first 14 assumptions listed in Table 1.1 are analyzed in those chapters. Chapter 5 explores the final assumption, equity and redistribution, a topic of tremendous importance to policy but one that has been given insufficient attention by health economists. Chapter 6 is new to this edition of the book, and provides a discussion of potential problems with government involvement in markets in general, different ways and degrees in which government can be involved in the health services sector, some cross-national empirical evidence, and tentative lessons from this evidence. Chapter 7, the conclusion, offers some final thoughts concerning the role of competition in health services. The Appendix provides a brief overview of the health services systems in ten developed countries, to aid in the understanding of Chapter 6.

Chapters 2 through 5 share a similar format. First, they present the traditional economic model, so that readers not familiar with intermediate microeconomics will find the remaining material accessible. Readers already familiar with the core concepts of microeconomic theory can skip these sections (Sections 2.1, 3.1, 4.1, and 5.1) and go directly to the two remaining parts of these chapters: problems with the traditional model (Sections 2.2, 3.2, 4.2, and 5.2), and implications for health policy (Sections 2.3, 3.3, 4.3, and 5.3).

Chapter 2

Market Competition

THE ECONOMIES OF nearly all developed countries are based on market competition. In health, the extent of reliance on private markets varies from country to country, with the United States generally being viewed as more "market like" than others. In recent years, however, many (but not all) developed countries—not just the United States—have moved to instill more market competition and less government into national health systems. Several examples are provided in Chapter 6. This chapter, after presenting the reader with background on competition, addresses whether economic theory provides a strong enough justification for enacting competitive policies in the health services area.

Section 2.1 summarizes the traditional model of competition, including some of the standard tools of microeconomic analysis. Section 2.2 explores three of the most critical assumptions used in justifying the advantages of a competitive marketplace. Section 2.3 draws a number of implications for health policy.

2.1 THE TRADITIONAL ECONOMIC MODEL
The field of microeconomics is devoted to the study of competition—mainly its virtues, but also some of its pitfalls. Although many of the techniques economists use are fairly new, the emphasis on competition—dating back to the writings of Adam Smith (1776) more than 200 years ago—is not. Smith believed that people driven by their own economic interest in the marketplace are guided by an "invisible hand" to act in a manner that ultimately is most beneficial to society at large.

The notion of competition is intuitively appealing. In a competitive market, people are allowed but not compelled to trade their wealth,

9

including their labor, if they find it beneficial to do so. Figuratively speaking, once everyone stops trading because no additional advantage is apparent, the market is in *equilibrium*. Such an outcome is desirable on two fronts: (1) people are making their own choices; and (2) by not engaging in any more trades, people *reveal themselves*[1] to be as satisfied as possible with their economic lot, given the resources with which they began.

This section outlines the economic theory of competition, what competition can and cannot achieve, and the assumptions on which this theory is based. It is divided into four subsections: consumers, producers, the economy as a whole, and Pareto optimality and social welfare. The presentation is informal and brief, providing just enough information to support the remaining material in the chapter. Those familiar with standard microeconomic theory can proceed immediately to Section 2.2, and those seeking more detail on the material presented may wish to consult any of a number of microeconomics textbooks.[2]

2.1.1 Consumers

In consumer theory, people seek to maximize their *utility* (i.e., happiness), which is largely determined by the bundle of goods and services that they possess. To do so, they purchase their ideal bundle based on their desire or *taste* for alternative goods, and on the prices of these alternatives, subject, of course, to how much income they have available to spend.

We will define U as the level of utility that a representative consumer receives from the consumption of alternative quantities of "n" different goods and services, indicated as X, Y, Z, and so on.

$$U = f(X, Y, Z, \ldots, n) \tag{2.1}$$

The utility obtained from consumption of one more unit of any good is called its *marginal utility*.

It is further assumed that consumers prefer more of a good to less of it, but that at some point, additional units of a particular good bring less utility than previous units; this is known as *diminishing marginal utility*. These concepts can be represented graphically by an *indifference curve*, which shows alternative combinations of two goods that result in the

---

1. Chapter 3, on the theory of demand, discusses the concept of revealed preference.

2. There are many good introductory microeconomics textbooks; Parkin (1999) is an example.

Figure 2.1: Consumer Indifference Curves

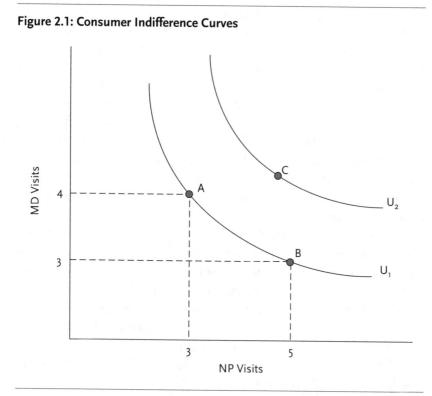

same level of utility. Indifference curves (examples of which are shown in Figure 2.1) tend to have a convex-to-the-origin shape because of diminishing marginal utility; once a person has a great deal of one good and little of another, that person has to receive a lot more of the former in order to give up even a little bit of the latter. The slope of the indifference curve is called the *marginal rate of substitution*. It is equal to the ratio of the marginal utilities of the two goods.[3]

---

3. This can be demonstrated as follows. Along an indifference curve, the consumer's level of utility is constant. Thus, any movement along the curve (which defines the curve's slope) represents a change only in the way in which the consumer achieves a given level of utility. If he or she has more of Y and less of X, the gain in utility from the former must equal the loss in utility from the latter. Specifically,

$$(\Delta Y) \times (MU_Y) = (\Delta X) \times (MU_X)$$

Rearranging these terms, we find that the slope of the indifference curve $(\Delta Y / \Delta X)$ equals the ratio of the marginal utilities of the two goods.

To make this less abstract, Figure 2.1 shows only two goods that might appear in a consumer's utility function: visits to physicians (MDs) and visits to nurse practitioners (NPs). (For expository purposes, it is also helpful to assume that all of a person's money is spent on these two services.) The quantity of nurse practitioner visits appears on the horizontal axis, and the quantity of physician visits, on the vertical axis. The consumer is indifferent to all points on curve U_1, since by definition all points bring equal levels of satisfaction. As drawn, three NP visits and four MD visits (point A) are equal in desirability to five NP visits and three MD visits (point B). The person would be even happier to have more (for example, point C on curve U_2), but that would involve spending more money than he or she has available.

The choice of how much of each type of visit to purchase depends not only on how much the person wants each type, but also on the respective price. The way in which consumers maximize utility is to spend each successive dollar in a way that brings about the most utility. This means that when they have spent their last dollar, consumers will, across all of the goods in their utility function, have equalized the ratio of the marginal utilities (*MU*) with the price of the good. If we define P_m as the price of MD visits, and P_n as the price of NP visits, then, for a consumer who has maximized his or her utility,

$$MU_m / P_m = MU_n / P_n \qquad (2.2)$$

By cross-multiplying and rearranging the terms, this can also be written and thought of in another way, where the ratios of the marginal utilities are equal to the price ratios of the two goods:

$$MU_m / MU_n = P_m / P_n \qquad (2.3)$$

It is easy to see why a consumer must fulfill Equation 2.2 (and therefore also Equation 2.3) in order to maximize utility. Suppose that the equality is not met, because the marginal utility of each good equals 1 but the price of MD visits is $50 and the price of NP visits only $25. In this case, the consumer would not be in equilibrium but, rather, would find it beneficial to buy more NP visits and fewer MD visits with his or her income. This will, however, result in lower marginal utility of NP visits, and higher marginal utility for MD visits. Only when both sides of Equation 2.2 (or 2.3) are equal will the consumer have nothing left to gain from trading.

Figure 2.2: The Consumer "Optimum"

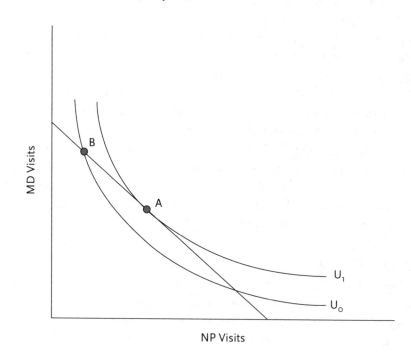

This concept is illustrated in Figure 2.2. Here, the straight line is the consumer's *budget constraint*, which shows how many of each type of visit the consumer can purchase with a given income. Its slope is the price ratio between NP and MD visits; the point at which the line intersects each axis shows how many of each the consumer could buy by spending all income on that single service. At point *A*, the slope of the consumer's indifference curve is tangent to (i.e., has the same slope as) the budget constraint. In contrast, at point *B* they do not have the same slope, and the consumer is on an indifference curve that conveys less utility, U_0. By trading MD visits for NP visits, it is possible to move down the budget constraint to point *A*, and thereby to increase utility by moving to the higher indifference curve, U_1.

What is remarkable is that the theory shows that *everyone* will have the same ratio of marginal utilities between any two goods and services. This is certainly clear mathematically; if everyone faces the same price ratio, the only way in which Equations 2.2 and 2.3 can hold is if everyone has the same ratio between their marginal utilities. How can that be achieved? Suppose a person really prefers NP visits and only wants an occasional MD visit. At the prevailing price ratio between the two services, the person will purchase a far greater quantity of NP visits. But at some point, the person will have so many NP visits that the utility brought about by the last one is very low—so low that the ratio of the marginal utilities between NP and MD visits becomes equal to the price ratio.

Broadly speaking, consumer theory concludes that people, taking into account their own preferences and market prices, can make choices that will make them best off. When they have done as well as they can do, given their resources, they stop trading, presumably to enjoy the mix of goods that they have acquired. These are strong conclusions; much of Chapters 2 and 3 will be devoted to examining and critiquing the assumptions on which they are based.

2.1.2 Producers

In production theory, firms seek to maximize profits in a way analogous to the way in which consumers attempt to maximize utility. To do so, they purchase inputs and transform them into outputs through the application of some sort of technology. This process is represented through a *production function.*

We will use one of the goods discussed above, MD visits, but this time will examine how it is produced by a firm. Assume that there are "m" ($a, b, \ldots, m$) inputs that are used in producing these visits through a production process "f." The production function therefore takes the form,

$$\text{Visits} = f(a, b, \ldots, m) \qquad (2.4)$$

The two most important classes of inputs are labor and capital.

Again, parallel to consumer theory, we assume that, given a fixed level of the other inputs, at some point additional units of a particular input will be less and less productive, a concept called *diminishing marginal productivity.* These concepts can be represented graphically by *isoquants,* as shown in Figure 2.3. Quantities of each of two inputs, *a* and *b*, are represented on the two axes; the isoquant labeled "visits" shows the alternative quantity of inputs required to produce a certain number of visits. The other isoquant indicates the inputs necessary for producing "more visits." The slope of an isoquant is called the *marginal rate of technical*

Figure 2.3: Producer Isoquants

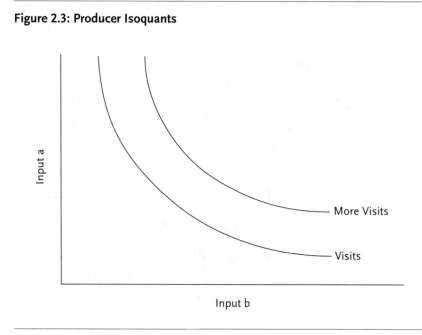

substitution and is equal to the ratios of the marginal productivities of each input.[4]

If, given the state of technology, a firm produces as much output as possible with a given amount of inputs, production is known to be *technically efficient*. That does not necessarily mean, however, that it is *economically efficient*; for economic efficiency, it is also necessary to use the mix of inputs that incurs the least costs. Only then can a firm maximize its profits. To produce in an economically efficient manner, a firm

---

4. This can be demonstrated as follows. Along an isoquant, the output level is constant. Thus, any movement along the curve (which defines the curve's slope) represents a change only in the way in which the inputs are combined to achieve a given level of output. If we use more of input *a* and less of input *b* in producing *X*, the total amount of *X* produced cannot change. Specifically,

$$(\Delta a) \times (MP_a) = (\Delta b) \times (MP_b)$$

where MP is the marginal product (i.e., amount produced) from the last unit of that input. Rearranging these terms, we find that the slope of the isoquant curve ($\Delta b/\Delta a$) equals the ratio of the marginal products of the two inputs.

must therefore take into account the prices of alternative inputs, which are shown by an *isocost* line in Figure 2.4. The isocost line indicates the price ratio of the two inputs. As in the case of consumer theory, the firm achieves its goal—here, profit maximization—at point *A*, where the iso-cost and isoquant lines are tangent. At point *B*, where the lines are not tangent, the production process would be economically inefficient. Although *B* is on an isoquant, that isoquant is associated with fewer visits being produced, as indicated by the dashed line.

Suppose we have two inputs, labor (*L*) and capital (*K*), with their respective prices defined as the wage rate (*w*) and the rate of return on capital (*r*). A firm will thus maximize profits in the following situation:

$$MP_L/P_L = MP_K/P_K \qquad (2.5)$$

By cross-multiplying and rearranging the terms, this can also be written in another way, where the ratios of the marginal products of the two inputs are equal to their price ratios,

$$MP_L/MP_K = P_L/P_K \qquad (2.6)$$

To see why a firm must fulfill Equation 2.5 (or 2.6) to maximize profits, imagine that the equality is not met: the marginal productivity of each input equals one, but the price of labor is $10 and the price of capital is $5. In such a situation, the firm will find it beneficial to buy or use more capital and less labor. Eventually, capital will become less produc-tive due to diminishing marginal productivity. Only when both sides of Equation 2.5 (or 2.6) are equal will the firm have no economic reason to change the ratio of inputs that it uses. And since all firms face the same input prices, they will all have the same ratio of marginal productivities.

After choosing the economically efficient mix of inputs, firms must decide how much output to produce and the price for which they will sell their output. In a competitive market, in which the products of al-ternative firms are indistinguishable, there really is no choice regarding price: a firm will lose its market if it charges more than the going price, and it will not maximize profits if it charges less. The rule of thumb for choosing the quantity to produce is to equate the *marginal cost* (MC) of production—that is, the cost of producing the last good—to the market price that can be obtained by selling the good. This is shown as point *A* in Figure 2.5, with a corresponding quantity *Q* produced at price *P*. In the figure, the firm faces a fixed or horizontal market price for selling the

Figure 2.4: The Producer "Optimum"

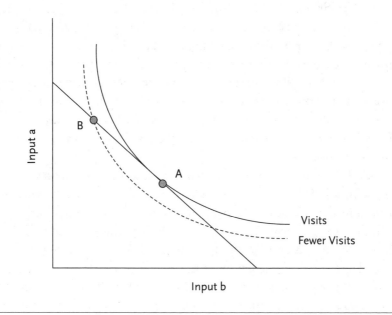

Figure 2.5: How Competitive Firms Choose Output Levels

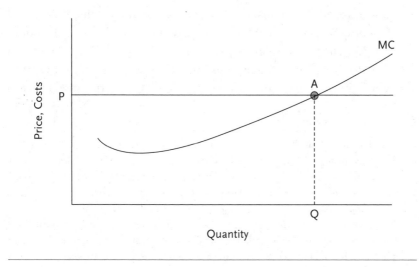

good, but the marginal cost curve slopes upward, reflecting the likelihood that it will cost more and more to produce successive units of output.[5]

The profit motive drives firms' decisions. If firms are able to make profits because, say, consumers suddenly want more of a particular product or because a new technology makes its production cheaper, existing firms will expand their output and/or other firms will enter the market, either of which will bring down the market price and eventually make profits fall back to a *normal*[6] rate of return. If firms incur losses, perhaps as a result of depressed consumer demand, they will cut back on production and/or some will leave the market, again until a normal rate of profits returns.

All of the above refers to *short-run* firm decisions. This period of time varies from industry to industry. The short run is a period in which the firm cannot vary its capital stock, but can vary labor inputs. In the long run, the firm can vary all of its inputs. The key long-run decision that a firm must make is how much capital to purchase, and this depends, to a large degree, on its anticipation of the size of its market.

In summary, production theory tells us that firms will seek to use their inputs most efficiently, and make their output choices in a way that maximizes their profits. In doing so, they also serve certain social purposes by (1) not wasting inputs, and (2) only producing those goods and services that consumers demand. Next, we describe the interaction of the many consumers and products that make up the economy as a whole.

2.1.3 The Economy as a Whole

Up until now, we have considered the consumer and producer sectors of the economy separately. This is inadequate, however, because the goods and services consumed in an economy must also be the exact ones that are produced, and consumers must purchase them at the same price for which firms sell them. Furthermore, changes in the market for a

---

5. As discussed below, the analysis being described here is called the short run, which is defined as the period of time over which capital inputs are fixed. Thus, to produce more output, the only choice is to use more labor. Eventually, however, too many laborers "crowd" the fixed amount of capital, making each successive laborer less productive. This will, in turn, raise the cost of production; thus, the marginal cost curve will slope upward.

6. A normal rate of return can be viewed as the rate of return on money invested in a different endeavor that has similar risk. If a firm does not earn at least a normal rate of return in an industry, it would do better to shut down and invest resources elsewhere.

Figure 2.6: Production Possibility Frontier

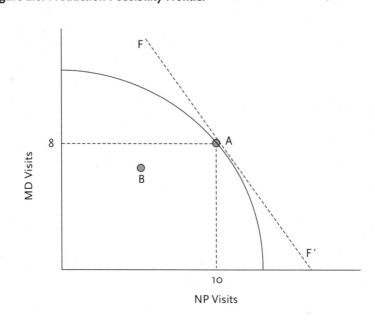

particular good or service may affect other markets as well. Viewing the consumption or production of a single good is called *partial equilibrium analysis*, while considering the economy as a whole is known as *general equilibrium analysis.*

Figure 2.6 illustrates a *production possibility frontier* (PPF), which shows the amount of each of two goods (NP visits and MD visits) that can be produced, given the amount of inputs that are available to the economy. Producing more MD visits will use scarce inputs that will no longer be available to produce NP visits. Hence, fewer NP visits will be produced. The slope of the PPF is called the *marginal rate of transformation*; it indicates how much of one good or service must be sacrificed to produce an extra unit of the other. The concave-to-the-origin shape indicates that costs increase as we shift production from one type of visit to the other. We will assume that our competitive market produces at point *A* on the PPF, that is, ten NP visits and eight MD visits.

Figure 2.7 uses the same information to produce an *Edgeworth Box*, named for economist Francis Edgeworth. It shows how the output at point *A* can be divided between two consumers, Paul and Jane. Paul's

Figure 2.7: Edgeworth Box

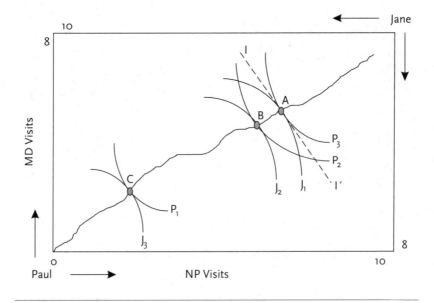

allotment of both types of visits is shown in the normal fashion: at point *A*, he has about six (of the ten) NP visits and five (of the eight) MD visits. Jane's allotment, on the other hand, is depicted by looking in the opposite direction (downward for MD visits and from right to left for NP visits). She therefore gets the remaining four NP visits and three MD visits.

The figure also shows various sets of indifference curves for each consumer. We saw earlier that equilibrium can occur only when consumers have the same marginal rate of substitution, which occurs where their indifference curves are tangent, along the *contract curve* O–A.

General equilibrium analysis shows that, for production and exchange to be efficient, consumers' marginal rates of substitution must be equal to the economy's marginal rate of transformation. That is, the slope of the consumers' indifference curves at equilibrium, indicated by the line *I–I'*, must be equal to the slope of the PPF at point *A*, indicated by the line *F–F'* in Figure 2.6.

Why must this be the case? Suppose that the marginal rate of substitution between NP and MD visits is one, but the marginal rate of transformation is two. If Jane, one of our consumers, reduces her consumption of MD visits by one, she needs to get one more NP visit to be indifferent.

But by producing one less MD visit, the economy would be able to produce two more NP visits. That leaves an extra NP visit available that could be given to Paul or to Jane. Thus, if the marginal rates of substitution and transformation are not equal, the economy is not in equilibrium, because it is possible to make one person better off without making another worse off.

2.1.4 Pareto Optimality and Social Welfare

When the consumption and production markets are in equilibrium, and when consumers' rates of indifference are equal to the economy's ability to transform one good into the others, we are in a position called *Pareto optimality*, named after economist Vilfredo Pareto. In an economy that is in a Pareto-optimal state, it is impossible to make someone better off (that is, increase that person's welfare) without making someone else worse off. Under such a situation, the economy has reached a state of *allocative efficiency*, although as we shall see in the next section, this rests on a number of assumptions.

How does an economy reach Pareto optimality? Economists have shown that if certain conditions are met, a free or competitive market operating on its own will reach a *competitive equilibrium* that is Pareto optimal. Thus, allowing competition to occur will result in a situation where it is impossible to make someone better off without making someone else worse off.

The concept of Pareto optimality, although useful from a theoretical standpoint, is rather weak from a policy standpoint: it provides little guidance. This is because of the difficulty of imagining even a single public policy that would make some people better off without making another person or persons worse off. Suppose, for example, that the government chooses to subsidize immunizations against chickenpox. Although seemingly benign, such a policy would make worse off a taxpayer with no children who had already had the disease as a child; there would be costs to this person but no benefits.[7]

If there are winners and losers associated with all policies, then deciding between policies to enact involves a value judgment, namely, who should benefit and who should lose? Making such a determination is beyond the realm of economic analysis.

---

7. Of course, if this person were benevolent, he or she might find the policy desirable. This issue is taken up below, where we discuss positive externalities of consumption.

Consequently, over the years, economists have tried to develop tools to make it easier for them to make policy recommendations that are not value laden. However, the two main examples of this—classical utilitarianism[8] and the Kaldor-Hicks criterion[9]—have been strongly refuted in the economics literature.

Market competition in general, and Pareto optimality in particular, does not address issues of equity or the desirability of the distribution of income that results from the workings of a competitive economy. Thus, a competitive equilibrium can occur in which one person has nearly all of the output, and another has almost none. In fact, this can easily occur if the former person begins with the vast majority of initial wealth or inputs. Amartya Sen (1970) makes this point graphically:

> An economy can be [Pareto] optimal . . . even when some people are rolling in luxury and others are near starvation as long as the starvers cannot be made better off without cutting into the pleasures of the rich. If preventing the burning of Rome would have made Emperor Nero feel worse off, then letting him burn Rome would have been Pareto-optimal. In short, a society or an economy can be Pareto-optimal and still be perfectly disgusting. (p. 22)

Although it might seem desirable to transfer wealth from the rich person to the poor person, doing so cannot be viewed as improving the economy from a Paretian viewpoint because the change will involve making the rich person worse off. Under the traditional economic model, competition is designed to enhance efficiency; it does not necessarily improve equity.

This point is critical because members of society do care about equity.[10] This means that a Pareto-optimal competitive equilibrium does

---

8. Utilitarianism is discussed at greater length in Sections 3.1 and 5.2.

9. The Kaldor-Hicks criterion states that an economic change is desirable if the "winners" can compensate the "losers" to get the latter to agree to the change—but they don't have to follow through with the compensation!

10. Blendon and colleagues (1994) report on U.S. survey results indicating a strong moral commitment to the uninsured. At the same time, only 23 percent of Americans agreed with the statement, "It is the responsibility of the government to take care of very poor people who can't take care of themselves"; this compares to 50 percent of Germans, 56 percent of Poles, 62 percent of British and French, 66 percent of Italians, and 71 percent of Spanish people (Blendon et al. 1995a).

not necessarily make society best off. In fact, it is highly plausible that a society will be better off with an inefficient use of resources (that is, at point B inside the PPF in Figure 2.6) *and* a more desirable distribution of income than it would be at point A with a poor distribution.

Thus, it is natural to ask whether some Pareto-optimal points (i.e., points on the contract curve 0–A in Figure 2.7) are socially more desirable than others. To figure this out, it is necessary to make value judgments about how each person's utility affects society's total welfare. This is often illustrated by a *social welfare function*, as shown in Equation 2.7,

$$W = W(U_1, U_2, \ldots, U_n) \tag{2.7}$$

where W is society's total welfare, U indicates individual utility levels, and the subscripts represent each person in the population.

Coming up with society's social welfare function is no easy task. It could be imposed by a dictator, of course, but if one prefers more demo-cratic means, a problem arises. The problem, which is proved in Kenneth Arrow's (1963a) *possibility theorem*, is that any method of aggregating in-dividual preferences into a social welfare function violates at least one reasonable and desirable ethical condition. Thus, it turns out to be quite hard to come up with a desirable consensus on how to confront distri-butional issues, an issue to which we will return in Chapter 5.

2.2 PROBLEMS WITH THE TRADITIONAL MODEL

Given that the above "textbook" model of competition forms the basis of economic training at both the undergraduate and graduate levels, it would appear that the traditional economic model of competition has a strong grip on economists in general. Only one study, however, has doc-umented the views of health economists on issues such as the desirability of market competition in the health services area. This was from a 1989 mailed survey of almost 300 individuals in the United States and Canada who consider themselves to be health economists, the results of which are summarized by Roger Feldman and Michael Morrisey (1990).

One of the questions asked in this survey was whether the respondent believed that the "competitive model cannot apply" to health. Interest-ingly, respondents were evenly divided on this question; half thought the model could apply, and half did not. More noteworthy, perhaps, were some of the response patterns to the question. Two-thirds of respondents who received their doctoral degrees from top economics departments thought that the competitive model could apply, versus 53 percent with degrees from other economics departments. Few of those who received their training in noneconomics departments believed that the competitive model could apply to the health system. Other patterns showed that younger respondents were more likely to believe in the competitive model, as were U.S. (versus Canadian) respondents.

In another survey that, among other things, sought to find out whether all health economists think alike, Victor Fuchs (1996) found a great deal of agreement on so-called positive (factual) issues, but very little on normative (opinion) ones[11]—which would presumably include whether health economists believe that the competitive model can apply to the health market.

The remainder of this section examines three reasons why the use of market competition may not lead to the highest level of social welfare. Section 2.3 will then provide some applications to health.

This critique of the competitive model is divided into three parts, in accordance with the first three of the assumptions listed in Table 1.1:

Assumption 1. There are no negative externalities of consumption.
Assumption 2. There are no positive externalities of consumption.
Assumption 3. Consumer tastes are predetermined.

The first two subsections deal with *externalities.* One of the key assumptions with regard to the advantages of competition is that there are no externalities of consumption—or alternatively, that any such externalities are explicitly dealt with through public policy. A consumption externality exists when one person's consumption of a good or service

---

11. For example, almost all health economists disagreed with the positive statements that: "the high cost of health care in the United States makes U.S. firms substantially less competitive in the global economy"; "widespread use of currently available screening and other diagnostic techniques would result in a significant reduction in health care expenditures 5 years from now"; and "differential access to medical care across socioeconomic groups is the primary reason for differential health status among these groups." However, opinions about normative issues were much less uniform. For example, about half of the health economists agreed with the statement, "The U.S. should seek universal coverage through a broad-based tax with implicit subsidies for the poor and the sick." Of the 13 normative questions, 11 of them showed substantial differences of opinion, which I define as between 25 percent and 75 percent of respondents agreeing with the statements. This was true of only one of the seven positive statements (Fuchs 1996).

has an effect on the utility of another person. There are positive and negative externalities of consumption. With a positive externality, one person's consumption of a good raises the utility of another person. With a negative externality, the consumption lowers another person's utility.

Certain consumption externalities have received much attention from health economists. Perhaps the classic example of a positive externality of consumption in all of economics, not just health, is immunizations. If I receive an immunization, I will not be the only beneficiary because my immunization also makes it less likely that others will get the disease, since they cannot catch it from me. But because, in a competitive market, an individual bears the full cost of the immunization, too few immunizations will be purchased. Recall that consumers purchase goods until the ratio of the marginal utility of each to its price is equal across all goods (Equation 2.2). When there is a positive consumption externality, society's marginal utility is greater than that of the individual, so that consumers, acting on their own, will not purchase a large enough quantity of such goods.

A parallel argument can be made about negative externalities such as smoking. If my smoking lowers your utility, then society's marginal utility from my smoking will be lower than my own. Hence, in making consumption decisions through equalizing the marginal utility and prices of all goods, people will smoke more than is in society's best interest.

The existence of important externalities like these means that the operation of a competitive market, by itself, will not result in a socially optimal outcome. One possible way to improve matters is through government intervention. In the case of a positive externality like immunizations, government can subsidize their provision, even providing them free of charge. By funding such a program through taxes, most taxpayers would help contribute, which would seem desirable, since so many people are benefiting. Dealing with a negative consumption externality like smoking is somewhat more problematic. Although it is easy to tax smokers by enacting special taxes on the production of cigarettes, it is much harder to ensure that this revenue is disbursed to those who are most affected by smoking. As a result, governmental bodies in the United States have taken an additional route by prohibiting smoking in many public places.

Here we deal with two different types of consumption externalities (one negative and one positive) that have received far less consideration from economists—and which, perhaps not coincidentally, cannot be easily rectified through simple taxes and subsidies. The negative consumption externality is concern about status and rank; the positive one is concern about the well-being of others. We will argue below that it is quite plausible that most people are simultaneously subject to both of these mental traits. The final subsection deals with a very different but equally important assumption: that consumers' tastes are predetermined—that is, shaped outside of the economic system.

2.2.1 Negative Externality: Concern About Status

In considering the problem to be examined in this section, recall Equation 2.1, in which a consumer's utility (U) was assumed to depend on the various quantities of the goods and services ($X, Y, Z, \ldots, n$) possessed:

$$U = f(X, Y, Z, \ldots, n) \tag{2.1}$$

It was also assumed that having more of each good was better.

What is more important is what is *not* in the equation: *there is no consideration given to how one's bundle of goods and services compares to, and affects or is affected by, the bundles of goods and services that other people possess.*

Let us for a moment suppose that a person's utility function is more complicated; it depends not only on the quantity of goods (X, Y, Z) a person has, but also on how this compares to how much other people have, on average (as indicated by the bars above the letters). We will denote this as follows:

$$U = f\left(X, Y, Z, X/\overline{X}, Y/\overline{Y}, Z/\overline{Z}\right) \tag{2.8}$$

This states that a person's utility is determined not only by what he or she has, but by how this compares to the average of the population. (A more realistic formulation might have as a comparison those people with whom a person has most contact, or those in the same social class.)

Alternatively, one could even imagine a utility function where *only* one's position relative to others matters,[12] as shown in Equation 2.9,

$$U = f\left(X/\overline{X}, Y/\overline{Y}, Z/\overline{Z}\right) \tag{2.9}$$

---

12. Yet another possibility is that one's absolute wealth matters up to a subsistence level, after which only relative wealth matters.

A few well-known economists have, over the years, noted the substantial implications for the competitive model if one believes that relative as well as absolute wealth matters. Lord (Lionel) Robbins (1984) writes that:

> If the remaining groups regard their position relatively, they may well argue that the spectacle of such improvement elsewhere is a detriment to their satisfaction. This is not a niggling point: a relative improvement in the position of certain groups *pari passu* with an absolute improvement in the position of the rest of the community has often been a feature of economic history; and we know that has not been regarded by all as either ethically or politically desirable. (pp. xxii–xxiii)

Similarly, Francis Bator (1958) states that,

> [M]arket efficiency is neither sufficient nor necessary for market institutions to be the "preferred" mode of social organization. . . . If, e.g., people are sensitive not only to their own jobs but to other people's as well, or more generally, if such things as relative status, power, and the like, matter, the injunction to maximize output, to hug the production-possibility frontier, can hardly be assumed "neutral," and points on the utility frontier may associate with points inside the production frontier. (p. 378)

We therefore need to ask which of the above equations is the best representation of people's actual behavior. Intuition tells us that Equation 2.1 is implausible, if not downright wrong. This equation implies that people are indifferent about their rank in society, have no concern about status, and do not worry about "keeping up with the Joneses." Rather, all that they care about is what they themselves have, irrespective of whether this is more or less, better or worse, than others with whom they have contact.

If this were true, then:

- How can one account for much if not most advertising, which tries to convey how favorably one will be viewed by others if one owns a particular car, wears a particular type of jeans, or drinks a particular brand of beer?
- How can one account for people's concern about their coworkers' salaries?

- How can one account for the following example, similar to one suggested by Robert Frank (1985): Give each of two siblings one piece of candy, and both children will be happy. But give two pieces to one child and three to another, and the child who receives the smaller share will be less happy than if each received only one. As Reinhardt (1998) quips, "the trait has its onset in early childhood and lingers until about, say, age 100, even among economists" (p. 28).

In this regard, A. C. Pigou (1932), one of the founders of modern economics, quotes and affirms John Stuart Mill's statement that "Men do not desire to be *rich*, but to be richer than other men" (p. 90). (In a lighter vein, Frank [1985] notes that "H. L. Mencken once defined wealth as any income that is at least one hundred dollars more a year than the income of one's wife's sister's husband" [p. 5].) Lester Thurow (1980) has stated that, once incomes exceed the subsistence level, "individual perceptions of the adequacy of their economic performance depend almost solely on relative as opposed to absolute position" (p. 18).

It is perhaps not unnatural to think that, while other people may behave in this manner, you and I are above such petty concerns about rank and status. Such a viewpoint is hard to hold, however, after giving consideration to the following thought experiment provided by Frank (1985):

In this experiment you are to imagine yourself in the following situation: As a high-income resident of the United States, you are suddenly confronted with an opportunity to be transported to a much richer planet. The trip will be free of charge, but with no option of return. You are a genuine standout here on Earth. You earn $100,000 per year and live in a tastefully decorated home in a quiet, fashionable neighborhood. Your children are enrolled in the best schools and are very popular among their classmates. You are happily married to a person you hold in high esteem, who regards you likewise. You are a person of integrity, a highly respected expert in your profession, and are in good health. You enjoy peace of mind and the admiration and affection of a large group of friends, who regard you as one of the most charming and caring people they know.

On the new planet your income would be $1,000,000 per year. But instead of being near the top of the income scale as you are here, you would be at the bottom. The home you would be able to afford there is much larger and better appointed than the one you live in here. Yet it is located in a marginal neighborhood, one that people urge their children not to venture into. You would pursue the same occupation there as you do here. But the people on the new planet are so skilled that they regard your profession in the way we think of repetitive, assembly tasks here. The schools your children would go to there compare very favorably with the ones they go to here, but among schools on the new planet they are thought to be ill-equipped and poorly staffed. Although your children will amass more knowledge in those schools than they do in the ones here, they will struggle there on the academic borderline, instead of bringing home A's as they do here. Although your children are much sought after by their classmates here, you will discover on the new planet that most parents attempt to steer their children to more suitable playmates. You will recount the same anecdotes there as you do here, but your friends there will regard them as simple and boring, instead of clever and erudite as your friends here regard them. Although your spouse will love you equally there as here, you know that, once there, he or she cannot fail to notice how the achievements of others surpass your own. (pp. 116–17)

Frank contends that you would be willing to give up $900,000 in income in order to retain your current status; it is hard to disagree.

The discussion up until this point has been intuitive, so it is natural to ask whether there is any evidence supporting the superiority of Equation 2.8 or 2.9 over Equation 2.1. Two classic studies are relevant here. James Duesenberry (1952) developed the *relative income hypothesis*.[13] Under this hypothesis, people's drive for self-esteem makes them wish to emulate the consumption habits of those who are on a higher socioeconomic rung of the ladder; he states that "this drive operates through inferiority feelings aroused by unfavorable comparisons between living standards" and is heightened with more frequent contact between "the quality of the goods he uses with those used by others" (p. 31). The theory predicts that people with lower incomes will save a smaller proportion of their income because they will have more frequent contact with those in the economic

---

13. As developed by Easterlin (1974), the relative income hypothesis was not about health, per se. In the 1990s, this same term was adopted to describe the theory (discussed in Section 2.3.1) that a more uneven income *distribution* may harm the health of a population.

Table 2.1: Percentage "Not Very Happy" in Lowest and Highest Status Groups, Seven Countries, 1965

Country	Number of groups	Lowest Status Group		Highest Status Group		n
		Designation	NVH (%)	Designation	NVH (%)	
Great Britain	3	Very poor	19	Upper, upper middle, middle	4	1179
West Germany	3	Lower middle, lower	19	Upper, upper middle	7	1255
Thailand	2	Lower/middle	15	Middle/upper	6	500
Philippines	2	Lower middle, lower	15	Upper, upper middle	5	500
Malaysia	2	Lower/middle	20	Middle/upper	10	502
France	3	Lower	27	Upper	6	1228
Italy	3	Lower middle/lower	42	Upper, upper middle	10	1166

NVH = not very happy.
Source: Easterlin, R. 1974. Nations and Households in Economic Growth: Essays in Honor of Moses Abramovitz, P. A. David and M. W. Reder, eds., (Academic Press, New York City), p. 101. Used with permission.

Table 2.2: Percent Distribution of Population by Happiness, United States, 1946–1970

Date	Very happy	Fairly happy	Not very happy	Other	n
April 1946	39	50	10	1	3151
Dec. 1947	42	47	10	1	1434
Aug. 1948	43	43	11	2	1596
Nov. 1952	47	43	9	1	3003
Sept. 1956	53	41	5	1	1979
Sept. 1956	52	42	5	1	2207
March 1957	53	43	3	1	1627
July 1963	47	48	5	1	3668
Oct. 1966	49	46	4	2	3531
Dec. 1970	43	48	6	3	1517

Source: Easterlin, R. 1974. *Nations and Households in Economic Growth: Essays in Honor of Moses Abramovitz*, P. A. David and M. W. Reder, eds., (Academic Press, New York City), p. 109. Used with permission.

class just above them, whose consumption patterns they will mimic. This prediction has been verified repeatedly through empirical studies.

Further evidence is provided in Richard Easterlin's (1974) classic study of human happiness in 14 countries, some of the results of which are reproduced in Tables 2.1 and 2.2 and Figure 2.8. He found that in a given country at a given time, wealthier people tend to be happier than poorer people (Table 2.1). However, in a given country over time, happiness levels are surprisingly constant, even in the wake of rising real incomes. (Table 2.2 shows data from the United States.) Furthermore, average levels of happiness are fairly constant across countries; people in poor countries and wealthy countries claim to be about equally happy (Figure 2.8). The only way such findings can be reconciled is if relative wealth rather than absolute wealth matters. From this, Easterlin concludes:

[T]here is a "consumption norm" which exists in a given society at a given time, and which enters into the reference standard of virtually everyone. This provides a common point of reference in self-appraisals of well-being, leading those below the norm to feel less happy and

Figure 2.8: Personal Happiness Rating and GNP per Capita, 1960

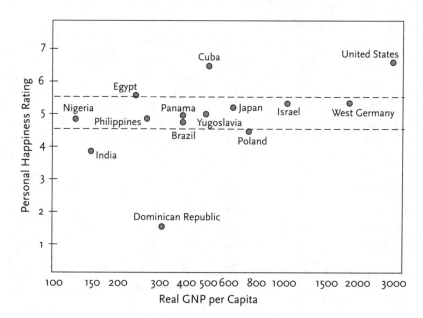

Source: Easterlin, R. 1974. *Nations and Households in Economic Growth: Essays in Honor of Moses Abramovitz.* Edited by P. A. David and M. W. Reder, p. 106. New York: Academic Press. Used with permission.

those above the norm, more happy. Over time, this norm tends to rise with the general level of consumption. . . . (pp. 112–13)

Curiously, the study seems to provide evidence that Equation 2.9 may be more in keeping with actual human behavior than Equation 2.8; in Equation 2.9, *only* one's relative standing matters. This is consistent with Easterlin's findings that wealthy people are about equally happy across countries, irrespective of whether the countries are richer or poorer, and that poor people are about equally happy across countries. If one's absolute possessions mattered as well, one would expect to see people in wealthy countries exhibit a greater level of happiness than those of similar rank in poor countries. In addition, over times of rising real income, people in a particular country should also become happier.

One has to be careful not to infer too much from cross-national comparisons of happiness, mainly because factors other than economic status are likely to play different roles in the happiness levels of people from different countries. Even so, accepting Equation 2.9, where the overriding determinant of happiness is one's relative rather than absolute standing, might seem a little hard. It implies that if I had more, but my relative standing remained the same, I would be no happier. This clearly contradicts the meaning of the indifference curves shown in Figure 2.1, in which it was assumed that more of each good would put a person at a higher level of utility.[14]

Although Easterlin's study does not explicitly attempt to refute the concept of the indifference curve, his research also helps provide an understanding of why people might behave in a way that is so contradictory to that predicted by traditional economic theory. He reports the results of a study by Hadley Cantril (1965) based on 1960s surveys of individuals living in the United States and India, concerning what makes them happy. Following are several quotations that strongly indicate that the things that make people happy vary dramatically with their circumstances:

India. I want a son and a piece of land since I am now working on land owned by other people. I would like to construct a house of my own and have a cow for milk and ghee. I would also like to buy some better clothing for my wife. If I could do this then I would be happy. [35-year-old man, illiterate, agricultural laborer, income about $10 a month]

India. I wish for an increase in my wages because with my meager salary I cannot afford to buy decent food for my family. If the food and clothing problems were solved, then I would feel at home and be satisfied. Also if my wife were able to work the two of us could then feed the family and I am sure would have a happy life and our worries would be over. [35-year-old sweeper, monthly income around $13]

India. I should like to have tap water and a water supply in my house. It would be able to have electricity. My husband's wages must be increased if our children are to get an education and our daughter is to be married. [45-year-old housewife, family income about $80 a month]

---

14. Easterlin does demonstrate, however, that the concept of happiness translates consistently into the different languages of different countries. He therefore argues that his findings are not the result of the vagaries of language.

India. I hope in the future I will not get any disease. Now I am cough-
ing. I also hope I can purchase a bicycle. I hope my children will study
well and that I can provide them with an education. I also would
sometime like to own a fan and maybe a radio. [45-year-old skilled
worker earning $30 a month]

United States. If I could earn more money I would be able to buy our
own home and have more luxury around us, like better furniture, a
new car, and more vacations. [27-year-old skilled worker]

United States. I would like a reasonable enough income to maintain
a house, have a new car, have a boat, and send my four children to
private schools. [34-year-old laboratory technician]

United States. I would like a new car. I wish all my bills were paid and
I had more money for myself. I would like to play more golf and to
hunt more than I do. I would like to have more time to do the things
I want to and to entertain my friends. [24-year-old bus driver]

United States. Materially speaking, I would like to provide my family with an income to allow them to live well—to have the proper
recreation, to go camping, to have music and dancing lessons for the
children, and to have family trips. I wish we could belong to a country
club and do more entertaining. We just bought a new home and expect to be perfectly satisfied with it for a number of years. [28-year-old
lawyer] (Cantril 1965, as quoted in Easterlin 1974, pp. 114–15)

These quotations, which are rather poignant in their own right, provide a glimpse of why two people in two cultures can be equally happy
with very different quantities of goods: people's utility depends not so
much on what they have as on what they have relative to the social norm.
    Interestingly, since the 1990s the issue of relative income has become
a major area of research in the area of health. Although controversial, the
notion is that relative income—and in particular, how well or poorly income is distributed within and between countries—has a major effect on
the health of the population. This discussion is deferred to Section 2.3.1,
as the first of six implications for health policy drawn from the critique
of traditional theory provided in this chapter.

Suppose that one accepts the notion that people care about how they compare with others, as well as what they themselves have irrespective of others (i.e., Equation 2.8). It could still be argued that, even if concern about relative position does exist, it is irrational or a character flaw that should not be respected by the analyst or policymaker. But this argument does not hold up for two reasons. First, the traditional economic theory does not evaluate where preferences come from or whether they are good or bad. Instead, it views them as what has to be satisfied for an individual, and ultimately a society, to be in a best-off position. Although this notion will be disputed in Section 3.2, economic theory does not view any individually held preferences pejoratively—and that would include the likes of envy, rank, or status.[15]

Second, it is not at all obvious that concern about one's status compared to others is an irrational or even undesirable character trait. Tibor Scitovsky (1976) makes a strong argument to the contrary:

> The desire to "live up to the Joneses" is often criticized and its rationality called into question. This is absurd and unfortunate. Status seeking, the wish to belong, the asserting and cementing of one's membership in the group is a deep-seated and very natural drive whose origin and universality go beyond man and are explained by that most basic of drives, the desire to survive. (p. 115)

Similarly, Reinhardt (1998) writes,

> Envy probably is among the most basic of all human traits. It is the very engine of economic growth. Normative economic analysis that

---

15. This tenet of modern theory also has its detractors. Joan Robinson (1962), for example, notes that under this theory, "Preference is just what the individual under discussion prefers; there is no value judgment involved. Yet, as the argument goes on, it is clear that it is a Good Thing for the individual to have what he prefers. This, it may be held, is not a question of satisfaction, but freedom—we want him to have what he prefers so as to avoid having to restrain his behaviour. But drug-fiends should be cured; children should go to school. How do we decide what preferences should be respected and what retrained unless we judge the preferences themselves? It is quite impossible for us to do that violence to our own natures to refrain from value judgments" (p. 49). This echoes the sentiments of Pigou (1932), who wrote, "Of different acts of consumption that yield equal satisfaction, one may exercise a debasing, and another an elevating influence" (p. 17).

abstracts from this common human trait, because it is deemed unsa-
vory, might be useful on other planets. It misses the core of the human
experience on planet Earth. (p. 28)

In this regard, what others have can also be viewed as necessary information for a person in formulating his or her individual desires. It shows
what can be had, and what is reasonable to expect.

Let us now return to the issue of how this negative externality—
concern about status and rank—affects the competitive model. Recall
that the advantage of competition is that it leads to Pareto optimality,
where it is impossible to make someone better off without making someone else worse off. In the absence of the human characteristics being discussed here, it is easy to see the appeal of relying on competition. Why
not let people engage in trade until they are satisfied with their lot and
no longer wish to engage in further trades? Similarly, why not enact policies that convey benefits to some people and no cost to others? Wouldn't
encouraging such trade, and enacting such policies, be in everyone's best
interest?

This section has tried to show that the answer to the last question is,
perhaps surprisingly, "not necessarily." This is because if people feel worse
off when they find themselves falling relative to others, then competition
is not necessarily the best means of improving societal welfare. If, for
example, by buying a fancy car, you make me unhappy because my car
no longer seems as appealing, then society's marginal utility from your
purchase of the car will be lower than your personal marginal utility. By
extension, if social competition leads to everyone purchasing fancier cars
than they need, society hardly will be better off, but the resources going
into them potentially could be used in other ways that most people would
find more useful.[16]

Without some sort of intervention (or intensive psychological therapy
to get me to stop caring about what you have), a competitive market will
overproduce goods and services that convey status.

When an externality exists, economists try to come up with taxes
or subsidies that can correct it. In this case, Frank (1999) suggests one

---

16. Frank (1999) suggests several things in which we could invest, where there are few if
any negative consumption externalities (because none of these is a status good): more vacation time, more leisure time (from less work) to spend with family and friends, and shorter
commute times from more investment in transportation.

possibility: a progressive consumption tax. For example, above a certain level of spending (say, $30,000 a year), government could charge a 20 percent tax on the next $10,000 in spending, a 21 percent on the next $10,000—up to, say, a tax of 70 percent on annual spending above $530,000.[17] The idea is that if everyone has to pay much higher taxes as they spend more, they will have more of an incentive to seek out non-status goods such as greater leisure time from not working as many hours or taking more vacation time. Whether such a plan is politically feasible, however, is an open question.

Where does all this leave us? It is my hope that the reader now has some appreciation for the notion that an economic system based on competition and that encourages production, but not necessarily the redistribution of more and more wealth, does not always make society better off. How this applies to the field of health will be covered in Section 2.3. First, however, we consider two more key assumptions in the competitive model, beginning with the one concerning positive consumption externalities. As will become clear, those arguments will bear close resemblance to the ones just made.

2.2.2 Positive Externality: Concern About Others

In this section we deal with a different type of consumption externality: *concern about the well-being of others.* If we care about other people's needs as well as our own—be they specific needs like food or medical care, or somewhat more vague concerns about how happy the people are—then a positive externality of consumption exists. As noted earlier, a competitive market, by itself, will not provide enough of the goods and services for which there is a positive externality.

The previous section argued that people are concerned about their status relative to others. But accepting this does not mean that people cannot also be concerned about others' well-being at the same time. People might have both a concern that others should have certain things like adequate food or medical care or even happiness, but might also feel envy when others have things that they themselves do not possess. Most plausible, perhaps, would be that people want those who have less than they

---

17. Frank argues that this could be carried out without explicitly keeping track of expenses, and by just adding a single line to the federal income tax form. Essentially, taxable consumption would simply be income earned minus how much of this income was saved. Thus, the system would have the added advantage of encouraging more savings.

have to have more—although not as much as themselves, as evidenced by the Mencken quotation—and, at the same time, want to have as much as those who have more.

Even though we are talking about concern for others, our focus here is also on issues of *economic efficiency*. We noted earlier that a competitive market is not designed to improve the distribution of resources among the population, so one might ask how its failure to deal with distributional issues can be raised as an efficiency problem.

The answer to this question is that there are, in actuality, two distinct reasons for redistributing income.[18] The one that might be most familiar to readers concerns issues of *social* or *distributive justice*—in essence, that redistribution is the "right thing to do." John Rawls's (1971) famous book, *A Theory of Justice* (discussed further in Chapter 5), provides a strong philosophical foundation for such a belief.

The economic tools provided earlier help illustrate the concept of social justice. Refer back to the Edgeworth Box in Figure 2.7. Suppose we are at economically efficient point *C*, where Jane has most of the wealth and Paul has little. If one views this situation, for some reason, as unfair, a possible justification for redistributing income from Jane to Paul would be to correct this inequity. Much of Chapter 5 will be devoted to examining these issues.

However, a second possible reason exists for redistributing resources: to improve economic efficiency. Suppose that I care about poor people and want them to have more food and medical care. To increase my own utility, I would want to give some of my resources to the poor, stopping at the point that the marginal utility that I gain from contributing the last dollar equals the marginal utility I attain from spending it on something else.

The obvious question that arises is, why doesn't everyone just donate their optimal amount to charity, which in turn should maximize their personal utility? The problem is that many, if not most, people will attempt to become free riders, which in turn will result in less redistribution than is optimal. Assume again that people care about others and want the poor to have more food, housing, medical care, and so forth. If this is done through a competitive model, an unfortunate thing happens. The Joneses will recognize that the poor will do about as well if everyone

---

18. A good discussion of the distinction can be found in Wagstaff et al. (1992).

except the Joneses provides donations. But if many or most people act in this way, too little money is redistributed. The outcome therefore remains inefficient; society would be better off if there were a way to redistribute the optimal amount of resources rather than the lesser amount that occurs under competition.

The standard "answer" to this problem in traditional economics is to rely on a competitive marketplace to allocate resources efficiently, and then to employ just the right amount of special kinds of taxes and subsidies to redistribute income. These are called *lump-sum* taxes and subsidies.

The idea of these lump-sum transfers is to come up with a way to tax, say, the wealthy, to subsidize, perhaps, the poor, without changing in any important way the efficiency-enhancing incentives of a competitive market. If no such methods are feasible, then use of market competition becomes problematic when there are consumption externalities: if we do not redistribute income, the market is inefficient because people want poorer people to be better off than they are. But if we do redistribute income, we damage the efficiency that the marketplace is designed to create.

The problem with this "lump-sum solution" is the virtual impossibility of establishing true lump-sum taxes and subsidies. We would need to come up with a way of transferring income that does not affect the incentives of either the payer of the tax or the recipient of the subsidy.[19]

Dealing first with alternative taxation schemes, the taxes that we use most commonly do not meet this requirement because they will alter incentives. An income tax, for example, results in a reduction in net wages from the provision of additional labor. In standard theory, laborers are assumed to work until their *opportunity cost*—forgone leisure—equals the wage rate. If net wages go down from the imposition of an income tax, workers are likely to substitute more leisure for labor because the value of labor will be lower. This results in a lower overall production of goods and services. The other common tax employed is a sales tax. The problem with a sales tax is that it results in the consumer paying a higher price than will be received by the producer. A condition of Pareto optimality is that consumers' marginal rates of substitution must be equal

---

19. For further discussion on problems in enacting such taxes and subsidies, see Graaff (1971), pp. 77–82; and Samuelson (1947), pp. 247–49.

to the economy's marginal rate of transformation. This is no longer the case when there is a sales tax; allowing competition to take place with sales taxes in place will not result in an economically efficient allocation of resources (Nath 1969).

Regarding the receipt of subsidies, it is equally difficult to come up with an incentive-neutral method. A typical way of transferring money to the poor is through welfare payments, but providing welfare payments to the poor results in a work disincentive. Receiving a smaller welfare check when your income rises is no different than facing an income tax; as we just saw, a competitive market with income taxes is not economically efficient. (This, it turns out, is one of the reasons that we will argue for the superiority of in-kind over in-cash transfers for the poor in Chapter 5.)

In theory, one sort of tax and subsidy might work, but it has no practicality. This is a *poll tax*—a tax that is levied irrespective of income. But as Graaff (1971) writes,

> [a poll tax] is not very helpful in securing desired redistributions unless we tax different men differently. But on what criteria should we discriminate between different men? Ethical ones? And what if a man cannot pay the tax? If we start taxing the poor less than the rich, we are simply reintroducing an income-tax. If we tax able men more than dunderheads, we open the door to all forms of falsification: we make stupidity seem profitable—and any able man can make himself seem stupid. Unless we really do have an omniscient observing economist to judge men's capabilities, or a slave-market where the prices they fetch reflect expert appraisals of their capacities, any taxing authority is bound to be guided by elementary visible criteria like age, marital status and—above all—ability to pay. We are back with an income tax. (p. 78)

The problem gets even more ticklish when we consider issues of fairness. Suppose we decide to tax people based not on their income, per se, but rather on their *ability* to generate income. This would mean that those who are least able to earn would be taxed less than those more able. As Paul Samuelson (1947) notes,

> Analytically, the problem resembles that of determining . . . a fair "handicap" for golfers of different ability. We wish to equalize opportunity for all contestants, but we do not want them to hold back

from playing their best because of a fear of losing their favorable handicap. . . . Thus, we might decide that everyone should have at least a minimum income, that Society will make up the deficiency between what the less fortunate can earn and this minimum. Once this is realized by those who fall below the minimum, there is no longer an incentive for them to work at the margin, at least in pecuniary material terms. This is clearly bad social policy. . . . (pp. 247–48)

The foregoing discussion has been aimed at showing the near impossibility of devising workable lump-sum taxes and subsidies—which are necessary if we are to retain economic efficiency in the wake of externalities of consumption. What, then, are the implications of this dilemma? Simply this: in making policy, it is impossible to separate issues of resource allocation from issues of resource distribution. Rather, they both must be dealt with simultaneously.[20] Thurow (1980) states this nicely:

Decisions about economic equity are the fundamental starting point for any market economy. Individual preferences determine market demands for goods and services, but these individual preferences are weighted by incomes before being communicated to the market. An individual with no income or wealth may have needs and desires, but he has no economic resources. To make his or her personal preferences felt, he must have these resources. If income and wealth are distributed in accordance with equity (whatever that may be), individual preferences are properly weighed, and the market can efficiently adjust to an equitable set of demands. If income and wealth are not distributed in accordance with equity, individual preferences are not properly weighted. The market efficiently adjusts, but to an inequitable set of demands. . . . One way or the other, we are forced to reveal our collective preferences about what constitutes a just distribution of economic resources. (pp. 194–95)

This anomaly—the impossibility of separating allocative and distributional activities of the economy—has been raised in a variety of contexts

---

20. This is one of the key points of Rawls's (1971) book, *A Theory of Justice*. He argues that we must start with an allocation of "primary goods" that is based on principles of fairness. Once that is achieved, it is not inappropriate to use the market mechanism to achieve an efficient allocation of resources. Section 5.2 discusses these issues in more detail.

by several economists, but has received little attention from the profession at large.[21] If this is the case, then the traditional economic method, in which competitive forces are allowed to prevail and distribution is only done afterward, is not necessarily appropriate—especially in the presence of consumption externalities.

An example will help clarify why this is so. Suppose that a market economy reaches a Pareto-optimal state, but that this does not result in society's ideal distribution of income. (We might, for example, be at point C in Figure 2.7 but prefer to be at point B.) Consequently, it is necessary to employ taxes to redistribute income, but recall from the above discussion that there are no feasible lump-sum taxes. Instead, we use the conventional method—an income tax.

If an income tax (or, for that matter, any feasible tax) is used to redistribute income, the economy would no longer be in an optimally efficient state. If the allocation of resources was efficient before the redistribution, it would no longer be afterward. However, without carrying out the redistribution, society would still have a suboptimal income distribution—which would mean that social welfare would be lower than it could be.

This concern would be eased if income were redistributed to the degree desired by members of society. If such redistribution does not occur, then other strategies are necessary to deal with both the inefficiencies and inequities that arise when there are positive externalities of consumption. One of the best ways to deal with Thurow's concern is to enact policies that ensure that those in need obtain goods and services even if they do not have the economic resources to purchase them in the marketplace. Programs like Medicare and Medicaid in the United States—which are

---

21. Arrow (1963b), for example, has stated that, "If . . . the actual market differs significantly from the competitive model, or if the assumptions of the two optimality theorems are not fulfilled, the separation of allocative and distributional procedures becomes, in most cases, impossible" (p. 942). The two optimality conditions referred to by Arrow are that (if certain assumptions are met): (1) a competitive equilibrium is Pareto optimal; and (2) any Pareto optimum can be reached by a competitive equilibrium corresponding to a particular initial distribution of resources. Similarly, Mishan (1969a) writes, "Far from an optimum allocation of resources representing some kind of an ideal output separable from and independent of interpersonal comparisons of welfare, a particular output retains its optimum characteristics only insofar as we commit ourselves to the particular welfare distribution uniquely associated with it" (p. 133). Finally, Blackorby and Donaldson (1990) note that separating allocative and distributive decisions "require[s] a notion of efficiency that is independent of the distribution of income—an idea that makes no sense in real-world economies" (p. 490).

not in keeping with some economists' recommendations to rely on competition and then redistribute resources through cash subsidies—offer good examples of how society grapples with problems like these. More health implications are provided in Section 2.3.

2.2.3 Consumer Tastes Are Predetermined

Of all of the assumptions in the traditional economic model, perhaps the one that is most often forgotten is the notion that consumers' tastes are already established when they enter the marketplace. This assumption is extraordinarily important. This section will attempt to show that ignoring established taste is not realistic, and that when this assumption is not taken into account, the competitive model loses some of its advantages.

Economics is almost universally viewed as a social science. The common element among all social sciences is that they seek to understand how individuals and/or groups of people behave. But each social science has its own way of viewing human behavior. Sociology, for example, focuses on how behavior is affected by society's organization, social stratification, group dynamics, and the like (Mechanic 1979). Political science examines how individuals and groups attempt to obtain what they want through such means as "conflict, influence, and authoritative collective decision making in both public and private settings" (Marmor and Dunham 1983, p. 3). Social psychology attempts to understand "the influences that people have upon the beliefs or behavior of others" (Aronson 1972, p. 6).

One facet of these other social sciences is that, in general, they seek to determine how people and groups *actually* behave. In contrast, Thurow (1983) contends, "while the reverse is true in the other social sciences that study real human behavior, prescription dominates description in economics" (p. 216). In this regard, in economics one commonly sees the word "ought" (e.g., people ought to maximize their utility, or otherwise they are being "irrational"; to maximize social welfare a society "ought" to depend on a competitive marketplace).

According to Gary Becker (1979), three things distinguish economics from the other social sciences. First, economics assumes that people engage in "maximizing behavior"; that is, individuals strive to obtain the most utility possible, firms work for the greatest profits, and so on. Second, the milieu in which people operate is the market. And third, according to Becker, is that "preferences are assumed not to change substantially over time, nor to be very different between wealthy and poor persons, or even between persons in different societies and cultures" (p. 9). Similarly, Stigler and Becker (1977) go even further than this, claiming that,

> [T]astes neither change capriciously nor differ importantly between people. . . . [O]ne does not argue over tastes for the same reason that one does not argue over the Rocky Mountains—both are there, will be there next year, too, and are the same for all men. (p. 76)[22]

Not only are preferences assumed to be immutable, but they are also assumed to be predetermined, that is, determined outside of the economic or even social system in which the person exists. In economic theory, individual tastes and preferences "simply exist—fully developed and immutable" (Thurow 1983, p. 219). This is what Kenneth Boulding (1969) has referred to as the "Immaculate Conception of the Indifference Curve," because "tastes are simply given, and . . . we cannot inquire into the process by which they are formed" (p. 2).

Milton Friedman (1962) provides one explanation for this, which is consistent with the previous discussion of how economics differs from the other social sciences:

> [E]conomic theory proceeds largely to take wants as fixed . . . primarily [as] a case of division of labor. The economist has little to say about the formation of wants; this is the province of the psychologist. *The economist's task is to trace the consequences of any given set of wants.* (p. 13, emphasis added)[23]

Henry Aaron (1994) has pointed out one of the problems with this viewpoint—when individuals' behavior influences, and is influenced by, the community. He notes that,

---

22. Stigler and Becker (1977) also imply that there is no need for social sciences other than economics. Recall that demand is a function of prices, incomes, and tastes. If tastes do not differ between people or change over time, all consumer behavior can be determined simply by understanding changes in price and income. Indeed, they argue that "the economist continues to search for differences in prices or incomes to explain any differences or changes in behavior" (p. 76).

23. Becker (1979) provides a second explanation for this assumption: "The assumption of stable preferences provides a stable foundation for generating predictions about responses to various changes, and prevents the analyst from succumbing to the temptation of simply postulating the required shift in preferences to 'explain' all apparent contradictions to his predictions" (p. 9).

It is then essential to recognize how changes in individual beliefs and values alter the environment in which individual actions occur. The environment is important both because people's preferences are shaped by pressure from peers and neighbors and because community attitudes shape the actual payoffs to various kinds of individual behavior. (p. 7)

It is beyond the scope of this book to fully demonstrate that people's tastes and behaviors are mutable. Indeed, the field of social psychology is devoted, to a large extent, to this particular issue. Good overviews of the field, as well as evidence from some of the more noteworthy experiments, are provided in Aronson (1972) and Ross and Nisbett (1991).

Overwhelming evidence suggests that people's decisions—market-related ones and otherwise—can indeed be influenced by their environment. Consider the case of advertising. The reader, who is likely well-versed in the tactics of the media, probably will admit that most consumer advertising is not aimed at providing objective information for the purposes of minimizing consumers' search for the best value. Rather, advertising is designed to (1) *minimize* the search process itself, and more generally, (2) change consumer tastes, in part by exerting social pressure. It is hard to claim that the tastes people come to have, as the result of exposure to this sort of advertising, are sacrosanct. In fact, people often make "bad" or nonmaximizing decisions by acting on the message—the hallmark of a successful advertising campaign!

Although it does not deal with market behavior directly, one particular set of social psychology experiments are reviewed here because they show, so graphically, how people's beliefs and behaviors can be so distorted by their environment. These are Stanley Milgram's (1963) renowned studies of obedience in the face of authority.[24] These results have been used to explain, among other things, the behavior of Nazi officials during the Holocaust (Ross and Nisbett 1991).

In one version of the experiment (Milgram 1963), 40 male volunteers ages 20 to 50 are solicited to participate in a study of memory and learning

---

24. According to Lee Ross (1988), "Perhaps more than any other empirical contribution to the history of social science, [Milgram's] have become part of our society's shared intellectual legacy—that small body of historical incidents, biblical parables, and classic literature that serious thinkers feel free to draw on when they debate about human nature or contemplate human history" (p. 101).

at Yale University. An "experimenter" has two other individuals—one a naive subject and the other an imposter—draw lots to determine who will be the "teacher" and the other the "learner." By design, the naive subject always becomes the teacher, and is instructed to give electrical shocks to the learner (who is stationed in a different room) when the latter provides incorrect answers on a memory test. Although the shocks are, of course, fake, participants apparently believe that they are real, being told that "although the shocks can be extremely painful, they cause no permanent tissue damage" (Milgram 1963, p. 373). The experimenter tells the teacher to administer a shock of 15 volts for the first wrong answer, and to increase this by 15 volts each time a subsequent wrong answer is given, up to a maximum of 450 volts. The apparatus that supposedly gives the shocks has been labeled to indicate their severity, going from as low as "slight shock" to as high as "danger: severe shock." At a purported shock of 300 volts, the victim starts banging on the walls, begging that the experiment be discontinued. After 315 volts, even these protests stop, at which point the victim no longer provides any answers. But the subjects are urged by the experimenter to continue because no answer is to be construed as a wrong answer, until the maximum 450 volts is administered.

Not surprisingly, as the experiment proceeds, some subjects question the experimenter about whether they should go on, and/or whether the recipient of the shocks is all right. When this occurs, the instructor insists that they continue to participate, although no loud voice or threats are used.[25]

Much to the surprise of the researchers (and subsequently, to much of the civilized world as well), most people continued to administer shocks all the way to the maximum level. In the study referred to here, all 40 participants continued to shock the victim up to a level of 300 volts, and 35 continued even after the wall banging. A full 26 (65 percent) continued to the maximum 450 volts.

It is especially curious that subjects continued to administer the shocks, given that they were clearly not predisposed to such behavior. As Milgram (1963) reports,

---

25. When questioned, the experimenter would say "please continue." If the subject balked, he would then say, in order, "the experiment requires that you continue," "it is absolutely essential that you continue," and "you have no other choice, you *must* go on" (Milgram 1963, p. 374).

Many subjects showed signs of nervousness in the experimental situation, and especially upon administering the more powerful shocks. In a large number of cases the degree of tension reached extremes that are rarely seen in sociopsychological laboratory studies. Subjects were observed to sweat, tremble, stutter, bit their lips, groan, and dig their fingernails into their flesh. . . . One sign of tension was the regular occurrence of nervous laughing fits. . . . The laughter seemed entirely out of place, even bizarre. . . . In the post-experimental interviews subjects took pains to point out that they were not sadistic types, and that the laughter did not mean they enjoyed shocking the victim. (p. 375)

Why people can be influenced to behave in a way that so contradicts their personal values has been debated for years and has still not been satisfactorily explained (Ross 1988). Milgram himself offered 13 reasons in his 1963 article. Some of the reasons clearly reflect the peculiar nature of the situation in which subjects found themselves.[26] The point being made here is that people's behaviors are not predetermined or fixed, but rather are subject to innumerable cognitive and social forces.

Why, then, does economics consider tastes predetermined and fixed rather than subject to the forces of change? Readers who are most familiar with economic theory will understand one possible reason. The primary tenet of modern economics is the sanctity of consumer choice. Most economists believe that the consumer is the best judge of what will maximize his or her utility. Consequently, to maximize overall social welfare, we should set up an economic system that is best at allowing consumer choices to be satisfied. Where these choices come from, as Friedman said, is beside the point.

But if what you want depends on what you had in the past, or on the influence of peers or advertisers, then it is not clear that a competitive marketplace is the best way to make people better off (Pollack 1978). True, if certain conditions are met, a competitive market will result in allocative efficiency; however, a major caveat is attached to this—the things people

---

26. The experiment was sponsored by a noted university; it was purportedly for a worthy purpose—to study how to enhance learning; the "victim" supposedly volunteered and was randomly chosen to be the recipient of the shocks; the experimenter did not bend in his conviction that the subject continue administering the shocks; the subject was told that no permanent physical damage will result from the shocks, and so forth (Milgram 1963).

demand are really the ones that will make them best off. We pursue this issue more broadly in Chapter 3. Here we focus on the specific issue of whether satisfying consumers' tastes, as indicated by their demand for particular goods and services, will necessarily maximize their utility.

In the paragraphs below, three examples are provided in which people's market behaviors are not predetermined but rather are a result of their past or present environments. In each case, it is not clear that fulfillment of their personal choices would make them best off.

The first example, and perhaps the least important of the three given, concerns addiction. Suppose that, while growing up, you are in a peer group that smokes cigarettes and you become addicted. Once you leave that peer group, you will still have a "taste" for cigarettes and are more likely to demand them than someone who is not addicted. Can we really say, in such an instance, that satisfying this "taste" through the marketplace is efficient from a societal standpoint—in the same way as satisfying the demand for bread or literature? Might not you be better off if cigarettes were taxed so prohibitively (or even banned) that you stopped smoking?[27]

A second and much more general application is habit formed by past consumption patterns.[28] Suppose you live in a community that has not discovered the joys of music. A resident of such a place will therefore not have developed a taste for music. But, as Alfred Marshall (1920), another of the fathers of modern economics, once noted, "the more good music a man hears, the stronger is his taste for it likely to become" (p. 94). The aforementioned resident might likely be better off with music than without, but he or she has not been sufficiently "educated" to know this.[29,30]

---

27. Note that this argument does not hinge on the negative externalities associated with smoking. Prohibitive taxes could also be enacted so that fewer negative side-effects on others result from your smoking.

28. For a good discussion of these issues, see Hahnel and Albert (1990).

29. Stated in economic terms, the tangency between their indifference curve and budget constraint is not utility maximizing.

30. The idea of having the economic system not only reflect given preferences, but also nurture "more refined" preferences, has been a theme of some radical economists. Herbert Gintis (1970), for example, has said that a person can use his existing preferences to demand what he has demanded before, or alternatively, "*improve* his preference structure so as to be capable of increased satisfaction based on available material goods" (p. 12). Gintis believes that the commodities that are contained in people's utility functions should not be viewed as ends

This is a very big problem for competitive markets. If people demand goods based on their prior experience—as they certainly must—and furthermore, if their prior experience is colored by the economic environment in which they live, then they will demand the things that tend to be characteristic of that environment. That implies a strong advantage for whatever is the status quo; familiarity breeds preference (as opposed to breeding contempt), so what exists now will be demanded in the future.[31]

If one believes that tastes are determined in such a way, then it becomes clear that a society might be better off pursuing some goods and services that are not demanded most strongly by the public. This is because people might not know what alternatives are available that will make them better off, but to which they have not be exposed in the past. But if consumer tastes are viewed as predetermined, as they are in the economic model, people become "stuck" with whatever they demand because they are assumed always to know best.

The third example concerns occupational choices. In the traditional economic model, it is assumed that people make occupational choices based on weighing all alternatives; factors considered would include how much satisfaction they obtain from the work and the wages that it offers. Whatever choice is made in a competitive labor market is assumed to be utility maximizing. But this might not be the case if tastes are a product of one's environment.

Suppose, for example, that a person grows up in a factory town and later decides to work in the factory. This might not necessarily be utility maximizing; it is possibly a poor choice, made because of the person's limited horizons. As another example, imagine that one person works to perform house-cleaning services for another. This may not reflect the personal preferences of the worker as much as lack of good alternatives (Buchanan 1977). In this regard, John Roemer (1994) states that "people learn to live with what they are accustomed to or what is available to them. . . . Thus the slave may have adapted to like slavery; welfare judgments based on individual preferences are clearly impugned in such situations" (p. 120). The status quo would be favored by competitive

---

in themselves, but rather, as instruments for obtaining higher welfare; he attacks conventional welfare economists as "commodity fetishists."

31. For a review of health studies that show a preference for the status quo, see Salkeld, Ryan, and Short (2000).

markets, even though people might be better off if society, in some way, intervened in these choices. (A public job-training program would be an example.)

In summary, this discussion has tried to show that encouraging consumer choice through competitive markets might not always be the best way of raising people's and society's welfare, if people have strong positive or negative feelings about the possessions of others, or if their tastes are malleable rather than predetermined. The next section considers some examples of how these assumptions affect health policy.

2.3 IMPLICATIONS FOR HEALTH POLICY

This chapter has attempted to show that economic theory does not provide a strong justification for the superiority of competitive policies in the health services area. This is because the competitive model is based on certain important assumptions that, we argued, do not appear to be met. This section provides some implications of these conclusions for health policy.

2.3.1 Does the Distribution of Income Affect the Health of the Population?

Economic theory focuses on absolute, not relative, relationships. An individual, for example, is assumed to care only about the bundle of goods he or she possesses, not about what others have. A natural extension of this theory is the belief that absolutes are the things that matter when it comes to the population as a whole. A wealthier nation, for example, should be a happier nation if, as is assumed by theory, utility is determined by the value of the goods possessed. It was shown earlier in the chapter, however, that this does not appear to be the case.

What about health? Nearly all research shows that more wealth improves most measures of health among the poor, but has a much smaller effect as incomes rise. This is true not only at the individual level, but in the aggregate as well. Wealthier countries tend to exhibit better population health up to a certain income threshold, but above some point little relationship is apparent (Daniels, Kennedy, and Kawachi 2000). This relationship is illustrated by the curved line in Figure 2.9.

The issue addressed here is whether there is also a relationship between health and the *distribution* of income. That is, at any given level of wealth, do countries (or states or cities) where the wealth is spread more evenly among the population exhibit better health outcomes? If so,

Figure 2.9: Relationship Between Health Status and Income

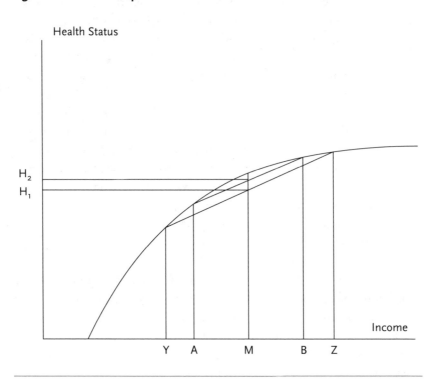

then narrowing the distribution of income would be a way to make the populous healthier.

It is natural to wonder why such a relationship might exist. Proponents point to a number of possible pathways, three of which are noted here (Kawachi and Kennedy 2001; Wilkinson 1999). The first relates to stress. In an inegalitarian society, it is hypothesized, those that are on the bottom of the income distribution are more likely to feel under pressure—which in turn can have both negative physiological and psychological consequences. This can be the result of various factors, such as being unable to make ends meet, feeling anger at one's lot, or being "picked upon," either directly or indirectly, by those in higher social classes.

One noted research endeavor supportive of how social standing affects health is the Whitehall studies of British civil servants (Marmot et al. 1997), the first of which began in the 1960s and the second in the 1980s.

The first study found that over time, lowest-level civil servants, such as clerks, had twice the mortality as those in the highest level, such as administrators. The second study found differences of about 50 percent in coronary heart disease, much of which was the result of how much control workers felt they had over their work. But why does control matter? Michael Marmot and his coauthors (1997) write:

> The putative pathophysiological mechanisms by which psychosocial factors cause [coronary heart disease] involve activation of the autonomic nervous system and the hypothalamic pituitary adrenal axis, which in turn leads to metabolic changes that increase cardiovascular risk. Work conditions are not the only way to activate these neuroendocrine pathways: low control in other areas of life, a self-image of low efficiency, and hostility may be other social or psychological factors that activate these pathways. (p. 239)

Researchers have not confined their inquiry to homo sapiens. Studies of other primates, such as wild baboons (Sapolsky, Alberts, and Altmann 1997) and captive monkeys (Shively and Clarkson 1994), show how low social standing among these species can also lead to a greater risk of coronary disease and other health risks, apparently as a reaction to continual stress. As interpreted by Robert Evans (1999):

> If you are constantly under the pressure of fight or flight, slowly you will, in fact, find your health deteriorating in various ways. [One study] found that the sub-dominant animals were in a state of permanent arousal—partly because of constant threats from the dominant animals and partly because once that state was triggered, physiologically they were changed in ways that made it difficult for them to turn off that fight-or-flight switch. In other words, they were physiologically changed by the experience of their rank and position. (p. 17)

Although difficult to demonstrate directly, the analogous theory is that humans who find themselves on the lower rungs of employment and social structures will experience similar reactions.

The second pathway relates to how income distribution may affect the resources available to those in lower classes. In a nearly egalitarian society, people are more likely to feel empathy toward others because most everyone is in a similar position. Of course, some people will be more disadvantaged than others, but when less of a bridge across classes exists, more societal resources are likely to be transferred to those who are more in need. In contrast, a society with a large gulf between classes is less ripe for such feelings of empathy, and in fact may exhibit overt hostility. In such a situation, the well-to-do may provide fewer resources to help others. In this regard, it has been hypothesized that, "political units that tolerate a high degree of income inequality are less likely to support the human, physical, cultural, civic, and health resources needed to maximize the health of the population" (Daly et al. 1998, p. 319). This theory has garnered some empirical support (Kaplan et al. 1996). Related research indicates that social investment in disadvantaged children is particularly important to their development (Hertzman 2001); areas with greater income inequality tend to provide fewer such investments.

A third and closely related pathway concerns some potential deleterious effects of a more stratified society, including a lack of trust, less individual investment in personal capital, and more violence—each of which may affect health. These issues are discussed briefly in Section 5.3.3, where the term *social capital* is introduced.

Unfortunately, it is very difficult to construct an unambiguous test of whether income distribution does affect health status through some of the causal mechanisms noted above. The main problem is specifying and collecting data on all of the factors that are likely to affect health status. The distribution of income in an area is related to many other characteristics—social, environmental, perhaps even behavioral—that may also affect health outcomes. If all of these are not controlled for, then empirical analyses of such data can inappropriately attribute causal effects to the distribution of income rather than to other, unmeasured factors.

Another difficulty with conducting this research is that we would expect to find a correlation between health and income distribution—even if none of the causal factors mentioned above matter.[32] This may seem counter-intuitive, but is illustrated in Figure 2.9.[33] Now suppose that each point on the curve shown represents a particular person in an area. Further suppose two areas each have the same average income, but one

---

32. For a fuller discussion of a number of conceptual problems in distinguishing between alternative hypotheses, see Wagstaff and van Doorslaer (2000).

33. Although this graph is similar to one provided by Kawachi (2000), the argument is based on a critique of the literature by Gravelle (1998).

exhibits a narrow distribution of income, ranging from A to B, whereas the other has a wide income distribution, ranging from Y to Z. Mathematically, the average health status is shown as the midpoint (M) of a line segment connecting these points. In the area with more equal incomes, average health status will be H_2, which is higher than health status (H_1) where there is greater income inequality. This means that "[o]verall population mortality increases when inequality increases, even though every individual's risk of mortality depends only on their own income level and not on the income level of anyone else" (Gravelle 1998, p. 383). This would hardly be supportive of the viewpoint that relative income matters through the pathways outlined above.

A substantial body of literature reports on whether income distribution affects health status, but unfortunately, there is little agreement among researchers and the issue is far from settled. One of the earliest studies was conducted by Rodgers (1979). Using data from 56 countries, he found that, controlling for the level of income, measures of income distribution had a large effect on infant mortality and life expectancy. Compared to an inegalitarian society, societies that are relatively egalitarian have lifespans of five to ten years more. Using data from the United States, Kennedy, Kawachi, and Prothrow-Stith (1996) found that states with the greatest distribution of income had higher total mortality and infant mortality rates. A number of other studies have also found evidence that narrower income distributions improve health.[34]

Significant literature, however, criticizes the studies that have found a relationship between income inequality and health and provides some counter-evidence. One of the main criticisms is that the above studies, and ones like them, do not adequately control for other factors that are related to both income distribution and health status (and thus suffer from "omitted variables bias"). Judge (1995) finds no relationship between several alternative measures of income inequality and life expectancy among developed countries. Mellor and Milyo (2001) find little evidence for the hypothesis using data from several dozen countries at a particular time period as well over time, nor do they find evidence of it when looking at nine different measures of health status across the different states in the United States. Similarly, Deaton (2001) finds no evidence of a relationship between income inequalities and health, although he does posit

---

34. For a collection of such studies, as well the views of a few dissenters, see Kawachi, Kennedy, and Wilkinson (1999).

that other types of inequalities between people other than income might be important. In a review of the literature, Wagstaff and van Doorslaer (2000) conclude that little convincing evidence exists that income inequality affects health.[35]

In summary, although many have explored how income distribution affects health, the literature demonstrates no consensus of findings. Fortunately, this issue continues to attract much research; its resolution has key implications for health policy. Many of the world's developed countries, including the United States and United Kingdom, Australia, and Canada, are showing greater income inequality over time (*Economist* 2001; Coburn 2000)—a trend certainly correlated and probably a result of a renewed focus on markets. A natural (although not necessarily inevitable) consequence of greater reliance on markets is a concomitant reduction in the role of the welfare state (Coburn 2000). One reason is that greater use of markets goes hand in hand with lower tax rates; with lower tax revenues, less money is available to finance welfare-related programs. If, as some have argued, income inequality reduces population health—and especially that of the poor—then a pull-back in welfare-related policies is likely to worsen these health-related consequences.

2.3.2 Equalizing Access to Health Services

Market forces operate through individuals' desires to gain from trade. If someone wishes to enter the marketplace to engage in such trading, economic theory shows that allowing that person to do so will increase his or her welfare without reducing that of others—which, in turn, will make society better off. This is true, however, only if there are no significant negative consumption externalities associated with the person's consumption.

At first glance, it might appear that most developed countries embrace this individualistic viewpoint when it comes to health policy. Practically all countries with comprehensive universal health insurance programs still allow their citizens to spend their own money on additional health services if those citizens wish to go outside of the government-sanctioned program. But on closer examination, health policy has been conducted

---

35. The January 5, 2002 issue of the *British Medical Journal* includes several more studies that find little or no evidence of this phenomenon (see Osler et al. 2002; Shibuya, Hashimoto, and Yano 2002; Sturm and Gresenz 2002; and Muller 2002).

on quite contrary principles. This is true even in the United States, where, it will be argued, society has up until now tried to minimize large differences in access to care.

One concern, however, is whether future health policy in developed countries will embrace the competitive ethic too literally. In the United States, the uninsured rate among the nonelderly population has risen considerably over the past decade, in part because of competitive pressures on providers and insurers. As yet, no parallel trend is apparent in other countries, although some observers are concerned that the movement toward more market involvement in general, and private insurance in particular, will erode public insurance programs and leave those who are in such programs with inferior access to care (Morone 2000). Lack of—or inadequate—insurance coverage can lead to a situation in which people see themselves as disadvantaged in comparison with others. A continuation of this trend will result in even more of the negative externalities that previous policy has tried to reduce.

Evidence supporting the viewpoint that U.S. health policy has eschewed the competitive prescription dates back many years. Beginning with the post–World War II period, the subsidization of the building and expansion of hospitals under the Hill-Burton Act (1948) and subsequent subsidization of physician training costs directly reflected a belief that poorer, rural areas of the United States should not be disadvantaged *relative to* wealthier, urban areas of the country. By defining the need for hospitals based on the per capita availability of beds, the philosophy behind Hill-Burton was that no areas of the country should be given greater access than others to hospital care.[36]

More recent evidence is provided by state mandates concerning the content of health insurance coverage. An implication of the competitive model is that insurance companies are allowed to provide whatever health insurance coverage they wish. Economists have argued that these mandates have a number of potentially deleterious consequences, including raising insurance costs, lowering wages, and lowering health insurance coverage rates (Jensen and Morrisey 1999).

---

36. In fact, because of greater driving distances in rural areas, subsidies were aimed at giving them higher bed-to-population ratios than urban areas. The construction and expansion of hospitals was subsidized up to a level of 5.5 beds per 1,000 people in areas where there were fewer than six persons per square mile, versus only 4.5 beds per 1,000 in area exceeding 12 persons per square mile.

Public policy makers have followed this advice, however. States, which have almost all regulatory authority over the sale of insurance, have enacted numerous "mandates" concerning the eligibility for, and content of, health insurance policies. One study found that by 1988, there were more than 730 mandates across the different states (Gabel and Jensen 1989). It reported, for example, that 37 states require insurers to cover alcohol treatment, 28 require that mental health services be covered, and 18, maternity care. A more recent study found that the number of state mandates had grown to about 1,000 by 1997 (Council for Affordable Health Insurance 1997). In 1996, the most common mandates were for mammography screening (46 states), alcohol treatment (43 states), and services provided by psychologists and chiropractors (41 states each) (Jensen and Morrisey 1999). Special interest groups provide much of the support for these mandates; nevertheless, consumer groups, and particularly people who need certain services (or know someone who does), also tend to support them—indicating a viewpoint that the public does not want insurance coverage decisions left solely to the marketplace.

Similar evidence can be seen by examining the political fallout that arose from the Oregon proposal for Medicaid reform, which was dubbed as requiring "rationing" of services. Early versions of the proposal engendered a great deal of opposition, mainly because program beneficiaries would not be able to receive coverage for the same services as the rest of the population. Rather, what services would be paid for would depend on how much money was available. Less cost-effective services would not be covered if program money was exhausted after paying for more cost-effective services. This prompted Bruce Vladeck (1990), who later became director of the federal government's Health Care Financing Administration (currently, the Centers for Medicare & Medicaid Services), to write,

> [T]his will be the first system in memory to explicitly plan that poor people with treatable illnesses will die if Medicaid runs out of money or does not budget correctly, and providers will be excused from liability for failing to treat them. The Oregonians argue that it is healthier for society to make such choices explicitly, but it is hardly healthy to establish rules of the game that require such choices. (p. 3)

In fact, the proposal was cleared by federal officials only after the methodology was revised to ensure that disabled individuals would not face discrimination in coverage (Fox and Leichter 1993), and after the state made it clear that all essential services would be provided.[37] After the modified proposal had been implemented, a survey of Medicaid beneficiaries in the state found that one-third had needed a service that was not covered. In 38 percent of these cases, it was because the service was "below the line"—that is, a service that was not covered because funding was insufficient. About half of these people obtained the service with their own money. Among the other half, 60 percent said that their health had deteriorated as a result (Mitchell and Bentley 2000).

A final example of how U.S. health policy operates in conflict with the competitive model concerns coverage for new technologies. Imagine that a new technology becomes available that can help save lives, but is very expensive. Is society better off if we allow only the very rich to purchase it, as the Pareto principle would imply? It might seem that the answer is "yes," because we do allow people to spend their own money for such procedures so long as the procedures are not illegal. But on further reflection, it becomes clear that something quite different is going on.

Traditionally, when new and potentially effective technologies become available, they are viewed as experimental until their safety and efficacy are established. Once established, insurers almost always cover them; failure to do so results first in strong pressure from policyholders and eventually in lawsuits that the insurer is withholding necessary medical care. Having these technologies covered by public and private insurance ensures that access to them is available to the large majority of the population that has health insurance. In this regard, Uwe Reinhardt (1992) writes,

> Suppose [that a] new, high-tech medical intervention [is available] and that more of it could be produced without causing reductions in the output of any other commodity. Suppose next, however, that the associated rearrangement of the economy has been such that only well-to-do patients will have access to the new medical procedure. On these assumptions, can we be sure that [this] would enhance overall

---

37. Politics undoubtedly entered the decision as well. The first Bush Administration had blocked approval of the plan, but soon after taking office, the Clinton Administration approved it. See Pollack et al. (1994).

social welfare? Would we not have to assume the absence of *social envy* among the poor and of guilt among the well-to-do? Are these reasonable assumptions? Or should civilized policy analysts refuse to pay heed to base human motives such as envy, prevalent though it may be in any normal society? (p. 311)

If public policy were based on market competition, then we would see a gap between the services that are available to the wealthy and those available to the rest of the insured population. We do not see such a gap; once a procedure is found to be safe and effective, everyone with private health insurance is potentially eligible to receive it.[38] And, if insurers are not sufficiently quick to adopt new procedures, states can and do mandate their provision.[39]

This is not to say that policy has ensured equal access for all Americans. In fact, the uninsured population tends to use few services and to benefit from fewer new medical technologies than others (Institute of Medicine 2001). Up until now, however, most have been able to benefit from a safety net of public hospitals and community clinics, as well as "cross-subsidization" of uninsured patients by their insured counterparts.

One consequence of the increasingly competitive medical marketplace in the United States is a breakdown in the public health system, coupled with reduced cross-subsidization of the uninsured. To keep costs down, private hospitals are sending more of their sickest indigent patients to public hospitals, which in turn find themselves in increasing financial distress (Thorpe 1997). Private insurers (spurred in part by employers, who foot much of the bill) are less willing to pay providers enough to allow them to care for those without coverage. Thus, although U.S. public policy has tried in the past to keep differences in access to care from becoming large, increased competition in the health services sector appears

---

38. Some HMOs have tried to ration the use of medical technologies, with varying degrees of success. This is one of the primary reasons for the so-called "consumer backlash" against managed care, a consequence of which has been a movement away from some of the heavy-handed cost-control techniques that had previously been used (Gabel et al. 2001).

39. States cannot currently mandate provision of services under employer-sponsored health plans that fall under the jurisdiction of the Employee Retirement Income and Security Act (ERISA). Although this has effectively reduced the strength of state mandates, there is little doubt that such mandates would still exist if ERISA were repealed.

to be working in the opposite direction—which, we have argued, is not consistent with raising social welfare in the presence of externalities of consumption. Chapter 6 discusses some similar trends in other developed countries.

2.3.3 What Comes First: Allocation or Distribution?

As noted above, in the traditional economic paradigm, a competitive market is used to ensure that resources are allocated efficiently. But if there are positive externalities of consumption—for example, if society wants poorer people to have more resources—then the free-rider effect will prevent a competitive economy from achieving allocative efficiency. The solution to this problem under the economic model is to institute lump-sum taxes and subsidies, because they do not distort incentives and reduce efficiency; but in practice, no such mechanisms are available.

A more reasonable approach to dealing with this problem is for society to grapple with allocative and distributive issues concurrently. Rather than saying, "we will take whatever the competitive market gives us, and then institute the necessary taxes and subsidies," a reasonable society might contend that "we will start with certain redistributive principles, and once they are established, allow the market to operate around these principles."

Reinhardt (1992) provides a similar philosophy:

> [T]o begin an exploration of alternative proposals for the reform of our health system without first setting forth explicitly, and very clearly, the *social values* to which the reformed system is to adhere strikes at least this author as patently *inefficient*: it is a waste of time. Would it not be more *efficient* merely to explore the *relative efficiency* of alternative proposals that do conform to widely shared *social values*? (p. 315)

This method—rather than the method advocated through the competitive model—is how policy has traditionally been made in the United States as well as almost all developed countries. In the United States, public programs like Medicare and Medicaid were established *outside* of the competitive marketplace to ensure that our priority—access to medical care services for the elderly and the poor—was met.

The belief that we should start with principles of fairness, and then proceed to considerations of efficiency, is also the foundation on which most other health systems have been built. In their comprehensive study of financing and equity in nine health systems in Europe and the United States, Adam Wagstaff and colleagues (1992) found that:

> [t]here appears to be broad agreement . . . among policymakers in at least eight of the nine European countries [studied] that payments towards health care should be related to ability to pay rather than to use of medical facilities. Policymakers in all nine European countries also appear to be committed to the notion that all citizens should have access to health care. In many countries this is taken further, it being made clear that access to and receipt of health care should depend on need, rather than on ability to pay. (p. 363)

The United States has seen a resurgence of late in reliance on health maintenance organizations (HMOs) and other competitive policies in both the Medicare and Medicaid programs.[40] Although such policies may bring about cost savings, there is concern that their enactment will reduce access for some of the poor and elderly—which, as was argued, has up until now increased social welfare because of the positive externalities associated with coverage for these groups. This is not because they would lose coverage; rather, it stems from a concern that the two groups that may be least able to "navigate" their way through HMOs' gatekeeping systems are poor and elderly persons (Ware et al. 1986; Ware et al. 1996; Goldstein and Fyock 2001). The overall concern is that the reliance on more competition will jeopardize the principles that formed the basis of these programs in the first place.

2.3.4 Competition and Prevention

Another manifestation of the problems associated with the free-rider effect concerns prevention. Traditionally, HMOs have encouraged preventive services both through low service copayments, and by covering services not traditionally included in many fee-for-service health plans, such as annual preventive examinations and diagnostic tests. One of the reasons HMOs have given for providing these services to members is that

---

40. Between 1998 and 2001, Medicare HMO enrollment actually declined; this was largely brought about by reductions in payments to these HMOs. Nevertheless, overall there has been substantial enrollment growth in the past decade.

such services will reduce future health-related costs. This will not be the case, however, if plan members regularly switch between competing (and often nearly identical) health plans. In this regard, Donald Light (1995) writes,

> [P]revention by any given [health] plan only makes economic sense within a contract year, or else one's competitors may benefit from one's efforts when subscribers switch plans in the next contract year. . . . Why should a given plan, for example, make efforts to reduce drug abuse or smoking at the schools of a given town when only some of the children are their customers, and their parents may move or switch plans next year? (p. 151)

Recent data show that individuals are willing to switch their health plans in the wake of very small premium differences—particularly when the discernible differences between these alternatives are few (Buchmueller 1998; Christianson et al. 1995).[41]

It is too early to know whether, in fact, the provision of preventive services is indeed declining as a result of this free-rider effect. Documentation of such an effect would provide further reason to consider limiting the number of health plan choices available to consumers, or to move toward a more publicly funded system.[42]

2.3.5 Government-Sponsored Health Education

The traditional economic model assumes that consumer tastes are predetermined. People come into the marketplace knowing what they want, and what they want is intrinsic to them; it is not shaped by past consumption or by external forces.

How does advertising fit into all of this? There are really two types of advertising: that designed to provide purely objective information (e.g.,

---

41. Individual practice associations and network-model HMOs often have very similar provider panels, so it would not be clear to most consumers that the plan they choose would make much of a difference. This may not be the case, however, because different plans might have different financial incentives for providers, employ different utilization monitoring techniques, and so forth. For a discussion of these issues, see Hibbard, Sofaer, and Jewett (1996).

42. In this regard, Robert Kuttner (1997) writes, "A purely privatized system is likely to be more fragmented, and less willing to pay for public health, or to grasp its logic" (p. 158).

prices, availability) and that aimed at shaping consumer tastes. Advertisers may pass along information to the consumer that, if accepted, will not necessarily be in the consumer's best interest.

One policy implication of this concerns health education. Because economics concerns itself primarily with money-type variables (e.g., price, insurance, income), its practitioners tend to be less conversant about other policy interventions, such as education designed to change people's harmful habits. If, however, preferences are the product of advertisers' activities, medical education may have a role in undoing some of these deleterious effects.

Government has long been involved, for example, in trying to convince the public not to smoke. Part of this effort has been regulatory. Tobacco companies in the United States, for example, cannot advertise their products on television. Government has also been directly involved in antismoking campaigns, through explicit advertisements as well as requiring tobacco companies to put various health disclosures on their packaging. One wonders if more of this, extending into other consumer behaviors (e.g., nutrition, drinking) is not warranted. The need for these efforts is heightened if consumer tastes are malleable rather than predetermined.

2.3.6 Should Cost Control Be a Public Policy?

A larger issue that arises if consumer tastes are pliable concerns cost control. Health economists often point out that we cannot say that a country spends too much of its national income on health services. Who is to say that 14 percent or even 25 percent is "too much"? It is contended that nothing is necessarily wrong if a society wants to spend more of its money on, say, expensive technologies. In fact, survey data show that about two-thirds of all Americans believe that the country spends *too little* on medical care (Blendon et al. 2001). But this viewpoint is harder to justify if one views consumer tastes not as predetermined, but rather as the product of previous experiences.

Take the example of the use of medical technology. People are likely to demand the fruits of new technologies in part because they come to expect them. Later in the book we present data on the use of so-called "high-tech" procedures in ten different countries. As shown in Table 6.8, the U.S. utilization rate is almost four times the average of the other countries for coronary bypass operations and almost five times as high for angioplasty. Furthermore, much of the difference is due to considerably higher rates among the "oldest old" (Verrilli, Berenson, and Katz 1998).

Because of the availability of high-tech equipment in the United States, the public is likely to have developed greater expectations of their use. Some analysts argue that it is the growth of these technologies—or, as Joseph Newhouse (1993) termed it, "the enhanced capabilities of medicine" (p. 162)—that is primarily responsible for rising health costs in the United States.

The point that maybe people would be equally well off without so many expensive (not to say duplicative) lifesaving interventions is made only tentatively. One would not want to claim that people want to live longer because they are inculcated into believing that is desirable. Clearly, though, quality-of-life issues become relevant to such a discussion, as does the fact that the United States ranks near the top of the world in only one major vital statistic category—life expectancy after reaching age 80.[43] One must take pause when considering Easterlin's results that were presented earlier—that people in poor countries seem to be equally happy as those in wealthier ones—or, perhaps more relevant to health, the fact that citizens of other countries, which spend far less money on medical care, tend to be much happier with their medical care systems. This latter point is supported by the data later in the book (Tables 6.5 and 6.6), which show that satisfaction among citizens with their medical systems in other developed countries is no lower than in the United States.

This belief, that more and more spending on technologies does not seem to be increasing utility levels very much, is consistent with a rather sober quotation[44] from E. J. Mishan (1969a):

---

43. Data from 24 developed countries show that life expectancy in the United States at age 80 is rivaled only by Canada and Iceland. In contrast, more than 15 of the countries exceed the United States in life expectancy at birth. See Schieber, Poullier, and Greenwald (1994).

44. Similarly, Kuttner (1997) discusses the book, *The Overworked American* by Juliet Schor (1993), which he describes as pointing "to a vicious circle in which the pursuit of material satisfactions promised by advertising leads Americans to work more hours than they really want, in order to have money to buy the products that never quite yield their promised fulfillments. Over time, people internalize two contradictory conclusions—a cumulative cynicism combined with an unquenchable hunger that perhaps the next product will somehow yield the elusive satisfaction" (Kuttner 1997, p. 57). This theme is echoed by Frank (1985, 1999), which is discussed above.

As I see it, the main task today of the economist at all concerned with the course of human welfare is that of weaning the public from its post-war fixation on economic growth; of inculcating an awareness of the errors and misconceptions that abound in popular appraisals of the benefits of industrial development; and also, perhaps of voicing an occasional doubt whether the persistent pursuit of material ends, borne onwards today by a tidal wave of unrealisable expectations, can do more eventually than to agitate the current restlessness, and to add to the frustrations and disillusion of ordinary mortals. (p. 81)

Let us end the chapter on a more encouraging note, however. In two books discussed earlier in the chapter, Robert Frank (1985, 1999) argues that consumer behavior is badly skewed away from the things that would bring the most benefit because people care so much about how their possessions rank compared to those of their peers. As a result, people spend far more of their resources on consumables that bring about (in their minds) status, and less on arguably more valuable things, such as additional leisure time or travel—or perhaps health. To provide a single example, he argues that a 4,000-square-foot house, compared to one with 3,000 square feet, will do little to make a person happier, but constitutes a considerable increase in resources. He further argues that people buy houses of this size, along with expensive cars, clothes, and the like, to distinguish themselves from others. But if everyone else does so, overall societal happiness is no higher, and thus, much of a country's wealth has been expended needlessly.

One might argue that expenditures on improving health are the type that Frank would want to encourage. Generally, these are not done to "keep up with the Joneses," nor does better health usually connote higher social status. If everyone were healthier, society would be better off; your better health does not detract from mine.

This has an important implication: additional societal spending on health services—*if* it leads to better health—might to be an attractive investment. Thus, research should focus on such things as the types of medical spending that have the best opportunity for improving health, as well as the preferences of individuals and communities in this regard.

Chapter 3

Demand Theory

JUST AS MARKET competition represents the core concept in micro-economics, demand theory is the key to understanding market competition. Demand, which economists often define as how many goods and services are purchased at alternative prices, is the mechanism that drives a competitive economy. Under demand theory, the amount of a commodity that is produced and consumed is determined by people's demand for it. If people's tastes change for some reason, and they want more of one good and less of another, prices will change, prompting firms to adjust their production. Unless some sort of constraint on obtaining the necessary inputs for production exists, in the long run supply adjusts to satisfy demand.

But demand theory means more than just this. It also forms the basis by which economic theory evaluates social welfare. If people demand a certain bundle of goods and services, it means that they prefer that bundle to all other ways in which they could spend their money. In other words, the things people demand are, by definition, those things that put them at the highest level of welfare, given the resources available. If all people act in a way that maximizes their utilities, given their available income, society will also be at a welfare maximum.[1]

Section 3.1 contains a brief summary of the traditional demand theory; readers already familiar with such concepts as social welfare, revealed preference, and consumer surplus can move on to the following section.

---

1. This assumes that society is satisfied with the distribution of income, which will be discussed further in this chapter as well as in Chapter 5.

Section 3.2 provides a critique of demand theory; this critique is based, to a large extent, on questioning the validity of some of the assumptions of demand theory that were listed in Chapter 1. Section 3.3 applies this critique to a number of health economic issues and tools that are used to draw policy conclusions about health policy.

3.1 THE TRADITIONAL ECONOMIC MODEL

This discussion is divided into four subsections: utility and social welfare; revealed preference; demand curves and functions; and the meaning of demand and consumer surplus.

3.1.1 Utility and Social Welfare

In Section 2.1.1, we saw that under traditional economic theory, consumers are assumed to make choices about the goods and services they purchase in ways that will maximize their utility. How do we determine whether these choices will also be best for society as a whole?

Some early theorists, who collectively are known as the *classical utilitarians*, believed that total social welfare was simply the numerical sum of all individuals' welfare. The question naturally arises about how it was possible to quantify such measures. Perhaps the leading early advocate of classical utilitarianism, Jeremy Bentham (1791), thought that it was possible to measure utility through its manifestations of pleasure and pain. Of these, he writes:

> Nature has pleased mankind under the governance of two sovereign masters, *pain* and *pleasure*. It is for them alone to point out what we ought to do, as well as to determine what we shall do. On the one hand the standard of right and wrong, on the other the chain of causes and effects, are fastened to their throne. They govern us in all we do, in all we say, in all we think: every effort we can make to throw off our subjection, will serve but to demonstrate and confirm it. (Bentham 1968, p. 3)

If everyone has the same capacity to experience pleasure and pain, and if we also assume the existence of diminishing marginal utility, then an interesting policy prescription arises under classical utilitarianism: social welfare is maximized when everyone has the same income. It is easy to see why this is the case. Suppose one person has $10,000 in income and another $5,000. If an additional dollar is spent by the former person, it will bring less utility than if spent by the latter. Only if everyone has the same income will total welfare be maximized.

Although some "radical utilitarians" were comfortable with this implication, others—some of whom presumably would have lost a great deal through the equalization of incomes—were not. And it was not hard to poke holes in the theory. Classical utilitarianism is based on two important assumptions: (1) utility can be quantified, and (2) it is possible to add utilities across different individuals.

Modern economists tend to eschew both of these assumptions and have made a great deal of progress without them. (As noted in Section 5.2, economists still employ a utilitarian viewpoint, but one that makes much weaker assumptions.) The works of Pareto and Edgeworth, discussed in Section 2.1, were instrumental in this regard, as was the more recent work of Paul Samuelson. Microeconomics now proceeds under the Pareto principle, where a policy is desirable if it makes someone better off without making anyone worse off. But to go further—say, to advocate one program or tax over another, when there will be both winners and losers, as being better for society as a whole—explicit value judgments are necessary.

3.1.2 Revealed Preference

In Section 2.1.1, we introduced indifference curves but did not discuss where they came from. One way to derive them is to ask people which alternative bundle of goods they would prefer. This technique has two problems. First, it is difficult to imagine administering such a population survey given the nearly countless possible bundles of goods from which people can choose. Second, it is entirely possible that people will not tell the truth, or even if they do, their responses may not predict their actual behavior when faced with such market choices.

The concept of *revealed preference* is designed to eliminate these problems. Under this theory, pioneered by Samuelson (1938), people are simply assumed to prefer whatever bundle of goods they choose to consume. If they purchase one bundle but could afford another one, we can say that they have revealed themselves to prefer the former. One significant aspect of this theory is that it does not rely on understanding the psyche of the individual. Rather, as Robert Sugden (1993) has noted,

> [T]he most significant property of the revealed preference approach . . . is that we do not need to enquire into the reasons why one thing

Figure 3.1: Derivation of Demand Curve, Step 1

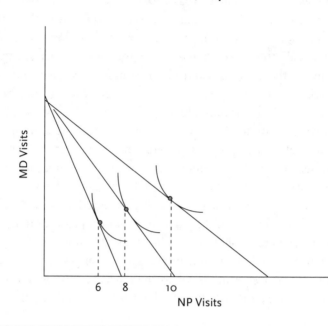

is chosen rather than another. We do not look into the factors that go into the deliberation which leads to a choice; we look only at the results of that process. (p. 1949)

Indifference curves may be derived through the theory of revealed preference; all one has to do is witness actual consumer behavior over different sets of prices and income. In doing so, economists are making an important assumption, to which we will return in Section 3.2: whatever bundle people choose is the bundle that, at least before the fact, is expected to make them best off.

3.1.3 Demand Curves and Functions

It is not hard to go from the concept of indifference curves and revealed preference to the concept of demand. Following the example given in Chapter 2, Figure 3.1 shows three indifference curves for nurse practitioner (NP) and physician (MD) visits for a particular consumer. We then vary the price of NP visits from P_n to $P_n/2$ to $P_n/4$ but do not change the price of MD visits (P_m) or income. The result is that the budget line

Figure 3.2: Derivation of Demand Curve, Step 2

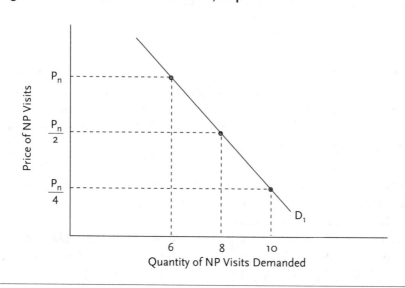

pivots outward. Under these three alternative sets of prices, suppose that the consumer chooses to purchase six, eight, and ten NP visits per year, respectively. These points are then plotted as a *demand curve* labeled D_1 in Figure 3.2. A demand curve shows how much of a good is purchased at alternative prices. Although one needs actual data on consumer behavior to draw such a curve accurately, in general it exhibits a downward-sloping-to-the-right direction, indicating that people will demand more when the price is lower.

We already saw that a demand curve is drawn under the assumptions that neither the price of other goods nor the person's income changes. It is further assumed that a person's tastes are also unaltered. In functional form:

$$D = f(P, P_a, I, T) \tag{3.1}$$

where D is demand for a particular good or service, P is its price, P_a is the price of alternatives, I is income, and T is tastes. *Aggregate* demand—how much is demanded by all individuals combined—is simply the sum of individual demands.

Alternative goods can be categorized two ways: *complements* and *substitutes*. Complements are goods that are used in conjunction with the good being studied, and substitutes are ones that are used instead.[2] We can therefore refine Equation 3.1 as follows:

$$D = f(P, P_s, P_c, I, T) \qquad (3.2)$$

where P_s is the price of substitutes, and P_c, the price of complements.

What is perhaps most noteworthy about these equations is the unobtrusive role played by T, tastes. This one variable represents much of what it is to be a human being. Much of the research in the fields of psychology and sociology has been devoted to addressing how individual tastes are formed and the ways in which they are manifested. But as we noted in Section 2.2.3, economic theory takes the taste variable as predetermined and unaffected by the person's environment.

In the health services area, perhaps the major component of T is health status. If people are sick, they are obviously more likely to use medical care than if they are well. In that one sense, they have more of a "taste" for health. This would not seem to be a very good way to classify your desire for medical services if, say, you are hit by a car, but there is no other place to put it if one uses Equation 3.2. As a result, sometimes one sees the demand for health written as:

$$D = f(P, P_s, P_c, I, HS, T) \qquad (3.3)$$

where HS is the patient's health status. In Equation 3.3, tastes no longer capture health status, but rather only the non–health-related determinants of demand.

As we saw, a single demand curve can be used to illustrate any relationship between the quantity and price of a particular good. It is assumed, however, that the other determinants of demand—the prices of alternative goods, income, health status, and tastes—remain unchanged. If they do change, then the demand curve must also shift. For example, when a person gets sick, his or her demand curve is likely to shift outward and to the right, indicating that he or she will demand more medical care at

---

2. The technical definitions are somewhat more involved. Goods are complements if their cross-price elasticity of demand is negative; they are substitutes if it is positive. The cross-price elasticity of demand is defined as the percentage change in the quantity demanded of a particular good, divided by the percentage change in the price of another good (the complement or substitute).

all price levels. Nevertheless, the amount demanded is still expected to depend, in part, on the price of medical care.

The exact relationship between the quantity of a good purchased and its price is represented by the *elasticity of demand*. This is defined as the percentage change in the quantity of a good demanded, divided by the percentage change in its price. If the elasticity of demand equals −0.5, when the price of the good changes by, say, 10 percent, the quantity demanded changes by 5 percent, but in the opposite direction. Much health economic research has been devoted to determining various demand elasticities for medical services.[3]

3.1.4 The Meaning of Demand and Consumer Surplus

The derivation of demand curves through indifference curves, which in turn can be derived from revealed preferences, leads to an important implication: the goods and services that people demand are the ones that, at least before the fact, are expected to make them best off. That is to say, the act of demanding one set of goods, given prevailing prices and incomes, implies that a person is likely to be better off with that set than with any other set of goods that he or she can afford. If this is the case, it is a fairly small leap to say, then, that an economic system that allows people to choose their bundles is best for society. Critiquing this proposition will be the primary purpose of Section 3.2.

An understanding of exactly what a demand curve means will provide insights into the important concept of consumer surplus. As indicated by revealed preference, when a person demands a good, he or she prefers it to all alternatives. One of these alternatives is, of course, not spending the money in the first place.

The theory therefore implies that the utility obtained from purchasing a good or service is at least as great as the price paid—or it would not have been purchased in the first place. What a demand curve therefore shows is the *marginal utility* of a particular purchase. If a person buys six apples when they are priced at 50 cents each but buys seven when they are priced at 40 cents, then the marginal utility derived from the purchase of the seventh apple is at least 40 cents.

We saw in Section 2.1.1 that consumers are assumed to try to maximize their utility through the bundle of goods that they purchase. They would

---

3. For a review of this evidence, see Feldstein (1998) or Phelps (1997).

therefore seek only those goods whose marginal utilities exceeded the market price. Consumers are often fortunate enough to be in a position where the market price of a good they seek is less than the maximum amount they would be willing to pay. The difference between how much consumers are willing to pay for something, and what it actually costs, is called *consumer surplus*. The concept, first used in the mid-1800s by Jules Dupuit, a French engineer, to determine the value of railroad bridges, was popularized by Alfred Marshall to the English-speaking world (Ng 1979; Parkin 1999).

The calculation of consumer surplus is illustrated in Figure 3.3. Suppose that the market price of an NP visit is $30, at which price our consumer Paul is willing to purchase four per year (point B on demand curve D_1). Note, however, that he was willing to pay much more for the first three visits: $40 for the third visit, $50 for the second, and $60 for the first. Thus, in purchasing four NP visits, Paul has earned a surplus. He was willing to pay $180 for the four visits but only had to pay $120 (4 × $30), so he has earned a consumer surplus of $60. This is illustrated by the triangle ABC in Figure 3.3.[4]

The concept of consumer surplus comes into play not so much at the individual level, but in the aggregate. If we add together all of the surpluses received by all consumers, we obtain the total consumer surplus, which is the difference between the value consumers receive from a good, and how much they have to pay for it. Economists use this tool for such matters as determining whether society should embark on a publicly financed investment or project, and in other applications such as calculating the "welfare loss" from excess health insurance, which is discussed later in Section 3.3.1.

3.2 PROBLEMS WITH THE TRADITIONAL MODEL

In *Candide*, the philosopher Dr. Pangloss attempts to prove that the obviously flawed state of nature and society is, nevertheless, the best of all possible worlds. Voltaire (1759) quotes his character as stating,

> It is demonstrated that things cannot be otherwise: for, since everything was made for a purpose, everything is necessarily for the best

---

4. The size of the triangle ABC equals $80 rather than $60 because, as drawn, Paul could purchase fractions of visits as well.

Figure 3.3: Derivation of Consumer Surplus

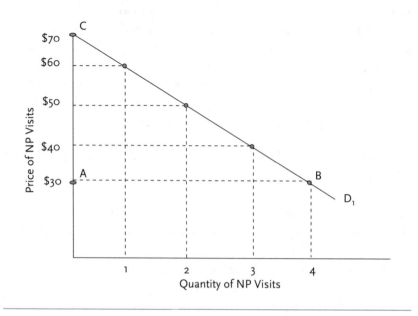

purpose. Note that noses were made to wear spectacles; we therefore have spectacles. Legs were clearly devised to wear breeches, and we have breeches. . . . And since pigs were made to be eaten, we have pork all year round. Therefore, those who have maintained that all is well have been talking nonsense: they should have maintained that all is for the best. (p. 18)

Although perhaps not recognized by most economists, the theory of revealed preference in particular, and consumer theory in general, bears a striking resemblance to Pangloss's philosophy.[5] By choosing a particular bundle of goods, people demonstrate that they prefer it to all others; consequently, it is best for them. And, if all people are in their best position, then society—which is simply the aggregation of all people—is also in its best position. Therefore, allowing people to choose in the marketplace results in the best of all possible economic worlds.

---

5. Other economists have also employed Dr. Pangloss in their critiques of contemporary economics. See, for example, Culyer (1982) and Evans (1983).

The purpose of this section is to demonstrate that this sort of syllo-gism (which will be made more explicit below) is tenuous at best because it is based on assumptions that are difficult to support, particularly in the health services area. We will question the conventional meaning of the demand curve where it purports to show the marginal utility obtained by consumers through the purchase of alternative quantities of a good. Accepting the arguments presented in this section has profound implica-tions concerning the wisdom of relying on competitive markets in health system financing and medical care delivery. Some of these applications are provided in Section 3.3.

In the process, we will question six of the assumptions of the compet-itive economic model presented earlier:

Assumption 4. A person is the best judge of his or her own welfare.

Assumption 5. Consumers have sufficient information to make good choices.

Assumption 6. Consumers know, with certainty, the results of their consumption decisions.

Assumption 7. Individuals are rational.

Assumption 8. Individuals reveal their preferences through their actions.

Assumption 9. Social welfare is based solely on individual utilities, which in turn are based solely on the goods and services consumed.

3.2.1 Social Welfare and Consumer Choice: A Syllogism

As we saw in Section 2.1.4, it is typically argued that an economic system that allows for consumer choice will, subject to some caveats,[6] result in Pareto optimality. Then, if society can reach some agreement on its social welfare function, redistribution can be implemented in ways that will maximize social welfare.

In this chapter, we will make the assumption that such a redistribution does occur. (Problems with this assumption were introduced in Section 2.2.2, which concerned positive externalities of consumption; Chapter 5 will elaborate on those problems.) By making this assumption, we im-plicitly assume that reaching Pareto optimality will ultimately lead to the

---

6. The primary caveat is that externalities are unimportant. That is why economists often say that the presence of important yet uncorrected externalities results in "market failure."

maximization of social welfare. This allows us to explicitly examine the assumptions under which allowing consumers to choose in the market-place will be best for society as a whole.

With this assumption in hand, we can form the following syllogism:

If
A. Social welfare is maximized when individual utilities are maximized,

and
B. Individual utilities are maximized when people are allowed to choose,

then:
C. Social welfare is maximized when people are allowed to choose.

This is obviously a strong conclusion because it implies that the type of consumer choice brought about by market competition will result, as Dr. Pangloss would say, in the best of all possible worlds. In the health field, the argument would provide strong ammunition for the superiority of competitive approaches. But if either proposition A or proposition B does not hold, then such a conclusion about the superiority of choice through competition is not warranted. In the next section, we will attempt to cast serious doubt about the validity of both propositions A and B—first proposition B, and then A. Because proposition B encompasses five of the assumptions on which the advantages of competition are based, most of the emphasis will be on it.

3.2.2 Are Individual Utilities Maximized When People Are Allowed to Choose?

One of the basic tenets of market competition is that people are best off when they are allowed to make choices. If, instead, some entity such as government makes the choices for them, it is extremely unlikely that consumers will fare as well; each person is different, and it would seem to be impossible for an outsider to appreciate an individual's exact desires. True, sometimes people are poorly informed about a particular good or service and must rely on the advice of an *agent* such as a physician. But even then, they still choose whether to seek that advice, as well as the particular agent from whom the advice is sought.

In a world such as ours, where high-paid consultants abound and access to more information seems to be the key to success, economists often consider an individual consumer to be the world's greatest expert in one particular area. That area, of course, is what he or she wants. This viewpoint is nicely stated by economist Friedrich Hayek (1945), another of the founders of modern competitive theory:

> Today it is almost heresy to suggest that scientific knowledge is not the sum of all knowledge. But a little reflection will show that there is beyond question a body of very important but unorganized knowledge which cannot possibly be called scientific . . . : the knowledge of the particular circumstances of time and place. It is with respect to this that practically every individual has some advantage over all others in that he possesses unique information of which beneficial use might be made, but of which use can be made only if the decisions depending on it are left to him or are made with his active cooperation. . . . If we agree that the economic problem of society is mainly one of rapid adaptation to changes in the particular circumstances of time and place, it would seem to follow that the ultimate decisions must be left to the people who are familiar with these circumstances. (pp. 521–22, 534)

This is indeed a persuasive argument. Nevertheless, this section will attempt to demonstrate that, at least in the health services area, allowing people to make their own choices does not necessarily make people best off.

Is a Person the Best Judge of His or Her Own Welfare?
The first question that needs to be addressed when considering whether sovereignty is best for consumers is whether consumers are the foremost authority of what is in their best interest. As Hayek pointed out, in many instances they unquestionably are. Nevertheless, they may not be in all areas. If, in some instances, consumers are not the best judge of what is in their interest, then choices in such areas can perhaps be relegated to some other entity.

Of the several assumptions that we question in this chapter, this is perhaps the most difficult because of the seeming impossibility for empirical testing. Obviously, no direct source of information on what is best for a particular person exists. Consequently, there is no way of objectively testing who—the individual or some other entity—is the better agent for obtaining what is best for the person. We must therefore rely on indirect methods to further our inquiry.

To demonstrate that the individual is not necessarily the best judge, we will examine how society goes about making allocation decisions about particular goods and services. What we will try to show is that most societies set rules that are explicitly designed to thwart the sanctity of individual choice.

Below is a list of practices that a libertarian—that is, a person who believes in the sanctity of individual sovereignty—would likely believe should be left up to the individual rather than be proscribed by society:

- personal use of narcotic drugs;
- gambling;
- prostitution;
- riding a motorcycle without a helmet;
- selling one's own organs; and
- suicide.

This list was chosen specifically because these are all decisions that mainly affect the individual in question rather than others. Other illegal activities, such as requiring one's child to work rather than go to school, were left out because they have a direct negative effect on someone other than the decision maker. The first three examples may contain some indirect externalities—for example, drug use or gambling leading to more robberies, or prostitution leading to more sexually transmitted diseases. But these are indirect consequences, and regardless, the last three would result in harm almost entirely to the individual.[7]

Why would society act in a way to abridge individual choice when consumer theory indicates that people can make welfare-maximizing choices themselves? Robert Frank (1985) suggests an interesting possibility: people are overly concerned with their status and will make the wrong economic, social, and/or moral decisions to enhance this status. One way that young people might do this is to try to "look cool," for instance, by smoking, using drugs, not wearing seat belts or helmets, or spending $200 on a pair of athletic shoes. Some of these practices are easy to outlaw, although rules against them cannot necessarily be enforced. But even the more vexing behaviors, such as excessive spending

---

7. It is true that there is an indirect effect on others in that health-related costs might be higher—and, particularly in the case of suicide, high psychological costs for the living—but these are not the primary reasons why such activities are illegal.

on status-building clothing, are not beyond society's grip. Many public schools have adopted uniform requirements as a way of reducing the negative manifestations of status seeking.

Even adults might be lured by choices that, in the long run, are bad for them. Frank suggests that this tends to manifest itself when adults make shortsighted decisions to obtain quick income to have money available to spend on consumables that ostensibly are status enhancing (e.g., trendy clothing or cars or new electronic equipment). People engaging in heavy gambling are likely doing it not to make money to save for their children's college education, but rather, to go on a spending spree. Similarly, one would imagine that an individual who sells one of his or her internal organs is doing so for reasons that an objective observer would say are not in that individual's best interest.

But trying to cut down on harmful status seeking does not seem to fully account for laws abridging personal choice. An American going to Mexico to purchase a supposed cure for cancer does not seem status raising; another reason for paternalistic laws that limit individual choice is that some types of spending decisions are simply a waste of money. Society is protecting people against their own foolishness.

A related reason for paternalism—one that is frequently cited in the health field—is that there are "experts" who know more than consumers, and can thus make better choices. In this regard, Tibor Scitovsky (1976) has written,

> The economist's traditional picture of the economy resembles nothing so much as a Chinese restaurant with its long menu. Customers choose from what is on the menu and are assumed always to have chosen what most pleases them. That assumption is unrealistic, not only of the economy, but of Chinese restaurants. Most of us are unfamiliar with nine-tenths of the entrees listed; we seem invariably to order either the wrong dishes or the same old ones. Only on occasions when an expert does the ordering do we realize how badly we do on our own and what good things we miss. (pp. 149–50)

It would seem clear, then, that society does not always judge people's decisions to be in their best interests. In making this judgment, society often acts to prevent people from engaging in some activity. The main pattern in this regard is that society often tells people what they cannot do; less often do we see situations in which people are told what they must do. This is certainly the case in health. People are told, for example, that they cannot purchase pharmaceutical drugs without a prescription. However, they are not told that they must take such drugs. To determine whether people do have the ability to make choices that are in their best interest, three other questions must be answered in the affirmative: (1) Do consumers have enough information to make good choices?, (2) Do consumers know the results of their consumption decisions?, and (3) Are individuals rational?

Do Consumers Have Enough Information to Make Good Choices?

Even if people know what they want and can pursue it in a rational manner, they may face another impediment—insufficient information about various alternatives.

Economic theory pins much responsibility on the role of good consumer information. Consumers, for example, need good information to make utility-maximizing product choices, firms need good information to choose a product niche and obtain the necessary inputs to maximize profits, and workers need good information to obtain a job that satisfies their joint desires for professional satisfaction and good wages.

Indeed, in the health services area, one frequently reads journal articles by economists calling for more information. In discussing whether a welfare loss is associated with excess amounts of health insurance—a topic considered in Section 3.3.1—Roger Feldman and Bryan Dowd (1993) state that, "if there is an inefficiently low level of information in medical care markets, the solution is to inform consumers, not to insure them fully" (p. 199). A contrasting viewpoint is offered by Reinhardt (2001), who writes:

> [I]magine a patient beset by chest or stomach pain in Anytown, USA, as he or she attempts to "shop around" for a cost-effective resolution to those problems. Only rarely, in a few locations, do American patients have access to even a rudimentary version of the information infrastructure on which the theory of competitive market and the theory of managed care rest. The prices of health services are jealously guarded proprietary information. . . . Information on the quality of care is generally unavailable or not trustworthy. Not even the infection or complication rates experienced in hospitals are publicly known. Such

information on quality as is made available in the media or on Web sites typically consist of mysteriously weighed aggregate indexes that obscure the detailed information patients would need in a competitive market. Much is made now of the ability of Web-enabled healthcare consumers to view physicians as full partners or mere ordering clerks. Perhaps the typical American patient will fit that image one day. In the meantime, the image will remain the stuff of futurist tracts and of conference circuit fantasy. (pp. 986–87)

The standard rallying cry to allow for more competition as long as better information is available is not viewed sympathetically by some noneconomist observers. Sociologist David Mechanic (1990) has stated,

> To many economists, purchasing healthcare is fundamentally no different than purchasing carrots or cameras, and many of the uncertainties or imperfections of medical care markets can be accounted for by "information costs," the residual category of economic analysis that seemingly explains away many of the core concerns of the other social sciences. (p. 93)

The question we need to consider, then, is whether people have enough information available to them to make the right choices. This obviously depends on the type of health service being considered, and unfortunately, very little research is available on the subject. Most work on the adequacy of consumer information has examined physicians.

An intriguing debate on how much information consumers need was carried out in a now almost-legendary 1977 conference sponsored by the U.S. Federal Trade Commission.[8] Mark Pauly (1978) argued that we need to consider separately three kinds of services:

1. those purchased relatively frequently by the typical household;
2. those provided frequently by a physician, but used infrequently by a patient; and
3. services that even a physician provides infrequently.

---

8. Ten years later, the summer 1988 issue of the *Journal of Health Politics, Policy and Law* (volume 13, number 2) was devoted to a follow-up of these issues. The fall 1989 issue of the journal included a critique of some aspects of this follow-up (see Rice and Labelle 1989; and Wedig, Mitchell, and Cromwell 1989).

The first group would include pediatric care, dental care, prescription drugs, and the like. The second would include most surgical procedures, and the third, unusual and experimental procedures. Although Pauly thought that current information should be sufficient for consumers to make good choices in the first category of services, he estimated that three-fourths of expenditures would fall into the second and third categories.

In another conference paper, Frank Sloan and Roger Feldman (1978) argued that "standard [economic] theory does not require that *everyone* possess perfect information—only that there be a sufficient number of marginal consumers both able to assess output and willing to seek it out at its lowest price." They quote Pauly in this regard:

> I know even less about the works of a movie camera than I know about my own organs; yet I feel fairly confident in purchasing a camera for a given price as long as I know that there are at least a few experts in the market who are keeping sellers reasonably honest. (Sloan and Feldman 1978, p. 61)

Uwe Reinhardt (1978) criticized this viewpoint by presenting two "rather bewildering" sets of specifications for stereo amplifiers. He then notes:

> Consider now a consumer without knowledge of electronics, with an only moderately sensitive ear. It can be wondered how our consumer would necessarily be driven to select the right model from these and other models *for his or her particular circumstances* simply because true experts in the market have established reasonable prices for these models, *given these experts' predilections and circumstances.* Chances are that our consumer would rely on expert advice in making the selection; chances are that the *vendor* would offer much advice freely; and chances are that the consumer will take home a model that may not be the most appropriate for his or her particular circumstances, especially if the vendor is overstocked on a particular model or if profit margins differ among models. It could happen even to an economist! (p. 165)[9]

---

9. This issue about what economists often call "asymmetric information" between the provider and patient will be taken up again in Chapter 4, where we consider supply-side issues in health economics.

Some empirical research has been conducted on how consumers go about trying to collect information on the alternatives they face in the health market. A number of fairly old studies found relatively little evidence of "consumerism" in the health services area, with one physician observer sardonically noting that consumers "devote more effort selecting their Halloween pumpkin than they do choosing their physician."[10] A more recent study, by Thomas Hoerger and Leslie Howard (1995), examined how pregnant women search for a prenatal care provider. The sample included women from Florida who gave birth in 1987. Women who believed that they had a choice of prenatal providers were asked, "Before you selected your actual prenatal care provider, did you seriously consider using another prenatal care provider?" If they answered that in the affirmative, they were further queried, "Did you actually speak with or have an appointment with another prenatal care provider?" Curiously, only 24 percent of the respondents seriously considered using another provider, and only 14 percent actually had contact with another provider. The authors conclude:

> This amount of search is surprisingly low, given the importance of childbirth, the ample opportunity for choice, and the relative surplus of information about prenatal care providers compared to providers of other physician services. Recall that we expected the choice of prenatal care providers to establish a benchmark or *upper bound* on the extent of search for other physician services. (p. 341, emphasis added)

Interestingly, experience from previous births did not explain the results. For most women, the birth examined was the first child; furthermore, women with previous births were more likely to search for a provider than those who were having their first child. Thus, the little we know on the topic indicates that consumers often do not seek out information to choose a physician. But another, equally important question needs to be addressed: Are consumers able to successfully use the information that *is* made available to them? Judith Hibbard and Edward Weeks (1989a, 1989b) conducted studies of how information about physician

---

10. This quotation, from Dr. Harvey Mandell, is from Hoerger and Howard (1995). The Hoerger and Howard article contains a good review of the literature on consumers' search for physicians.

fees affects consumers' knowledge levels and their use of services. Using data from random samples of state government employees and Medicare beneficiaries in Oregon during the mid 1980s, the researchers divided sample members into experimental and control groups. The experimental group received a directory listing the fees for common procedures among area physicians, as well as a summary chart showing the ranges. Although receiving the directory resulted in increased knowledge levels among the government employees (but not the Medicare beneficiaries), the authors found that it did not result in changed behavior. The behaviors examined included asking about the costs of visits, procedures, tests, or medications; or changing physicians or insurance plans (Hibbard and Weeks 1989a). They also found that receipt of the information had no effect on costs per physician visit, the number of visits, or on annual health expenditures (Hibbard and Weeks 1989a). Although some of the sample had multiple insurance policies that would have covered the cost-sharing requirements associated with higher physician charges, the authors found that cost information had no effect, even on those sample members who claimed costs to be a financial burden (Hibbard and Weeks 1989b).

The increased importance of managed care and capitation brings with it many challenges for consumers. To make the most appropriate choices about health plans, consumers need to understand such concepts as primary care gatekeeping, financial incentives to providers, and other plan characteristics that affect the type of care patients receive. Unfortunately, there is little evidence that consumers do understand these concepts.

When surveyed, most consumers do not understand the difference between fee-for-service medicine and managed care plans, even at a rudimentary level (Isaacs 1996). Consumers are particularly bad at understanding certain key features of their own health plans. One U.S. survey, for example, found that whereas 62 percent of plan members believed that plans had to approve specialty referrals, the actual figure was just 28 percent (Cunningham, Denk, and Sinclair 2001).

One possible explanation for consumers' lack of understanding of their health plans is that most believe that the health plan they choose is not an important determinant of the quality of care they will receive (Hibbard, Sofaer, and Jewett 1996; Jewett and Hibbard 1996). Such a belief indicates a lack of awareness of the many levers health plans have available to them to affect the types and quantity of services provided to plan members.

An important area in which consumers need to be skilled at using information is with *report cards* on their health plans. People may obtain these report cards from their employer and then are supposed to choose a health plan by weighing such factors as quality, convenience, flexibility, and costs. Currently, no one standard report card format is used.

Good report cards should be easy to understand. Some items, such as satisfaction ratings, are comprehensible to most people, but other elements are more problematic. Whether consumers know how to make effective use of information on utilization rates for alternative services is not clear; neither is whether they understand the relative importance of survival rates from high-incidence versus low-incidence procedures.

Most of the current quality measures on report cards are based on the Health Plan Employer Data and Information Set (HEDIS), sponsored by the National Committee on Quality Assurance. HEDIS includes various measures of health plan performance in such areas as provision of preventive care to members and the appropriateness of care for particular problems, as well as patient satisfaction. When asked what they would expect to learn from different HEDIS measures, consumers typically ignore the data elements that they do not understand—which tend to be the "objective" measures of quality such as various utilization rates. Similarly, they overinterpret what can be learned from simple satisfaction data, the one element that they do tend to understand. Hibbard and Jewett (1997) report that,

> Interestingly, consumers perceive that patient ratings of overall quality give more information about the monitoring and follow-up of a condition than do the HEDIS indicators designed specifically for this purpose (such as rates of eye examinations among diabetic members, asthma hospitalizations, and low-birthweight infants). . . . These findings suggest that consumers are unsure of what many indicators are intended to tell them. (pp. 224–25)

Marc Rodwin (2001) notes a number of problems with the report cards in use today. One problem is that they ignore key aspects concerning how health plans operate, such as the stringency of utilization review and the financial incentives that providers face. Another is that many of the tasks previously performed by health plans have now devolved to capitated physician groups, whose performance is only occasionally available from report cards. A third is that report cards—to simplify—tend to be aggregated and not focused on performance for particular medical conditions, even though the management of chronic conditions is perhaps the most important barometer of the success of a health plan.

Not surprisingly, a study of managed care in 15 representative communities during 1995 concluded that, although much competition exists on the basis of price, "in general, there was almost no competition on the basis of measured and reported technical quality process or outcome measures" (Miller 1996, p. 116). How, then, can consumers get the information that they need? In another study of this problem, Rodwin (1996) concludes that this can come about only through a large-scale organized consumer movement:

> Effective consumer protection requires organized consumer groups that are strong enough to make plans respond to their interests. . . . Consumers need organized groups to ensure the presence of and to monitor traditional government oversight; to help define policies and practices within managed care organizations; to monitor the performance of managed care organizations and private accrediting groups; to marshal political resources; and to form strategic alliances. (p. 112)

Thus far, few systematic efforts of this kind of have been undertaken in the health services area.[11]

Do Consumers Know the Results of Their Consumption Decisions?

Another concern about whether consumers can make appropriate choices involves a special characteristic in health known as the *counterfactual*. Counterfactual questions are those that are hypothetical in a special way: they concern what would have happened if history had been different. To illustrate, some economists have tried to determine how quickly the western United States would have developed in the absence of railways (Fogel 1964; Fishlow 1965). Questions such as these can never be answered with certainty because the future is impossible to ascertain if past activities are (artificially) altered.

The health services area poses many counterfactual questions. Suppose a person seeks care from a primary care physician and tries to

---

11. For a review of alternative ways of increasing "consumer voice" in the managed care market, see Rodwin (2001).

determine what he or she learned from the experience. It turns out to be very difficult for the person to determine whether he or she made the right decision in seeking care from that provider, because to do so would involve answering several counterfactual questions, such as:

- Would the problem have gone away if I had left it untreated?
- What would have happened if I had sought the care of a specialist instead of a primary care physician?
- Would the result have been different if I had seen a different primary care physician than the one I sought?

In this regard, Burton Weisbrod (1978) has written that,

> For ordinary goods, the buyer has little difficulty in evaluating the counterfactual—that is, what the situation will be if the good is not obtained. Not so for the bulk of health care. . . . Because the human physiological system is itself an adaptive system, it is likely to correct itself and deal effectively with an ailment, even without any medical care services. Thus, a consumer of such services who gets better after the purchase does not know whether the improvement was because of, or even in spite of, the "care" that was received. Or if no health care services are purchased and the individual's problem becomes worse, he is generally not in a strong position to determine whether the results would have been different, and better, if he had purchased certain health care. And the consumer, not being a medical expert, may learn little from experience or from friends' experience . . . because of the difficulty of determining whether the counterfactual to a particular type of health care today is the same as it was the previous time the consumer, or a friend, had "similar" symptoms. The noteworthy point is not simply that it is difficult for the consumer to judge quality before the purchase . . . but that it is difficult even after the purchase. (p. 52)

Weisbrod concludes that "when buyers have difficult quality-evaluation problems, the theorem of economics that more information . . . is always preferred to less need not hold" (p. 54).

Are Individuals Rational?
We must also consider whether consumers act rationally. This question is really very different than whether people are the best judge of their own

welfare. Even if people know what will make them best off, it does not necessarily mean that they will make choices that are consistent with this knowledge.

Before addressing this, consider the meaning of "rational." Economists typically use a rather technical definition, whereby a person is rational if his or her other choices are consistent and transitive (Mishan 1982). Consistency can be thought of as meaning that, if a person faces the exact same circumstances more than one time, he or she will make the same choice. Transitive means that if a consumer prefers (and therefore chooses) good A over good B, and good B over good C, then he or she would also prefer (and choose) good A over C.

Although this definition will not be employed here, it is noteworthy that research on people's behavior has found numerous situations in which people do not act rationally in the economic sense. (See Thaler 1992, for a book full of such "anomalies.") Tversky and Kahneman (1981) provide a health example. In one experiment, they took two groups of people, asking the first,

> Imagine that the U.S. is preparing for the outbreak of an unusual Asian disease, which is expected to kill 600 people. Two alternative programs to combat the disease have been proposed. Assume that the exact scientific estimate of the consequences are as follows: If Program A is adopted, 200 people will be saved. If Program B is adopted, there is a 1/3 probability that 600 people will be saved, and 2/3 probability that no people will be saved. Which of the two programs would you favor? (p. 453)

Under this scenario, 72 percent chose Program A, indicating that they exhibit so-called risk-averse behavior.

The second group of people was asked the same question, but with two changes: "If Program C is adopted 400 people will die. If Program D is adopted there is a 1/3 probability that nobody will die, and 2/3 probability that 600 people will die" (Tversky and Kahneman 1981, p. 453). Under this scenario, 78 percent chose Program D. The authors conclude,

> The preferences . . . illustrate a common pattern: choices involving gains are often risk averse and choices involving losses are often risk taking. However, it is easy to see that the two problems are effectively identical. The only difference between them is that the outcomes are

described in problem 1 by the number of lives saved and in problem 2 by the number of lives lost. The change is accompanied by a pronounced shift from risk aversion to risk taking. We have observed this reversal in several groups of respondents, including university faculty and physicians. (p. 453)

The economic definition is not terribly useful to us because the term "rationality" means much more than that. Here we propose that rationality be thought of as indicating *reasonable* behavior.[12] An example will help illustrate what we mean by this term. If an adult in a developed country smokes cigarettes, we do not necessarily regard this as irrational. This is because there are several potentially reasonable bases for some people to smoke. They may derive pleasure from smoking, they may feel that it enhances their image among a certain social group, or perhaps most importantly, they may be physically addicted. Thus, smoking can be a reasonable decision if the benefits outweigh the various costs. Now suppose that such a person also claims that smoking does nothing to harm health, and cannot point to a heavy-smoking aunt who lived to age 93 and died peacefully in her sleep. If the person is even minimally educated, that sort of behavior should be viewed as irrational because it is not based on reason. To deny that cigarette smoking can harm one's health simply does not make sense.

Economists, in contrast to social scientists in other disciplines, sometimes suppose that consumers must be rational and must therefore act to maximize their utility, but that supposition would seem to be false. In this regard, Harvey Leibenstein (1976) has noted that "the idea of utility maximization must contain the possibility of choice under which utility is not maximized" (p. 8). Similarly, Lester Thurow (1983) writes,

---

12. Not all economists would agree with this. In fact, some practitioners have tried to show that many seemingly self-destructive human behaviors, such as drug addiction and even suicide, are the result of utility-maximizing decisions! There is a body of literature— known as "rational addiction" theory—that purports to show drug and alcohol addiction to be consistent with rationality. Becker and Murphy (1988), for example, claim that "addictions, even strong ones, are usually rational in the sense of involving forward-looking maximization with *stable preferences*" (p. 675, emphasis added), and that even though unhappy people often become addicted, "they would be even more unhappy if they were prevented from consuming the addictive goods" (p. 691). Such a viewpoint flies in the face not only of common sense, but of the professional opinions of the vast majority of health professionals. Thus, this view of rationality is rejected here.

Revealed preferences . . . is just a fancy way of saying that individuals do whatever individuals do, and whatever they do, economists will call it "utility maximization." Whether individuals buy good A or good Y they are still rational individual utility maximizers. By definition, there is no such thing as an individual who does not maximize utility. But if a theory can never be wrong, it has no content. It is merely a tautology. (pp. 217–18)

This book is not the appropriate place for a thorough consideration of the validity of the rationality assumption. Indeed, much of the field of psychology, and some of the sociology literature, has been devoted to this issue. We will discuss only one such issue here because it has been well-researched in the field of social psychology but only touched on by economists—cognitive dissonance.

The theory of cognitive dissonance concerns a central aspect of human behavior—self-justification or rationalization. As explained by Elliot Aronson (1972),

Basically, cognitive dissonance is a state of tension that occurs when an individual simultaneously holds two cognitions (ideas, attitudes, beliefs, opinions) that are psychologically inconsistent. . . . Because [its] occurrence . . . is unpleasant, people are motivated to reduce it. . . . To hold two ideas that contradict each other is to flirt with absurdity, and—as Albert Camus, the existentialist philosopher, has observed— man is a creature who spends his entire life in an attempt to convince himself that his existence is not absurd. (pp. 92–93)

Whether people act in a way that we might define as rational or irrational depends on how difficult it is to change the behavior in question versus the cognition. Smoking offers one of the best examples. Suppose that a person smokes but knows that smoking is very dangerous to health. This causes cognitive dissonance; how can you continue to do something that is so self-destructive? If the person is not addicted or has a particularly strong will, he or she may quit. But an addict or a weaker person will typically find it easier to change the cognition rather than the behavior, either by attributing more pleasure to smoking than is truly obtained, or by denying that it is dangerous (Aronson 1972). Although this latter type of behavior has been repeatedly confirmed and is certainly understandable, it would seem to be a violation of the English language to deem it as "rational."

Economists George Akerlof and William Dickens (1992) have used cognitive dissonance to explain various economic behaviors. Examples include explaining the choice of risky jobs, technological development, advertising, social insurance, and crime. Regarding social insurance, they write:

> If there are some persons who would simply prefer not to contemplate a time when their earning power is diminished, and if the very fact of saving for old age forces persons into such contemplations, there is an argument for compulsory old age insurance. . . . [They] may find it uncomfortable to contemplate their old age. For that reason they may make the wrong tradeoff, *given their own preferences*, between current consumption and savings for retirement. (p. 317, emphasis added)

Note that saving is what would make people best off in their own eyes, but they fail to do it anyway. Hence, society makes the decision to override individual choice by establishing social insurance programs—like Social Security and Medicare.

In summary, when cognitive dissonance is important, there is little reason to suppose that people will act in a rational manner—that is, make decisions that truly maximize their utility.

Do Individuals Reveal Their Preferences Through Their Actions?

Amartya Sen (1982, 1987, 1992) has written a number of persuasive essays and books on this issue. The basic problem concerns an issue addressed earlier, in Section 2.2—interdependencies in people's utility functions. If people make their choices based not only on their own preferences but on the preferences of others as well, then these choices will not necessarily reflect their personal preferences. This becomes extremely important because it casts doubt on the conventional meaning of demand curves, which purport to show the marginal utility that people obtain from additional units of consumption.

This viewpoint is supported by Frank (1985), who writes,

> The economist's most favored methods for measuring benefits are all based on the theory of revealed preference. This theory says that when a person buys one combination of goods when he could have bought

another, he reveals by his action that he prefers the first combination to the second. This is a truism where individually defined preferences are concerned. But it is false when there are important interdependencies between people. (pp. 205–06)

Sen and Frank both illustrate this point by bringing up the well-known "prisoners' dilemma." In this example, two prisoners are each faced with the decision either to confess or not to confess to a crime for which they are jointly guilty. If one confesses and the other does not, the former goes free and the latter receives a long prison term (say, 30 years). If both confess, they receive a much shorter term (five years). If neither confesses, they can be prosecuted only for a lesser crime and would receive only one year in prison.

It would seem to be rational for each prisoner to confess. Imagine that you and I are the prisoners, and suppose first that you confess. If I confess, I go to prison for five years, versus 30 years if I do not confess. Now suppose that you do not confess. If I confess, I get no prison time, versus one year if I do not. Thus, it would seem to be in my interest (and therefore yours since you face the same schedule of penalties as I) to confess. But this, of course, is not the case. If we both confess, we get five years of prison; but if neither of us confesses, we serve only a year.

Sen points out that this outcome can be arrived at if each prisoner tries to mimic the preferences of the *other* prisoner, rather than himself. Suppose I try to minimize your prison term. Knowing that you are rational and would confess, I would not confess, and in that way you would get no prison (and I would get 30 years). And if you act the same way—in my interests rather than in your own—we will jointly reach the optimal strategy. Neither of us will confess, and we will each get only one year in prison.

In this regard, Sen (1982) writes:

Each [prisoner] is assumed to be self-centered and interested basically only in his own prison term, and the choice of non-confession follows *not* from calculations based on this welfare function, but from following a moral code of behaviour suspending the rational calculus. . . . And it is this difference that is inimical to the revealed preference approach to the study of human behaviour. . . . The interest in the prisoners' dilemma lies not in the fiction which gives the problem its colour, but in the existence of a strictly dominant strategy for each person which together produce a strictly inferior outcome for all. . . . The essence of the problem is that if both prisoners behave *as if* they are maximizing a different welfare function from the one that they actually have, they will both end up being better off even in terms of their *actual* welfare function. . . . This is where the revealed preference approach goes off the rails altogether. The behaviour pattern that will make each better off in terms of their real preferences is not at all the behaviour pattern that will *reveal* those real preferences. Choices that reveal individual preferences may be quite inefficient for achieving welfare of the group. . . . I would argue that the philosophy of the revealed preference approach essentially underestimates the fact that man is a social animal and his choices are not rigidly bound to his own preferences only. I do not find it difficult to believe that birds and bees and dogs and cats do reveal their preferences by their choice; it is with human beings that the proposition is not particularly persuasive. An act of choice for this social animal is, in a fundamental sense, always a social act. (pp. 65–66)

On perhaps a less abstract level, Sen argues that much human behavior that we witness flies in the face of the notion that your actions indicate your personal preferences. He does this by distinguishing two concepts, sympathy and commitment. A person who acts on feelings of sympathy is indeed showing his personal preferences through his actions; you feel better if you help. Commitment, however, is different; you would rather do something else, but you do not because you are committed to a particular cause. Sen uses recycling as an example. He argues that people recycle not because they enjoy it or because they believe that their own recycling behavior will make a marked difference in the cleanliness of the environment, nor do they think that their own actions will convince anyone else to do it, but they do it because of their commitment to a cleaner environment. He summarizes this point, noting that "one way of defining commitment is in terms of a person choosing an act that he believes will yield a lower level of personal welfare to him than an alternative that is also available to him" (Sen 1982, p. 92). Sen notes further that this concept "drives a wedge between personal choice and personal welfare, [but] much of traditional economic theory relies on the identity of the two" (p. 94).

People's actions, at times, therefore seem to be motivated by things other than selfishness, and thus the choices one observes do not necessarily indicate the level of welfare derived by the individual or by society. (In this regard, Sen [1982] writes, "The *purely* economic man is indeed close to being a social moron" [p. 99].) But the results of this behavior can go in either direction: either choosing something that enhances social but not personal welfare (e.g., commitment); or choosing not to help others when it would be personally beneficial to do so. S. K. Nath (1969) provides a useful example of the latter behavior.

Suppose we observe a person *not* giving to a charity aimed at improving the health of the poor. Using revealed preference, one would conclude that the person would rather have something else—the good or service purchased with the money that could have been spent on the charity. This might not be the case, however. It may be that the person would benefit from providing such a donation because his or her utility function contains an element encompassing the health of the poor. But he may believe that his contribution will not be of much help because others are not compelled to follow suit.[13] Thus, the person would like the poor to have better access to health services, but this is not evidenced by his market behavior. Nath states that there is a "fallacy in the assumption than an individual's welfare function coincides with his utility function as revealed by his market choices. This is a very common fallacy in economic writings" (p. 141).

What we have tried to show in Section 3.2.2 is that proposition B in the syllogism presented above—that individual utilities are maximized when people are allowed to choose—often may not be met in the health services area. The next section examines the validity of the other proposition that must be met in order for consumer choice to result, of necessity, in what is best for society.

3.2.3 Is Social Welfare Maximized When Individual Utilities Are Maximized?

This section examines proposition A of the syllogism presented earlier, that social welfare is maximized when individuals maximize their own utility. This is essentially the same thing as Assumption 9 from Table 1.1:

---

13. This is called the *free-rider effect*. In this case, I would like to give to charity if it makes a difference to the poor, but my contribution, by itself, will make almost no difference. If everyone contributes, it will make a difference, of course. I may realize that the poor would be just about as well off if I were a free rider, that is, if I did not contribute but everyone else did. The problem is that, if everyone acts this way, little will be contributed to the poor.

Assumption 9. Social welfare is based solely on individual utilities, which in turn are based solely on the goods and services consumed.

Recall that in this chapter, we are making the assumption that society can and does redistribute income. (Problems with this assumption can be found earlier in Section 2.2, which concerned externalities of consumption, and in Chapter 5.) This allows us to examine explicitly the advantages of allowing for consumer choice in the health market without worrying about issues of equity.

Although the proposition that social welfare is based solely on individuals' welfare is a philosophical issue and cannot be proved true or false, two reasons call to question its validity. The first of these arguments is also from Sen (1982, 1987, 1992), who disputes this notion that individual welfare is the only legitimate component of social welfare. He calls such a philosophy "welfarism," which "is the view that the only things of intrinsic value for ethical calculation and evaluation of states of affairs are individual utilities" (Sen 1987, p. 40). Sen's arguments, which span several books, are too lengthy to be properly summarized here. One of the reasons that Sen rejects the welfarist approach is that it does not allow us to distinguish between different *qualities* of utility. An example he gives is that, if you get pleasure from my unhappiness, that counts as much under the welfarist approach as anything else. In contrast, one might believe that a society should devote its resources to meeting somewhat more lofty desires. Another reason is that the concept of individual welfare does not seem to be well-captured simply by the goods you have; other aspects of life, such as freedom, would also seem to be important. In this regard, Robin Hahnel and Michael Albert (1990) point out that conventional theory would make you equally well off if you are *assigned* a bundle of goods, versus a situation in which you *choose* the bundle. It does not take much introspection to realize that the latter may indeed result in higher utility.

A second reason to doubt that social welfare is not the sum of individual welfare is brought up by Frank (1985), who notes that much of what individuals seek out is status or rank. But these are relative things; if my status goes up, yours goes down by definition. This leads to a situation where people engage in consumption that does not add to the social welfare. For example, if I buy a fancy car, I get utility both from the various characteristics of the car, and from the fact that I have distinguished my-self from you. Once you (and others like us) buy the car, the latter part of my utility is canceled out. Total utility (or social welfare) is thus lower than the sum of our individual utilities.

3.3 IMPLICATIONS FOR HEALTH POLICY

This chapter has attempted to show the various problems with inferring that the goods and services people demand in a competitive marketplace will necessarily make them best off. We have attempted to show that such a supposition is based on several assumptions whose fulfillment in the health services area is open to serious question. This section provides a number of implications concerning the tools health economists use and the issues they study.

3.3.1 Is Comprehensive National Health Insurance Necessarily Inefficient?

Some health economists have long contended that people in the United States and other developed countries are "overinsured," which results in a societal *welfare loss*. That is, people have more insurance than is optimal for them or for society at large. To the noneconomist, this might seem like an odd belief, given the great concern about the number of uninsured people in the United States. In fact, nearly all economists would agree that a risk-averse[14] person would do better by purchasing fairly priced health insurance. Nevertheless, many economists contend that people with health insurance have too much coverage—that is, they do not have to pay enough of the costs of care out-of-pocket.

The Welfare Loss Argument

To better understand the welfare loss argument, it is necessary to review a concept in insurance called *moral hazard*. Moral hazard exists when the

---

14. A risk-averse person can be thought of as someone who prefers "a bird in the hand to two in the bush." The specific definition is that a person is risk averse if the marginal utility of additional income declines as income rises. In other words, if you make $30,000 a year, the last $1,000 you make brings about more utility than an additional $1,000 (that would make your income $31,000). It can be shown that such a person would generally want to buy insurance if the administrative or "loading" charges are small. For derivations of this, see Feldstein (1998) or Phelps (1997).

possession of an insurance policy increases the likelihood of incurring a covered loss, and/or the size of a covered loss. The term dates back to the purchase of fire insurance in the nineteenth century. It was recognized that a business or person that had fire insurance on a property might be more likely to incur a loss—either by deliberately setting a fire (hence, "moral" hazard) or by being less diligent in ensuring that a fire would not start in the first place. A quotation from a textbook on fire insurance dating back to 1877 will give some flavor to the term:

> We cannot too earnestly impress upon [insurance] agents, everywhere, the necessity of care. The agent who contributes, by over-insurance or in any way, to an incendiary fire, *endangers the common safety and commits a crime against society.** Constant supervision and watchfulness, with a keen judgment of men and values, are necessary. . . . It must be borne in mind that companies sometimes lose as much in consequence of *the indifference of honest men . . . as by the designing villainy of those who do not scruple to apply the match.*
>
> *While over-insurance causes fires, a proper amount of insurance may prevent them by teaching a malicious vagabond that he cannot harm his enemy by burning his property, as the insurance company's interposition restores the loss. (Moore 1877, p. 18)

In the health services area, the existence of moral hazard implies that people use more services when they are insured, or more fully insured. But as Mark Pauly (1968) pointed out in his famous essay on moral hazard, "the response of seeking more medical care with insurance than in its absence is a result not of moral perfidy, but of rational economic behavior" (p. 535). For a fully insured person, the cost of using an additional service will be shared by everyone who pays premiums. Thus, the person is likely to use more services than if he or she paid the full cost of the additional service.

In fact, the existence of moral hazard simply means that the demand curve for medical care slopes downward and to the right: people seek more services when their out-of-pocket payments are lower.

Despite the fact that moral hazard in medical care is an example of rational economic behavior, many economists are nevertheless troubled by its existence. This is because, when people are fully insured, they may demand services that only provide a small amount of benefit. But these services are likely to cost just as much as any other services. Thus, the benefits people derive from the purchase of these "marginal" services might be swamped by their cost.

In his article, Pauly tried to show that a country might be better off without compulsory, government-sponsored health insurance. This was in response to an article by Kenneth Arrow (1963b), who contended that government might be justified in providing such insurance out of tax dollars if a private market did not exist. Pauly's argument provides some useful guidance to the discussion that follows.

Suppose first that a person is uninsured, and has a 50 percent chance of staying well during a year, a 25 percent chance of being mildly sick, and a 25 percent chance of being very sick. Further suppose that his medical expenditures will be zero if he is well, $50 if he is mildly sick, and $200 if he is very sick. These expenditure levels are indicated by the vertical axis and vertical demand curves D_2' and D_3' in Figure 3.4. Consequently, the expected value of his annual medical costs will be $62.50 (0.5 × $0 + 0.25 × $50 + 0.25 × $200). Now suppose that the person has health insurance that pays 100 percent of costs. Assume that he continues to use no services if he is not sick, but spends $150 (instead of $50) if he is mildly sick, and $300 (instead of $200) if he is very sick. These expenditure levels are shown by the vertical axis and diagonal demand curves D_2 and D_3 in Figure 3.4. In this instance, the expected value of his annual costs will be $112.50 (0.5 × $0 + 0.25 × $150 + 0.25 × 300).

Pauly's point is that the person might be better off with no insurance, and paying $62.50 a year out-of-pocket, than having government-sponsored insurance, and paying $112.50 in taxes. The person may have used more services with the insurance, but the services used might not be of sufficient value to him to justify the additional $50 in expenditures.

Figure 3.4 can also be used to calculate the welfare loss of health insurance for this particular person. Recall that in conventional theory, a demand curve shows the marginal utility associated with alternative quantities purchased. A mildly sick person who is provided insurance coverage, and whose expenditures rise from $50 to $150, accrues benefits equal to the lower triangle AGB. However, the cost to society of producing these extra services is indicated by the square $AGBC$ (a constant marginal cost of producing services, MC, is assumed for convenience). Consequently, the upper triangle ABC provides an estimate of the welfare loss associated with health insurance. Adding this to the triangle DEF, which shows the welfare loss for very sick people, gives the total welfare loss. Pauly (1968) summarizes,

Figure 3.4: Pauly's Analysis of Welfare Loss

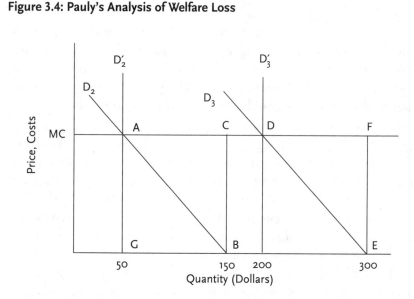

Source: Pauly, M.V. 1968. "The Economics of Morel Hazard: Comment." *American Economic Review* 58 (4): 531–37. Used with permission.

[T]he inefficiency loss due to behavior under insurance, if that insurance were compulsory, would then be roughly measured by triangles *ABC* and *DEF*. These areas represent the excess that individuals do pay over what they would be willing to pay for the quantity of medical care demanded under insurance. Against this loss must be offset the utility gain from having these uncertain expenses insured, but the net change in utility from a compulsory purchase of this "insurance" could well be negative. (p. 534)

The existence of moral hazard that results from the possession of health insurance has made many economists conclude that a societal "welfare loss" is associated with the ownership of too much health insurance. This is a very important conclusion; it implies that a society is not best off if its members have more health insurance than is deemed to be optimal. In a survey of U.S. and Canadian health economists conducted in 1989, 63 percent strongly or mildly agreed with the statement that health insurance causes societal welfare loss (Feldman and Morrisey 1990).

A number of researchers have computed the magnitude of this welfare loss for the United States as a whole.[15] One well-known set of estimates was calculated based on results of the RAND Health Insurance Experiment, which was conducted from 1974 through 1982. (This experiment is discussed in greater detail in Chapter 4.) In this study,[16] which constituted perhaps the most ambitious undertaking thus far in the field of health services research, individuals in six sites across the United States were randomly assigned to insurance plans that differed on the basis of patient coinsurance rates and some other factors. The effect of different coinsurance rates on annual expenditures is shown in the last column of Table 3.1. It was found that people who have to pay 95 percent of charges had annual expenditures that were 28 percent less than those who paid nothing. From a policy standpoint, perhaps more relevant is the finding that those facing a 25 percent coinsurance rate had expenditures that were 18 percent less than those with free care. Willard Manning and colleagues (1987) used these results to estimate a total welfare loss of $37 billion to $60 billion, which represented between 19 percent and 30 percent of total national health expenditures.

A more recent set of welfare loss estimates—also based on the RAND Health Insurance Experiment findings—come from a study by Feldman and Dowd (1991). This study provides a number of refinements over the previous one; in particular, it takes into account the fact that risk-averse individuals derive utility from being insured. It nevertheless concludes that the welfare loss associated with excess health insurance far outweighs the utility conveyed through owning insurance. Taking into account these conflicting components, the net welfare loss varied from $33 billion to $109 billion in 1984 dollars, depending on the assumptions employed, representing between 9 percent and 28 percent of health spending in the United States during that year.[17]

Critique of the Welfare Loss Argument

The argument supporting welfare loss from excess health insurance and estimates of the magnitude of that loss are based on the assumption that the demand curve shows the marginal utility that a person derives from an

---

15. The first such estimates were developed by Martin Feldstein (1973).

16. See Phelps (1997) for a summary of this experiment and its findings. The most detailed description and summary of the study is contained in Newhouse (1993).

17. This calculation is based on figures provided in Levit et al. (1985).

Table 3.1: Findings from the RAND Health Insurance Experiment

	Face-to-Face Visits (n)	Outpatient Expenses (1984 $)	Admissions	Inpatient Dollars (1984 $)	Probability Any Medical (%)	Probability Any Inpatient (%)	Total Expenses (1984 $)	Adjusted Total Expenses (1984 $)
Free	4.55	340	0.128	409	86.8	10.3	749	750
25 percent	3.33	260	0.105	373	78.8	8.4	634	617
50 percent	3.03	224	0.092	450	77.2	7.2	674	573
95 percent	2.73	203	0.099	315	67.7	7.9	518	540

Source: Manning, W. G., et al. 1987. "Health Insurance and the Demand for Medical Care: Evidence from a Randomized Experiment." *American Economic Review* 77 (3): 259. Used with permission.

additional service. In Section 3.2, however, we questioned that interpretation. For a demand curve to represent the marginal utility of purchases, several assumptions have to be met: consumers must act rationally (Assumption 7), they must have sufficient information to make good choices (Assumption 5), and they must know what the results of their consumption decisions will be (Assumption 6).

In essence, the welfare-loss argument says that consumers must be able to determine exactly how much an additional service is worth to them. Then they compare this to its price to determine if it is worth their while to purchase the service. If people have insurance, the price they have to pay will be less; consequently, they will be more receptive to purchasing a service that conveys little utility. The difference between the cost of the service, and the utility received, equals the welfare loss from the purchase of that service.

The question we need to consider, then, is whether information is available that allows us to determine whether consumers can accurately estimate the marginal utility they receive from additional services. Fortunately, a method of testing this exists; however, as noted later, some problems with this method have been identified.

Welfare loss occurs because consumers with health insurance have an incentive to purchase additional services (compared to what they would be purchasing without insurance) that provide little benefit to them. We can examine whether this occurs by observing the kinds of services that consumers forgo when they are provided with less comprehensive insurance coverage. The results from the RAND Health Insurance study show that utilization will go down in the presence of coinsurance. Welfare-loss theory tells us the types of services that ought to be forgone: those that provide relatively little utility.

The nature of this test is clarified in Figure 3.5, which is taken from an earlier work of the author (Rice 1992a). The horizontal line indicates the marginal cost (MC) of producing a service, which can be viewed as the cost to society—that is, the resources that have to be expended in providing a service. In a competitive market, that will also equal its price (P). The curved line, which is a demand curve, shows the marginal utility of each additional service. At a zero price—that is, with comprehensive insurance—the consumer will demand Q_0 services; the last such service provides very little utility.

Now suppose that two types of services are available—those that are highly effective (HE) and those that have low effectiveness (LE). Further

Figure 3.5: Change in Demand for Services of Differing Effectiveness

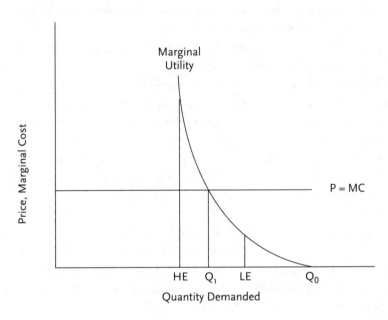

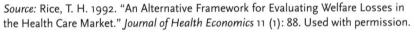

Source: Rice, T. H. 1992. "An Alternative Framework for Evaluating Welfare Losses in the Health Care Market." *Journal of Health Economics* 11 (1): 88. Used with permission.

suppose that the person no longer has health insurance, and his demand for care has declined from Q_0 to Q_1. Figure 3.5 demonstrates that the person would be expected to forgo the low-effectiveness service, *LE*, because its benefits are now outweighed by its costs. But service *HE* would still be purchased because its benefits exceed costs, even in the absence of insurance coverage. If people actually behaved as predicted, then we would have some confidence that the demand curve for medical care really shows the marginal utility consumers obtain from additional services. This, in turn, would provide support for the welfare-loss estimates discussed above.

A problem has been raised with this argument. John Nyman (1999a) notes that:

[E]conomic theory predicts that, if there were two procedures that were alike on every dimension except effectiveness (*and the effectiveness of the two procedures was known and greater effectiveness was valued*

by consumers), the quantity demanded of the more effective procedure would exceed the quantity demanded of the less effective procedure, at any given price. The empirical evidence supporting this
prediction is found in the many patients who bypass their local community hospital to travel to the Mayo Clinic (or any other similarly
highly regarded medical center) to receive their coronary bypass or
other procedure. . . . Given that the quantity demanded of high effectiveness procedures exceeds that of low effectiveness procedures other
things equal, economic theory would predict that as the price rises,
both quantities would decline, consistent with the Lohr et al. findings.
(pp. 811–12, emphasis added)

The key assumption made in the above quotation is buried in the
italicized parenthetical thought: when faced with choices between alternative medical procedures, consumers know the effectiveness of each.
Therefore, if they demand more of one than another, they either know
that the procedure with the greater demand is more effective or cheaper
than the other. The only evidence given to support this belief is that
consumers "bypass their local community hospital to travel to the Mayo
Clinic." Although undoubtedly true, this provides no evidence for believing that consumers can systematically compare the effectiveness of
alternative procedures with their cost. A more likely explanation, consistent with empirical evidence (some of which was discussed elsewhere in
this chapter), is that consumers were never aware of the fact that certain
procedures are less effective than others, and never were making utility-
maximizing comparisons between the effectiveness and prices of alternative procedures.

Returning to Figure 3.5, the problem with implementing this test, of
course, is coming up with a way of determining the marginal utility that
consumers receive from a service. The proxy used here is a measure of
the medical effectiveness of a service—as judged by medical experts. Although consumers and experts may differ in what they think is important, common sense tells us that consumers would prefer those services
that are thought to be the most effective.

As part of the RAND study, Lohr et al. (1986) grouped services into
categories based on their expected medical effectiveness:

Group 1. Highly effective treatment by medical care system;
Group 2. Quite effective treatment by medical care system;

Group 3. Less effective treatment by medical care system; and
Group 4. Medical care rarely effective or self-care effective.

The category into which a particular service falls is shown in Table 3.2, which is taken from the study. The authors found that,

> [C]ost sharing was generally just as likely to lower use when care is thought to be highly effective as when it is thought to be only rarely effective, [nor] was there any obvious trend suggesting that cost sharing would deter care seeking more as one moved "down" the effectiveness ranking. (p. S32)

They concluded that,

> [C]ost sharing did not lead to rates of care seeking that were more "appropriate" from a clinical perspective. That is, cost sharing did not seem to have a selective effect in prompting people to forgo care only or mainly in circumstances when such care probably would be of relatively little value. (p. S36)

Another component of the RAND study reached a similar conclusion regarding the effect of coinsurance on appropriate versus inappropriate hospitalization (Siu et al. 1986). What does all this mean for the theory of welfare loss from excess health insurance? The Lohr et al. study shows that consumers who face cost-sharing reduce demand across the board, both for care that is highly effective and less effective. But the welfare-loss argument rests on the supposition that the services forgone as a result of cost-sharing will be composed *entirely* of those that provide less utility; the Health Insurance study clearly shows this is not the case. At the very least, only services providing the lower level of benefits (such as service LE in Figure 3.5) should be included in the welfare-loss calculation. More generally, welfare-loss calculations are hard to defend when consumers cannot accurately value the benefits and costs of the medical services they consume (Rice 1992a, p. 89).

This view—that patient demand curves show how much consumers buy at different prices, but not necessarily the utility they derive from such services—runs very much against the grain of conventional economic theory. It is not, however, unique among economists. One noteworthy

Table 3.2: Medical Effectiveness Groupings in the Lohr et al. Study

Group 1: Highly Effective Treatment by Medical Care System
Medical care highly effective: acute conditions
Eyes—conjunctivitis
Otitis media, acute
Acute sinusitis
Strep throat
Acute lower respiratory infections (acute bronchitis)
Pneumonia
Vaginitis and cervicitis
Nonfungal skin infections
Trauma—fractures
Trauma—lacerations, contusions, abrasions
Medical care highly effective: acute or chronic conditions
Sexually transmitted disease or pelvic inflammatory disease
Malignant neoplasm, including skin
Gout
Anemias
Enuresis
Seizure disorders
Eyes—strabismus, glaucoma, cataracts
Otitis media, not otherwise specified
Chronic sinusitis
Peptic and nonpeptic ulcer disease
Hernia
Urinary tract infection
Skin—dermatophytoses
Medical care highly effective: chronic conditions
Thyroid disease
Diabetes
Otitis media, chronic
Hypertension and abnormal blood pressure
Cardiac arrythmias
Congestive heart failure
Chronic bronchitis, chronic obstructive pulmonary disease
Rheumatic disease (rheumatoid arthritis)
Group 2: Quite Effective Treatment by Medical Care System
Diarrhea and gastroenteritis (infectious)
Benign and unspecified neoplasm
Thrombophlebitis
Hemorrhoids
Hay fever (chronic rhinitis)
Acute middle respiratory infections (tracheitis, laryngitis)
Asthma

Chronic enteritis, colitis
Perirectal conditions
Menstrual and menopausal disorders
Acne
Adverse effects of medicinal agents
Other abnormal findings
Group 3: Less Effective Treatment by Medical Care System
Hypercholesterolemia, hyperlipidemia
Mental retardation
Peripheral neuropathy, neuritis, and sciatica
Ears—deafness
Vertiginous syndromes
Other heart disease
Edema
Cerebrovascular disease
Varicose veins of lower extremities
Prostatic hypertrophy, prostatitis
Other cervical disease
Lymphadenopathy
Vehicular accidents
Other injuries and adverse effects
Group 4: Medical Care Rarely Effective or Self-Care Effective
Medical care rarely effective
Viral exanthems
Hypoglycemia
Obesity
Chest pain
Shortness of breath
Hypertrophy of tonsils or adenoids
Chronic cystic breast disease (nonmalignant)
Debility and fatigue (malaise)
Over-the-counter or self-care effective
Influenza (viral)
Fever
Headaches
Cough
Acute URI
Throat pain
Irritable colon
Abdominal pain
Nausea or vomiting
Constipation
Other rashes and skin conditions
Degenerative joint disease
Low back pain diseases and syndromes
Bursitis or synovitis and fibrositis or myalgia
Acute sprains and strains
Muscle problems

Source: Lohr, K. N., R. H. Brook, C. J. Kamberg, et al. 1986. "Effect of Cost Sharing on Use of Medically Effective and Less Effective Care." *Medical Care* 24 (Supplement): S33. Used with permission.

example is from an article by Randall Ellis and Thomas McGuire (1993), who write,

> [W]e are skeptical that the observed demand can be interpreted as reflecting "socially efficient" consumption, [so] we interpret the demand curve in a more limited way, as an empirical relationship between the degree of cost sharing and quantity of use demanded by the patient. (p. 142)

As noted earlier, the argument against the welfare-loss calculations depends in part on the existence of a close correspondence between consumer preferences and experts' opinion of the medical effectiveness of alternative services. Intuitively, one would imagine that there would be such a correspondence, since consumers would seem unlikely to want to use services that experts find to be of little value. A related issue needs to be raised, however: the validity of the Lohr et al. categories shown in Table 3.2. Feldman and Dowd (1993) note one example of a potential problem: medical care is considered to be highly effective for the treatment of strep throat, but rarely effective for throat pain (although self-care is effective). Others have noted that it seems odd to include chest pain in the category where medical care is rarely effective. These concerns are indeed important ones, but no other study can be relied upon to inform us about the issue at hand. Until such a study exists, the Lohr et al. findings from the RAND study, in conjunction with the theory developed in Figure 3.5, must at the very minimum give us pause before accepting the conventional welfare-loss methodology and estimates.[18]

Where Is the Waste in Medical Care?

In 2000, the United States spent $1.3 trillion on health, with per capita expenditures exceeding $4,600 (Levit et al. 2002). This constituted 13.2

---

18. Nyman (1999b) argues that the benefits of health insurance are also severely underestimated, which implies that welfare-loss estimates are overstated. The traditional model presented in the text assumes that the benefits of health insurance are simply the result of risk-averse individuals deriving utility from being protected against unexpectedly high costs. Nyman posits another, potentially even greater, benefit of insurance: that it allows people to afford expensive procedures that otherwise would be too costly to obtain. This interpretation is disputed by Manning and Marquis (2001), however.

percent of national income, a figure about 30 percent higher than in any other country in the world (OECD 2001).

Economists are often quick to point out that the $1.3 trillion and 13 percent figures do not provide any direct evidence that we are spending too much for medical care in the United States. Maybe, they contend, people really get more out of this high level of medical care spending than they would from spending it in alternative ways.[19] Although this contention is very difficult to disprove, some circumstantial evidence indicates that the United States is not getting as much out of this extra spending as it might expect. Some of this evidence is discussed in Chapter 6, when we examine spending and outcomes in various developed countries.

In addition, since the early work of John Wennberg and colleagues,[20] experts have appeared to be in agreement that many of the services provided are not medically necessary. Although little agreement has been reached on the magnitude of unnecessary services used, for some procedures the rate has been estimated to be as high as 30 percent (Leape 1989; Schuster, McGlynn, and Brook 1998). As a result, probably the major research effort now being conducted by the health services research community at large is determining what services are and what services are not medically effective. This research is manifesting itself in two major ways: through the dissemination and use of practice guidelines for various medical conditions, and by "profiling" individual physicians' service provision rates. Managed care plans can then use the profiles in an attempt to assess physicians' medical decision making.

Where, then, is the waste in medical care? Under the traditional theory, the source of the waste is clear: patients demand too many services when they have complete or nearly complete insurance coverage. The alternative being presented here is that most of the waste is in the provision of services that do little or no good in improving the patients' health.[21]

---

19. As noted in Chapter 2, survey data show that about two-thirds of all Americans believe that the country spends too little on health (Blendon and Benson 2001).

20. Perhaps the best-known article is Wennberg and Gittlesohn (1982). For a thorough review of the early literature, see Paul-Shaheen, Clark, and Williams (1987).

21. Other writers have also advocated calculating welfare losses based on the provision of unnecessary services. See Phelps and Parente (1990), Phelps and Mooney (1992), Dranove (1995), and Phelps (1995).

These alternative theories are not totally contradictory—some services could be deemed wasteful under both approaches (e.g., a person with complete insurance demands a service that brings him or her little utility and that experts believe will have little or no effect on his health).

Nevertheless, the policy implications of the two approaches are *very* different. If one believes the conventional theory, policies should be enacted that make the user of services more sensitive to price. In contrast, if the problem is more in the area of the provision of services that are not useful, policies should target the provider of services.

The idea of pursuing supply-side rather than demand-side policies will be explored in greater detail in Chapter 6. The key point here is that most policies aimed at controlling costs in the United States—and practically all such policies in the rest of the world—are aimed at the supply side rather than the demand side. This contradicts conventional economic theory, in which consumers are the ones who should be in charge of deciding what services they should or should not receive, because only they can measure the utility that such services will bring.

The supply-side policies that are now most common—putting physicians at risk through capitation or other forms of incentive reimbursement, utilization review, and technology controls and global budgets in many countries—are designed to influence the types of services provided, without consulting the patient. Thus, the policies are based, in part, on the belief that someone other than the consumer is the best judge of what medical services should be delivered.[22]

Many analysts—economists as well as practitioners of other disciplines—believe that managed care strategies that are based on capitating health plans offer the best hope for controlling U.S. health costs. These strategies are aimed almost entirely at changing what services are provided by providers, rather than changing the demand by consumers. In fact, what is perhaps most noteworthy about the HMO approach to cost containment is that copayments are *lower* than the payments in fee-for-service medicine. If these strategies are designed to reduce waste, it would seem clear that the waste is thought to be generated through the provision of unnecessary services far more so than through excess demand by

---

22. This is not the only reason for such policies. Another important one is that fee-for-service medicine provides a strong incentive to overprovide services. But this also stems from consumers not being able to make effective decisions about the appropriate types and amounts of services they receive.

Figure 3.6: The Effect of Coinsurance on Welfare Loss

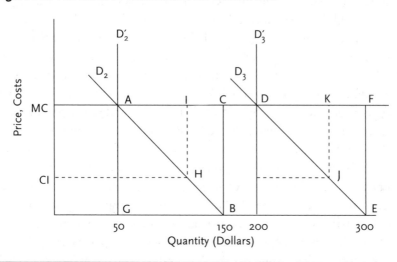

patients. And if this is true in the United States, it must be even more true in other developed countries, where, with a few exceptions, patient copayments tend to be lower, with almost all cost-control activities being focused on the providers of care.[23]

3.3.2 Should Patient Cost-Sharing Be Encouraged, or Should We Use Other Policies?

As indicated in Section 3.3.1, the thrust of the welfare-loss literature is that more patient cost-sharing will be beneficial to society. This argument can be demonstrated by modifying Figure 3.4 to show how institution of a patient coinsurance rate would reduce the welfare loss of complete health insurance coverage. In Figure 3.4, the triangles *ABC* and *DEF* showed the original welfare loss from full insurance. With the institution of coinsurance, *CI*, it would be cut to the sum of triangles *AHI* and *DJK* in Figure 3.6.

This sort of analysis contains a danger, which has been noted by Robert Evans (1984): "The welfare burden is minimized when there is no insurance at all" (p. 49). If one takes this reasoning very far, conventional

---

23. For more information on patient cost-sharing outside of the United States, see Section 6.2.2.

analysis will always find that the country with higher patient cost-sharing requirements will have the more efficient health system (Reinhardt 1992). Thus, the U.S. system would be deemed more efficient than the Canadian system or any of a number of European systems, not because of a comparison of outcomes to costs, but rather simply from the fact that the United States imposes patient copayments, which in turn reduces utilization. Although this conclusion might seem surprising, it follows directly if one holds the viewpoint that the demand curve provides our best estimate of the benefits derived from the use of additional services.

U.S. health economists, more so than those from other countries, seem to be inclined to believe that patient cost-sharing should be encouraged as a primary means of achieving efficiency in the health services area. Some of the most notable advocates of such a position were the researchers who conducted the RAND Health Insurance Experiment. One question these researchers asked was whether the experiment could justify its costs, which would exceed $200 million in today's dollars. They concluded that the experiment more than paid for itself because of its reduction in services that appeared to do little to improve health status:

> [W]e believe that the benefits of this particular experiment greatly exceeded the costs. . . . Between 1982 and 1984, there was a remarkable increase in initial cost-sharing in the United States, at least for hospital services. For example, the number of major companies with first-dollar charges for hospital care rose from 30 to 63 percent in those two years, and the number of such firms with an annual deductible of $200 per person or more rose from 4 to 21 percent. Although it is impossible to know how much of this change can be attributed to the experimental results, the initial findings of the experiment were published . . . and given wide publicity in both the general and trade press. In certain instances a direct link between changes in cost-sharing and the experimental results can be made. (Manning et al. 1987, p. 272)

Because the experiment showed that increased patient cost-sharing reduced medical expenditures, the researchers estimated that, under the most optimistic scenario, the eight-year experiment could have paid for itself in a week!

Non–U.S. health economists have been more amenable to the idea that a fee-for-service system could be efficient in the absence of patient cost-sharing. Robert Evans and colleagues (1983) argue that the case for patient cost-sharing is difficult to make if four questions can be answered in the affirmative:

- Is the service really health related?
- Does the service work?
- Is the service medically necessary?
- Is there no better alternative?

If a service passes all of these tests, "the standard argument against user charges, that they tax the sick, seems wholly justified" (Evans et al. 1983).

Two broad arguments can be made against employing patient cost-sharing as a cost-control technique. First, of course, is the issue of equity. Cost-sharing is more burdensome on people with lower incomes. In this regard, one of the key findings of the RAND study was that the health of the sick and the poor was most adversely affected by cost-sharing (Newhouse 1993).[24]

The other issue concerns efficiency—specifically, are there alternative ways of encouraging efficiency and containing health costs besides cost-sharing? Two U.S. health economists mentioned earlier, Ellis and McGuire (1993), have argued the benefits of what they deem to be a "neglected" area of reform, supply-side cost-sharing, "which seeks to alter the incentives of healthcare workers to provide certain services" (p. 135). (One could make a compelling argument that this has not been neglected by analysts in other countries, however.) With supply-side policies, Ellis and McGuire argue, it is possible to reach the same desired level of quantity as with demand-side levers. Furthermore, they claim that supply-side cost-sharing is clearly superior to traditional demand-side policies in one key respect: it does not result in a financial burden on patients.

Nevertheless, economists tend to focus most of their attention on the role of price. One possible reason, noted by Milton Friedman (1962), was given in Section 2.2: the focus on price is part of an overall division of labor between economics and the other social sciences. If each of the social sciences were equally influential in determining policy, this would not present a problem. But a strong case can be made that economics

---

24. For a summary of the literature on the effect of cost-sharing, see Rice and Morrison (1994).

seems to be paramount among the social sciences in its influence over health policy. Given that, it is incumbent on health economists to consider other health policy levers as well.

Although one could imagine many possible policy levers—and indeed, several supply-side levers will be discussed in Chapter 6—the focus here will be on a single, nonprice demand-side lever—influencing behavior. Curiously, economists who are concerned about the purported welfare loss due to excess health insurance often do not focus on more tangible losses such as the cost of "bad" behaviors from things like smoking, alcohol consumption, drug abuse, and so forth. This is not to say that health economists do not study such issues—they do—but rather that these costs are often not viewed as welfare losses for society. This is particularly curious given the estimated sizes of these losses: in the United States alone, an estimated $67 billion is lost annually for drug abuse, $99 billion is lost for alcohol abuse, and $91 billion is lost for smoking (Robert Wood Johnson Foundation 1994). These figures far exceed all estimates of the welfare losses from health insurance.

Sociologists and psychologists have been concerned about the factors that influence behavior and the ways in which it can be altered. The field of health education focuses, to a large degree, on how behaviors can be changed. Mechanic (1979) has stated that,

> Reducing needs involves the prevention of illness or diminishing patients' psychological dependence on the medical encounter for social support or other secondary advantages. Reducing desire for services requires changing people's views of the value of different types of medical care, making them more aware of the real costs of service in relation to the benefits received, and legitimizing alternatives for dealing with many problems. (p. 11)

The task of changing behavior is not easy, however. In this regard, Mechanic writes, "it is prudent to recognize the difficulty of the task, the forces working against change, and the depths of ignorance concerning the origins of these behaviors and the ways in which they can best be modified" (p. 12).

The point is not that economists need to be conducting this research. Rather, (1) policy levers like these need to be recognized by health economists who are proposing policy; and (2) relying on conventional tools such as demand elasticities to recommend policy is inappropriate once some of the special characteristics of the health market are recognized.

3.3.3 Should People Pay More for Price-Elastic Services?

Another generally accepted tool in the health economist's toolbox is that the magnitude of patient coinsurance rates should be directly related to the elasticity of demand. More specifically, services for which consumers show a high demand elasticity should have higher cost-sharing requirements than services for which consumers are less price sensitive. As we shall see, the basis for this argument is similar to the one used by economists in arguing a welfare loss associated with excessive amounts of health insurance.

Ellis and McGuire (1993) summarize the issue as follows:

> [T]he optimal insurance literature has been based on the assumption that the demand curve correctly reflects the marginal benefits of services. As a result, it has held that the greater the demand response to what consumers/patients must pay for health care, the higher should be demand-side cost-sharing. (p. 137)

Why is this the case? Suppose one views the demand curve as indicating the marginal benefits a consumer derives from a service. In Figure 3.7, point P_1 shows the price of medical care in the absence of health insurance, and point P_2, the price when a person has insurance that pays 80 percent of medical costs. Thus, at point C, which represents the quantity of medical care purchased with insurance, the marginal benefits derived from the last service are only one-fifth as great as at point A, where the person is uninsured.

As noted earlier, under the conventional theory this results in a societal welfare loss, which is equal to the difference between the costs of producing the last service Q_2—indicated by point B—and the benefits as shown at point C. But that is the welfare loss associated with only the last service. Welfare loss also occurs for all other services purchased between Q_1 and Q_2. The total welfare loss is therefore equal to the triangle ABC.[25]

---

25. As noted earlier, one needs to weigh this welfare loss in the conventional theory against the welfare gain from the reduction in risk brought about by the insurance. For convenience,

Figure 3.7: Relationship Between Demand Elasticity and Welfare Loss

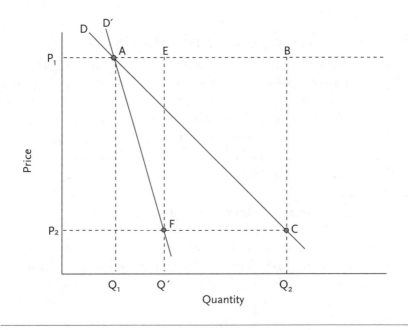

Now suppose that the demand curve is steeper, or less elastic (curve D'). In the figure, when the person obtains insurance, thereby lowering the price of care, his or her consumption increases only to Q'. Clearly, in this case, the welfare loss will be smaller, equaling the triangle AEF rather than ABC. Similarly, one can imagine that if the demand curve is more gently sloped (that is, more price elastic), health insurance will result in a larger welfare-loss triangle.

The intuition behind this result is straightforward. If the possession of insurance leads to a large increase in utilization, then welfare loss will be larger because more services will be purchased where the marginal costs exceed marginal benefits. Thus, one would improve social welfare by assessing higher patient coinsurance rates for such services, thereby reducing usage. In contrast, if utilization rates are not very sensitive to the possession of insurance, then there is little welfare loss, and less need to charge high coinsurance rates.

---

we do not consider the latter element here, but this does not affect the substance of the argument.

Table 3.3: Arc Price Elasticities of Medical Spending in the RAND Health Insurance Experiment

Range	Acute	Chronic	Well	Total Outpatient	Hospital	Total Medical	Dental
0%–25%	–0.16	–0.20	–0.14	–0.17	–0.17	–0.17	–0.12
25%–95%	–0.32	–0.23	–0.43	–0.31	–0.14	–0.22	–0.39

Source: Newhouse, J. P. 1993. *Free for All? Lessons from the* RAND *Health Insurance Experiment.* (Harvard University Press, Cambridge, MA), p. 121. Santa Monica, CA: RAND, 1988. Reprinted with permission.

Conventional theory calls for higher coinsurance rates when services are more responsive to out-of-pocket price. We therefore need to consider what services are the most price elastic, since those are the ones that the theory tells us should have the highest patient cost-sharing requirements.

The major source of data to answer this question is the RAND Health Insurance Experiment. Its results in this regard are somewhat ambiguous because the calculated elasticities vary depending on the level of coinsurance. In the study, patients were assessed 0 percent or 25 percent or 95 percent of the total charge.[26] Therefore, one can examine price responsiveness to alternative coinsurance rates only between these intervals.

These elasticities are shown in Table 3.3. In general, the elasticities do not vary a great deal by type of service. One noteworthy exception is "well-care services," which, while showing a comparable elasticity to other outpatient services (acute and chronic) in the 0 percent to 25 percent range, had a much larger one in the 25 percent to 95 percent range (Phelps 1997, p. 143). Dental services also showed a relatively high elasticity in the 25 percent to 95 percent range. The well-care services considered in the study would include preventive care, but other services as well. Other studies have found that mental health services tend to be far more price elastic than other types of care (Frank and McGuire 2000).

The implications of the standard economic model are clear: if mental health or preventive services are the most price responsive, they should

---

26. Some patients were charged 50 percent coinsurance rates, but they were not used in the analysis of demand elasticities.

have the highest patient coinsurance rates, which in turn will discourage their usage. This would be true even if some of these services were shown to be particularly effective in improving health and/or well-being.

Of course, alternative criteria could be used to determine the patient copayment levels that are in the best interest of society. One model would make preventive services free of any copayments—the *opposite* of what the economic model would recommend. Another might do the same for mental health services because the users of such services are, in many cases, least able to go through the rationality calculus of comparing marginal benefits and costs required in the standard economic model.

Several possible justifications exist for basing copayment rates on factors other than price elasticities, all of which have been discussed previously in other contexts. First is the issue of whether consumers have sufficient information. If they do not, then they are likely to underestimate the value of investing in such things as preventive services. Second, even if the appropriate information is available, consumers may not use it correctly. As noted, it is difficult for consumers to make choices based on counterfactual information. Furthermore, because of people's tendency toward cognitive dissonance, consumers may avoid seeking some types of services that are of value to them.

Third, medical experts may be better aware of the benefits of certain services than are individuals—and these experts routinely recommend more services than people are obtaining. Fourth, consumers might be shortsighted in their views, particularly when they are young. Fifth, both mental health and preventive care have a public-good aspect: "If it makes you healthy I want you to have it, but the free-rider effect (discussed in Chapter 2) will prevent me from subsidizing you." Subsidized low copayments therefore could meet this demand.

When one assumes that a demand curve for medical services represents the marginal benefits consumers receive from services, then certain policy implications follow. One such implication is that patients should be charged more for services that are price sensitive. But if one does not make such strong assumptions about the meaning of demand curves for health services, then a different set of policy prescriptions would seem to be more appropriate. One example is reducing patient prices for mental health and preventive services even if such services are more price responsive than others—a conclusion directly in conflict with that provided by conventional theory.

3.3.4 Defined Contribution, Premium Support, and MSAS
Defined Contribution

In general, health insurance can be provided to a group of individuals in two ways: through a *defined benefit* system or through *defined contribution*. More typical is defined benefit. Under such a system, the benefits of health insurance are legislated (e.g., all "medically necessary" services might be provided). In contrast, defined contribution programs do not establish the particular set of benefits. Rather, the entity funding health insurance, such as the government or an employer, provides a fixed monetary contribution toward premiums. Individuals and families use this contribution to purchase coverage. Such a system is used by about 20 percent of U.S. employees (Trude and Ginsburg 2000).

The defined contribution approach is based on the work of U.S. economist Alain Enthoven (1978, 1980, 1988; Enthoven and Kronick 1989). To illustrate the approach, suppose an employer provides a voucher worth $4,000 to an employee to purchase family coverage. Further suppose that the employer, as sponsor, offers a menu of four health plans, three HMOs and one fee-for-service. The HMOs cost $4,000, $4,500, and $5,000, respectively, and the fee-for-service plan costs $6,000. If the employee chooses the cheapest HMO, he or she pays no premiums. In contrast, the other two HMOs would cost the employee $500 and $1,000, and the fee-for-service plan, $2,000. Thus, the employee has a strong financial incentive to choose the cheaper plan. Nevertheless, he or she may choose another plan if its desirable features (perhaps fewer restrictions or better perceived quality) are worth the difference in premiums.

This is not the end of the story, however. By allowing choice on part of the employee, a "domino effect" could result that, proponents contend, will make the entire system more efficient. Because health plans must be attractive to employees, they have an incentive to keep costs down, but at the same time provide a quality product. Health plans, in turn, contract with providers such as hospitals and physicians. The latter must also strive to be attractive by keeping their fees reasonable and quality high, or else health plans will not select them into provider panels. This entire chain of events is known by the term *managed competition*.

Although aspects of managed competition have been adopted by some other countries (see Section 6.2.2), its closest incarnation is in the employment sector of the United States. As noted above, most employees do not find themselves under such a system, but a significant minority do. Many analysts believe that the primary reason that health costs were successfully controlled in the United States during the 1990s was the growth of managed competition as manifested through competing HMOs. Indeed, studies examining the institution of such a system have found the potential for considerable savings (Buchmueller 1998; Cutler and Reber 1998), although, as discussed below, serious problems may arise as well.

The description of defined contribution programs just presented refers to what has been tried in the past. More recently, defined contribution has been used in the United States to refer to a more fundamental reform of health insurance. Rather than providing a limited menu of choices, employees would be "empowered" to construct their own health insurance plans, usually through Internet-based tools or companies. Under one such system, employees are given a defined contribution and use it to select their particular primary care and specialist physicians from a large menu of participants. Every physician has an associated premium (which, in essence, is the capitation rate received by the provider). After the employee devises his or her own personal health plan, the component premiums are summed. The employee's share is simply the difference between the total of the premiums and the employer's defined contribution. Advocates believe that this system will also reduce intrusions of third parties into medical decision making. Physicians who provide more testing, for example, will simply charge a higher rate to consumers who choose those physicians. No regulator will tell the physician that they are providing too many services.

However, a number of concerns have arisen about defined contribution plans. One is whether consumers are able to make informed decisions about health plan choices. In particular, can consumers discern plan quality from the written materials that would be distributed through health plan report cards? Even if the information were collected by an independent organization—which is *not* the case currently—there is little evidence to indicate that consumers would be able to use such information effectively. As discussed earlier, researchers have found that consumers do not understand much of what is included on report cards (Hibbard and Jewett 1997).

Relevant here is a study by Judith Hibbard and Jacqueline Jewett (1996), which examined the type of information consumers look for on report cards. The authors found that most consumers indicate that the key types of information for them in choosing a health plan are "desirable events" such as utilization rates for mammograms, cholesterol screenings, and pediatric immunizations. Less important to consumers are "undesirable events" such as hospital death rates from heart attacks, rates of low birth weights, and hospital-acquired infections. Curiously, then, when given report cards on two alterative health plans—one with a better record on desirable events and the other with a better record on undesirable events—consumers overwhelmingly chose the latter.

In another study, Chernew and Scanlon (1998) examined data from 5,800 single employees at one large firm, who were given health plan report card information prior to choosing a plan during an open enrollment period. The authors were mainly concerned with whether employees used information that was provided to them on the quality and satisfaction of alternative plans. They found little relationship between these ratings and the plan chosen. Curiously, one measure of quality—consumer satisfaction—had an effect opposite of what was predicted. Plans that scored higher on satisfaction were *less* likely to be chosen, controlling for other factors.[27] Although far more research is needed in this area, this evidence casts doubt on how well consumers can use report card information to make the best choices for themselves. The mere existence and dissemination of information, even if objective and complete, does not guarantee that an individual will use it properly.

A second concern about defined contribution approaches concerns selection bias. Under competitive-based reform proposals, health plans are under intense pressure to attract enrollees by keeping premiums at a competitive level. One way to do this is through true efficiencies, but another is to try to obtain a *favorable selection* of patients. It is in the interest of plans to avoid groups whose costs are likely to be high, and individuals with chronic conditions (Light 1995).[28] Although, in theory, adverse selection could be ameliorated by risk adjusting premiums for

---

27. The authors are unable to determine the reason for this unexpected finding, but do offer one possibility: that the measure they use "incorporates both measures of satisfaction and of access, such as waiting times and the percentage of physicians accepting new patients. If popular physicians systematically are less likely to accept new patients and have longer waiting times for visits, employees systematically may prefer plans that score poorly on the satisfaction rating" (Chernow and Scanlon 1998, p. 18).

28. One way to deal with this problem would be to *risk adjust* payments to health plans—that is, to pay them more if they have sicker patients. Although health services researchers are devoting much attention to this problem, there are few instances in which health plan contributions use risk adjustment, and in most of those cases, adjustments are done based just on demographic characteristics of enrollees, such as age and sex.

the health status of enrollees, the current state-of-the-art system is not sufficient for doing so.

In addition, because enrolling in better health plans is likely to be more expensive, the lowest-cost plans in an area might possibly be the least desirable ones—for example, the ones having a limited provider network, offering little choice, paying for only the most basic services, making it difficult to obtain referrals, and so forth (Rice, Brown, and Wyn 1993). Indeed, to the extent that putting providers at considerable risk is effective in controlling costs, one would expect less expensive plans to employ more severe physician incentives to conserve resources.

One adverse and rather dramatic consequence of adverse selection is a premium *death spiral.* This occurs when one health plan is the recipient of sicker enrollees, which in turn results in higher costs, and, during the next open enrollment period, higher premiums. These higher premiums then dissuade all but the sickest enrollees to sign up; eventually, premiums can become so high that almost no one can afford them.

A dramatic example of a death spiral occurred in the University of California health benefits system. As reported by Buchmueller (1998), the university adopted a fixed contribution policy in 1994, whereas previously it essentially paid the costs of all plans except for a high-cost fee-for-service option. The new policy ultimately saved the university money, as plans had an incentive to compete with each other on the basis of premiums, and employees had an incentive to switch to lower-cost plans. A spill-over effect was that the only fee-for-service plan, Prudential High Option, experienced a premium death spiral resulting from an adverse selection of enrollees. In 1993, the year prior to the change, 10 percent of employees enrolled in this plan, paying $750 annually for single coverage. Just three years later, premiums had more than quadrupled to almost $3,300 and enrollment had fallen to 1 percent of employees. The death spiral continued unabated; in 2001, the annual premium had risen to almost $17,000 for single coverage, and over $40,000 for family coverage (University of California 2001). As a result, only a handful of members remained and new enrollment was barred.

The trade-off between cost savings and adverse selection is also illustrated in a study of Harvard University's health plans, reported by Cutler and Reber (1998). In this instance, a preferred provider organization (PPO) and several HMOs were offered, and until 1995, the PPO was heavily subsidized compared to the other plans. In 1995, Harvard adopted a fixed contribution policy. Because the PPO had an adverse selection of patients, out-of-pocket premium costs rose dramatically. A death spiral occurred as the people leaving the PPO each year were less costly than those who remained. By 1997, just three years after the fixed contribution policy was adopted, the PPO plan was driven from the market, and only HMO and point-of-service plans remained. Cutler and Reber note that even though Harvard saved some money from the policy, social welfare declined because people who wanted a PPO plan could no longer choose one.

A related and final concern about defined contribution concerns equity, particularly for those in poorer health. The fear is that those in poor health will not receive a sufficient amount of money to purchase adequate coverage—especially given the system's inability to adequately risk adjust premiums to account for sicker health status. It is possible to create a system in which this is not a problem—for example, having employers require that any insurers take all applicants. But as insurance becomes more individual in scope, where employees can choose, say, any health plan in their area, employers (and even government) will find it harder to successfully enforce these kinds of requirements.

Premium Support

Premium support is similar to defined contribution, so it will be discussed only briefly.[29] One of the main concerns about a defined contribution approach is that it shifts all financial risk from the employer or government to the enrollee. Suppose that health plan premiums rise precipitously. With a defined contribution approach, consumers would face the full cost increase if the payer did not increase the size of its contribution. This could make coverage increasingly unaffordable over time. Under a premium support system, the contribution made by the employer or government is fixed, but it is based on the premiums actually charged by competing insurers.

Premium support is a device for ameliorating (although not eliminating) this financial risk. The amount of contribution to enrollees is not determined in advance (as it would be under defined contribution) but rather is tied to the actual bids proffered by health plans. This is a key distinction because it means that if plans, on average, charge more, payers will *automatically* cover more, leaving a more manageable out-of-pocket

---

29. For a further discussion of the concept, see Aaron and Reischauer (1995) and Rice and Desmond (2002).

liability for individuals. Thus, under premium support individuals would still have an incentive to choose a cost-efficient plan, but at the same time financial protection would be afforded against overall inflation in premium costs.

The main area in which premium support is being considered is in the U.S. Medicare program. The proposal of most note, known as "Breaux-Frist I" after the senators who introduced it, was fashioned out of work on the part of the Bipartisan Commission on the Future of Medicare.[30] Under Breaux-Frist I, the current Medicare program is replaced by a system of competing health plans, one of which is the federally sponsored Medicare fee-for-service system. Beneficiaries can choose a health plan during an open enrollment period each year. The plan can be the traditional Medicare fee-for-service program offered by the government, or alternatively, a plan offered by a private organization. Each plan is paid its bid after some adjustment is made for the case-mix of enrollees as measured by their health status and geographic location. The Medicare contribution toward a beneficiary's coverage would be approximately 90 percent of the costs of providing benefits among the various competing insurers. Beneficiaries with incomes equal to or less than 135 percent of the official poverty level would not pay any premiums for the lowest-cost high-option plan that is available in their geographic area. If they choose another plan that is more expensive, then they are responsible for paying the difference in premiums.

Premium support proposals are designed to instill competition (and, it is hoped, increased efficiency) into the Medicare program, which is the main bastion of traditional fee-for-service medicine in the United States. More specifically, they are intended to enhance the plan choices available to senior citizens, encourage efficiency through price competition, and control Medicare costs. But in addition to some of the problems with defined contribution programs just discussed, premium support for Medicare also raises difficult issues concerning the ability of seniors to make informed choices about alternative health plan choices.

A premium support system depends much more heavily on Medicare beneficiaries' ability to use comparative plan information. The primary

---

30. The majority of Commission members voted in favor of reforming Medicare through a system of premium support, but not the number that was necessary for transmittal of an official recommendation to Congress and the President. Thus, no official recommendation stemming from the Commission's work was made.

reason is that staying in the Medicare fee-for-service system might entail substantial financial ramifications—particularly if the differences between fee-for-service and HMO premiums are considerable.

Seniors will present more of a challenge than those currently in the labor market for three main reasons: (1) cognitive functioning declines with age; (2) seniors have, on average, less experience with managed care; and (3) unlike in the employment-based insurance market, seniors have little opportunity to discuss their insurance options in a group setting. The second of these problems should become less of an issue over time as more seniors with experience in managed care age into the Medicare program, but the other two problems likely are more permanent.

Because cognitive ability tends to fall as people age, depending on seniors to use comparative plan information to make good choices under premium support raises major challenges. A number of skills are necessary for a person to make an optimal choice about the health plan in which they enroll: understanding the measures of benefits, costs, quality, and satisfaction; evaluating which are most salient for themselves; being able to compare ratings across several health plans; and appropriately weighing the advantages and disadvantages of each in light of their own priorities and situations.

In the nonsenior market, there is no consensus that most individuals can and do use such information effectively. Much less research has focused on the Medicare population. In one study, Hibbard and colleagues (2001) compared the ability of seniors against the working-age population in the use of comparative health plan information. The study examined 35 items that assess "the ability to accurately interpret comparative plan performance information when it is presented in tables, charts, and text [allowing a person] to identify optimal choices when viewing unambiguous data" (p. 199). The authors found "striking differences between the Medicare and younger sample in ability to use information accurately. Medicare beneficiaries made almost three times as many errors as younger respondents did" (p. 200). The authors conclude that:

> Given the population-related differences we observed, moving Medicare in the direction of mirroring the market approach used for the under-sixty-five population may not be feasible or desirable. The findings call into question a policy approach that relies on a level of consumer skill that more than half the population may not possess (p. 202).

Another study by Hibbard and colleagues (1998) tested Medicare beneficiaries on their knowledge of key aspects of HMOs and fee-for-service plans, including the role of primary care providers, physician networks, physician payment incentives, emergency care, appeal rights, and a variety of implications that arise from choosing one system over the other. The study was conducted in areas of the country with high managed care penetration, and included samples of both HMO and fee-for-service members. The authors concluded that only 11 percent of respondents had enough knowledge to make an informed choice about fee-for-service versus HMO coverage under Medicare. These findings are supported by another study, conducted by Stevens and Mittler (2000), which concluded that:

> [M]ost beneficiaries do not understand the basics of Medicare and M+C [Medicare+Choice] and are confused, regardless of whether they have choices. Beneficiaries seek information only when an event or crisis pushes them to do so [and] make decisions almost exclusively on the basis of cost, availability of prescription drug coverage, and inclusion of their own providers. They do not consider information about quality, at least as policymakers have defined it. (p. 27)

A final issue concerns the opportunity for seniors to discuss their health plan choices with others. In the employment-based insurance market, enrollees have more of a chance to discuss health plan options with benefit managers or with colleagues—either individually or in formal or informal group settings. This is not the case for Medicare beneficiaries unless they attend an informational seminar. This lack of discussion makes it more difficult to work through the implications of choosing one plan option over another. In addition, the literature on the nonsenior market demonstrates no consensus that most individuals can and do use such information effectively.

MSAs
Currently a great deal of policy interest in the United States has been directed toward *medical savings accounts* (MSAs), which rely heavily on patient cost-sharing. Under most MSA proposals, people (usually employees) would be able to choose a health plan with a very large annual deductible (often several thousand dollars), but that covers medical expenses above that amount in full. The (tax-favored) savings in premiums could be used

to make payments toward the deductible, or alternatively, to spend (or save) on anything that the consumer desires. Advocates suggest that MSAs have the advantage of offering protection against catastrophic health costs but provide strong incentives for people to think twice before using services needlessly.

We will focus on three issues that follow from the above discussion. The first issue is whether MSAs will indeed quell the demand for services. Although consumers with MSAs will likely forgo some minor services, the vast majority of medical spending goes toward "big-ticket items." For example, in a particular year, 2 percent of the U.S. population is responsible for 38 percent of expenditures (Berk and Monheit 2001). Because any hospitalization or procedure is likely to meet the annual deductible, patients will not have much of a financial incentive to curb medical spending. For that reason, MSAs would not result in depressed demand for expensive medical technologies.

Second, the idea behind MSAs is that individuals can make informed choices about whether treatment should be sought for a particular illness. It was shown earlier, however, that consumers' ability to perform this task well is questionable.[31] Findings from the RAND Health Insurance study indicate that patients are as likely to forgo effective medical services in the presence of cost-sharing as they are to forgo less effective care (Lohr et al. 1986; Siu et al. 1986).

Third, selection bias could cause various problems for a country embarking on MSAs. One would expect those who are less likely to need medical care to be the most likely to purchase the accounts. This would cause two problems. First, patients who are sicker—and who therefore might need more incentive to consider costs when making medical care decisions—would not tend to enroll in MSAs, and therefore would not

---

31. There is also concern whether consumers will make rational choices with regard to contributions to programs such as MSAs. In a study of university employees' contributions to tax-deductible flexible spending accounts, Schweitzer, Hershey, and Asch (1996) found that employees did not act rationally. Relatively few contributed to such accounts, even though it would have been in the best interest financially of most to have done so. And those who did contribute tended to give the same dollar contribution each year, even when their changing financial circumstances would have been expected to result in different contribution levels over time. The authors conclude that "[t]he pervasiveness of these patterns raises concerns that health care reform plans that rely on financial incentives at the consumer level—for example, proposed medical savings accounts—will be inefficient" (p. 583).

be subject to any efficiency-enhancing incentives that derive from cost-sharing. Second, the markets would be segmented, with healthier people in these less expensive plans and sicker people pooled together in non-MSA plans, making the non-MSA plans even more expensive.

Experience with MSAs has been minimal. The most well-developed model has been used in Singapore, but different analysts disagree on its effect. One common viewpoint is that although Singapore has had some success in controlling its health costs, this is not due to MSAs, but rather to supply-side controls such as the rationing of hospital beds and physicians, as well as regulating their fees (Yip and Hsiao 1997; Barr 2001).

There is little actual experience with MSAs in the United States. Research has instead relied on simulation techniques to predict the effect of MSAs. The most comprehensive study to date, conducted by Zabinski and colleagues (1999), used actual health spending from national surveys to simulate how individuals would respond if they were offered both traditional coverage and MSAs by their employers. The authors conclude that favorable selection into MSAs is likely; furthermore, under most scenarios this would lead to a premium death spiral in which traditional insurance coverage is driven out of the market. Those most affected would be poorer families in poor health. If such families stay in their traditional health plan, they would have to pay more in premiums, but if they switched to an MSA, they would have to pay much higher costs through the high deductible.

Chapter 4

Supply Theory

BESIDES DEMAND, THE other key element in understanding micro-economics is supply theory. Supply is usually defined as the amount of goods and services firms wish to sell at alternative prices. In a competitive market, the point at which demand and supply are equal indicates both the price at which goods and services will be exchanged, and the amount exchanged.

In most economic applications, supply plays a subsidiary role to demand. In general, if demand for a product changes because, say, people's tastes change, firms will produce less; similarly, if people demand more of a good, firms will tend to increase production and/or more firms will enter the market to meet this additional demand.

The health services market is different from others in this respect, however: supply considerations play a very important role in determining both prices and output. This is true primarily because suppliers are not just passive producers of whatever is demanded. Rather, as in the case of the physician who acts as the patient's agent, suppliers can play a major role in determining what services the consumer ultimately chooses to purchase. Because of this, the list of policy tools available in the health services sector is much more extensive than in most other aspects of the economy.

Section 4.1 briefly summarizes traditional supply theory; readers already familiar with the derivation and determinants of supply can skip this material. Section 4.2 provides a critique of supply theory based largely on doubts about the validity of the assumptions presented earlier. Section 4.3 then discusses several applications of this critique to the area of health policy.

4.1 THE TRADITIONAL ECONOMIC MODEL

Section 2.1.2 provided a brief summary of production theory. It showed how firms are expected to choose both the level of inputs and the level of outputs to maximize profits. In Chapter 4, we modify Figure 2.5 to indicate how a firm's supply curve is constructed; this is shown in Figure 4.1. As before, *MC* shows the marginal cost of production and *P* is the market price. The curve *AVC* is *average variable costs* of production; curve *ATC* shows *average total costs*.

To understand these curves, one needs to know that total costs are subdivided into variable and fixed costs. Variable costs are those that change as the level of output changes, whereas fixed costs are those—such as capital purchases and land—that do not. The *ATC* curve shows the average total costs of producing each level of quantity, whereas *AVC* shows the average of all costs except for fixed costs.[1] The reason the curves gravitate toward each other as quantity increases is because the difference between the two—*average fixed costs*—declines as quantity rises.[2]

At point *A*, the firm neither makes any economic profits nor suffers any economic losses because the price received for selling each unit of output is exactly equal to *ATC*. This lack of profits is not a concern to the economist, however, because the economic definition of costs includes an item for a "normal" rate of return on investment. Zero economic profits simply means that the firm is making a profit equal to the typical rate of return available on other investments. In a competitive market, firms are expected to have an economic profit rate of zero.[3]

Recall that to maximize profits, a firm produces at the point where the marginal cost of production equals the market price. As can be seen from Figure 4.1, all points on the *MC* curves that are below and to the left

---

1. These curves are drawn such that *MC* intersects both *AVC* and *ATC* at their minimum points. There is a mathematical certainty. When *MC*—the cost of the last unit—is higher than average costs *AVC* or *ATC*, it brings the average up. In contrast, when the last unit is less costly than the average, it brings the average down. Thus, the only point at which *MC* can be equal to *AVC* and *ATC* is at their minimum, where these curves are neither rising nor falling.

2. Average fixed costs are defined as total fixed costs (*FC*) divided by quantity produced (*Q*). By definition, *FC*, the numerator, does not change as output increases, but quantity, the denominator, obviously does. Thus, as quantity rises, average fixed costs decline, which means that *AVC* and *ATC* will converge.

3. This is because at positive profit levels, more firms will enter the market and/or existing firms will produce more, thereby raising market supply and depressing market prices until equilibrium is reached at the zero-profit level.

Figure 4.1: Economic Profits and Supply

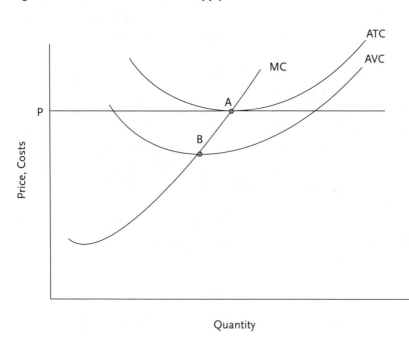

of point *A* are money losers, because at any corresponding level of quantity, *ATC* exceeds price. Note that between points *A* and *B*, the firm will lose money, but the market price still exceeds the firm's average variable costs. Thus, at least in the short run, the firm would be willing to stay in business because proceeds cover expenses. Below and to the left of point *B*, however, the market price does not even cover these variable costs. Unless the firm has some reason to believe that things will be different in the future, the sensible decision is to shut down.

The portion of the *MC* curve above point *B* is defined as the short-run *supply curve* for a competitive firm. All points on this curve show how much a profit-maximizing firm would be willing to produce at different price levels. This can be seen simply by drawing several horizontal lines, indicating alternative market prices that intersect *MC*. Each of the intersections represents a profit-maximizing level of output; the set of all such points above and to the right of point *B* is therefore the firm's supply curve. *Aggregate* supply—how much is supplied by the combination of all firms in a market—is simply the sum of each firm's individual supply.

We will not deal with the concept of the long-run supply curve here because it does not provide insights used later in the chapter. Briefly, in the long run, all costs are variable; the firm must choose not only the right level of variable inputs, but also its scale of operation (e.g., capital stock) to maximize profits.

A supply curve shows the relationship between different levels of market price and the amount of a good or service supplied by a firm. Its upward-sloping shape indicates that the firm would wish to supply more when the market price is higher and less when the market price is lower. Higher prices would result in more profits, and therefore an incentive to produce more. Lower prices, however, would result in lower profits. To maximize profits, the firm would cut back on its last, most costly units of production.[4]

Several factors can cause a supply curve to shift. Two notable ones are the prices of inputs and technology.[5] We can therefore write the firm's supply schedule as:

$$S = f(P, P_i, T) \tag{4.1}$$

where S is the amount of the good supplied, P is its market price, P_i is the price of inputs, and T is the level of technology.

Suppose that a technological breakthrough reduces the cost of production. This would mean that, at any price, the firm could profitably produce more; or alternatively, at any quantity, the costs of production would be lower. This means that the *supply curve* (examples of which are shown later in the chapter, in Figure 4.2) would shift outward. If the cost of inputs declines, the firm's supply curve would shift for the same reason. Note, however, that most analysts in the health services area find technology to be, on average, cost increasing rather than cost decreasing (Newhouse 1993). If this is true, the technologies being used are probably designed not to reduce cost so much as to improve people's health status and/or comfort.

The exact relationship between the quantity of a good supplied and its price is called the *elasticity of supply*. It is defined as the percentage change

---

4. See Chapter 2, footnote 5, for a discussion of why marginal costs are expected to rise as quantity increases.

5. Other factors sometimes listed in textbooks include expectations about the future market price level, taxes, and the prices of related goods produced by the firm.

in the quantity of a good supplied, divided by the percentage change in its price. A supply elasticity of +0.3 means that when the market price rises by, say, 10 percent, the quantity supplied increases by 3 percent.

The above model of supply depends on a number of assumptions. The validity of those assumptions that play an important role in health policy is assessed in the following section.

4.2 PROBLEMS WITH THE TRADITIONAL MODEL

In the traditional economic model, demand is key; supply is essentially along for the ride. Of course, to obtain the market price and quantity, one needs both. Beyond that, however, the role of supply is rather passive. If, for example, demand shifts outward, causing a short-run increase in prices, quantities, and profits, supply will increase to meet this demand. In contrast, a change in supply—perhaps due to a reduction in the cost of obtaining inputs—does not influence people's demand curve, which is a function primarily of tastes (or, in the health services area, health status).

If policymakers wish to alter a *competitive* market for some reason, traditional economic theory would suggest focusing on demand. Only a few limited tools are available for doing so, however. The main one, of course, is price. Taxes can be used to raise prices, thus suppressing the amount of a good that is demanded, and subsidies can do the opposite. A second policy lever might be to improve consumers' information so that they can make choices that are in their best interest. Beyond that, the list of demand-side tools is rather thin.

If, however, suppliers are not merely passive actors in the operation of the market, the list of policy tools available is considerably expanded. Among the most prominent set of these in the health services area are incentives designed to influence providers' behavior. Capitation, diagnosis-related groups (DRGs), and practice guidelines represent a few such examples. Thus, to determine which set of policy tools are most appropriate, in this section we examine the extent to which the assumptions of the competitive model in the area of supply are or are not met in the health services sector. The policy implications of this analysis are then provided in Section 4.3.

In this section, we critique five assumptions of the competitive model, which were presented in Table 1.1:

Assumption 10. Supply and demand are independently determined.
Assumption 11. Firms do not have any monopoly power.

Assumption 12. Firms maximize profits.

Assumption 13. There are not increasing returns to scale.

Assumption 14. Production is independent of the distribution of
wealth.

4.2.1 Are Supply and Demand Independently Determined?

The issue of the relationship between supply and demand, oddly enough,
is one of the most studied in all of health economics, but it is also
one in which there seems to be the least agreement. Most of the focus
has been on whether suppliers—particularly physicians—act totally in
their patients' interest, or if alternatively they can succeed in convincing
their patients to act in a way that also benefits them (the suppliers).
In the literature, this has been couched in terms of whether physicians act as *perfect agents* for their patients, or even more commonly,
in terms of whether physicians can *induce demand* among patients for
their services.

One reason that demand inducement has engendered so much interest among health economists is that its existence is so totally at odds
with the competitive model. Normally, an increase in supply would lower
price, but that is not necessarily the case if physicians induce demand.
Furthermore, physicians would be expected to supply fewer services if
they are paid less per service, but again, this would not necessarily be
true if demand inducement were present.[6]

As noted, there is little agreement on the issue, although most health
economists seem to believe that physicians are able to induce demand
to some extent. In a survey of almost 300 U.S. and Canadian health
economists, Roger Feldman and Michael Morrisey (1990) report that 81
percent of respondents believe that physicians generate *some* demand for
their own services. But many economists seem to have considerable doubt
concerning physicians' ability to go so far as to hoodwink patients into
demanding far more services than they really want.

This section is not intended to definitively answer any of the questions
that surround demand inducement. Rather, it tries to show that in spite
of the difficulty of testing for demand inducement, enough evidence is
available to make one doubt the independence of demand and supply

---

6. One possible exception to this is if physicians have a "backward-bending" labor supply
curve, which is discussed below.

curves in the physicians' services market. Readers wishing to examine both sides of the issue may wish to consult a published debate.[7]

This section is divided into four parts, the first three of which are devoted to different ways of testing for demand inducement, and the last of which provides some summary remarks.

Testing Demand Inducement Through Physician-Population Ratios

One of the earliest methods of testing whether physicians induce demand was to determine how a particular market measure, such as utilization or price, changes in response to a change in the number of physicians. The idea behind the test is straightforward: if there is an increase in competition among physicians and physicians can induce demand, they will do so to maintain their revenues. Many such studies have been conducted, some of which find evidence of demand inducement and others of which do not.[8] Because of inherent difficulties in conducting such studies, however, it is unlikely that they will ever reveal uncontestable evidence.

Some of the problems can be seen from Figure 4.2, which is taken from earlier articles by Uwe Reinhardt (1978) and by the author (Rice 1983).[9] D_0 and S_0 are the initial demand and supply curves, and S_1 reflects an independent or exogenous increase in the physician-population ratio. D_1 is the demand curve if physicians induce demand in response to the increase in competition. Clearly, just looking at whether utilization increases in response to more physicians does not distinguish between the competitive and demand-inducement hypotheses—both predict utilization to increase (from Q_0 to Q_c with no inducement, and from Q_0 to Q_i with inducement). But the problem goes beyond even that. Suppose that equilibrium price and quantity move from point A to point C. Although this would seem to be consistent with the inducement model, note that

---

7. For the anti-inducement side, see Feldman and Sloan (1988). For a contrasting opinion, see Rice and Labelle (1989).

8. A few notable studies that find evidence of inducement using physician-population ratios include Evans, Parish, and Sully (1973); Fuchs (1978); Hemenway and Fallon (1985); Cromwell and Mitchell (1986); and Tussing and Wojtowycz (1986). Some studies concluding that demand inducement is not terribly significant include Wilensky and Rossiter (1983); McCarthy (1985); Stano (1985); Escarce (1992); Carlsen and Grytten (1998); and Grytten and Sorensen (2001).

9. Reinhardt's article also shows that two other ways of examining inducement—output per physician and income per physician—also provide ambiguous results.

Figure 4.2: Effect of an Increase in the Number of Physicians in a Geographic Area

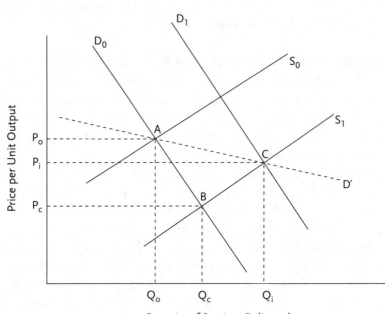

Quantity of Services Delivered

Source: Reinhardt, U. E. 1978. "Comment on Paper by Frank A. Sloan and Roger Feldman," In *Competition in the Health Care Sector: Past, Present, and Future,* W. Greenberg, ed., (Bureau of Economics, Federal Trade Commission, Washington, DC), pp. 156–90.

it would also be consistent with a no-inducement scenario if the initial demand curve were D' rather than D_0, as shown by the dotted line. Since it is very difficult to obtain data that tell us the exact shape of demand curves, it seems unlikely that examining changes in utilization can help us determine whether physicians induce demand in response to changes in the number of physicians in an area.

Another possibility is to look at what happens to price as evidence about demand inducement. But, as drawn, both models predict a decline in price. If physicians do not induce demand, market price will decline from P_0 to P_c, and if they do induce demand, from P_0 to P_i. This may seem a bit artificial, however, because one can imagine D_1 drawn in such a way that price would actually rise above P_0. Thus, it would seem that one way to determine whether physicians induce demand is to see if price *rises* in response to an increase in the number of physicians. If it does, then it would seem that physicians are inducing demand, although a decline in price, as just demonstrated, would not provide evidence one way or the other.

Unfortunately, this method also presents problems. The primary one is a statistical issue known as *omitted variables bias.* Suppose that we do indeed find that areas with more physicians have higher prices. This would seem to be consistent with the demand-inducement hypothesis, but only if we adequately control for all of the other factors that would make one area of the country more expensive than others. It might be that physicians gravitate to attractive urban and suburban settings with various cultural amenities, good schools, and the like—areas that tend to have higher price levels. If data are not available to capture all of these subtle yet important characteristics of an area, then we might incorrectly attribute higher physician prices to demand inducement.

Finally, Joseph Newhouse (1978) points out another problem with drawing conclusions about demand inducement by looking at the relationship between market price and physician supply:

> Recall that analysis of a competitive market assumes a fixed and homogeneous product. But physicians in areas with greater concentration of physicians spend more time with their patients and patients in such areas spend less time waiting for their physicians. More time with the physician and less waiting time are both desirable characteristics that lead to more physician time per visit. In a competitive market, visits using more physician time would be more expensive. As a result, even if the market were competitive, there could be a positive relationship between the physician/population ratio and the price of a (non-homogenous) physician visit. The test of demand creation based on physician prices also fails. (p. 60)

Testing Demand Inducement Through Physician Payment Rates

Perhaps a somewhat more promising method of testing for demand inducement is to determine how physicians respond to changes in the payments they receive. In general, one might expect that, without demand inducement, physicians would provide fewer services when they face a decline in payment—they would simply slide down the supply curve. But with demand inducement, they might behave differently—say, increase the provision of services in the wake of payment reductions to recoup lost income. Note that this sort of behavior is *not* consistent with the upward-sloping supply curve that is typically assumed in competitive markets.

Most, but certainly not all, of the evidence on demand inducement using these methods supports its existence.[10] In one of the earliest sets of studies, researchers from the Urban Institute found that California physicians increased the quantity and intensity of services provided to Medicare beneficiaries in response to a freeze in program payment rates during the early 1970s (Holahan and Scanlon 1979; Hadley, Holahan, and Scanlon 1979). In another set of studies, the present author found that physicians in urban areas of Colorado, who faced declines in their Medicare payment rates during the late 1970s compared to their nonurban colleagues, increased the intensity of medical and surgical services and the amount of surgery provided and laboratory tests ordered (Rice 1983, 1984). Other researchers have found that physicians responded to Medicare payment rate freezes during the mid 1980s by increasing the quantity and/or intensity of surgery, radiology, and special diagnostic tests (Mitchell, Wedig, and Cromwell 1989).

A study of the Canadian experience through the early 1980s showed that provinces that were least generous in raising physician payment rates over time experienced the greatest increase in the volume and intensity of services provided (Barer, Evans, and Labelle 1988). Unlike most other studies, this one could not be criticized for ignoring changes in patient out-of-pocket costs because during this period Canadians received services without any copayments. In contrast, one confounding factor in most U.S. studies is that reduced physician payment rates often result in lower patient copayments (e.g., the patient pays 20 percent of charges). Thus, if the physician provides more services after the payment reduction, it is possible that part of the reason is that patient demand increased as a result of lower copayments.

Some counterevidence has been published, however. A study using data from some of the Canadian provinces found little relationship over a dozen years between utilization of specific procedures and their fees (Hurley, Labelle, and Rice 1990). Some studies of Medicare payment rate

---

10. A review of much of the earlier literature (through the early 1980s) can be found in Gabel and Rice (1985).

reductions for "overvalued procedures" (mainly surgery and testing) in the late 1980s found little evidence that physicians increased the quantity of services provided (Escarce 1993a, 1993b). Other studies of the same payment reductions do find evidence of volume increases in the wake of Medicare payment reductions, however (Physician Payment Review Commission 1993).

Hurley and Labelle (1995) point out one problem with all of this literature. As in the case with testing demand inducement with physician-population ratios, results derived by examining response to physician payment rate changes may be consistent both with a demand inducement and with a competitive model of physician behavior (Hurley and Labelle 1995). Suppose that physicians have a normal, upward-sloping supply curve. If payment rates decrease, we would therefore expect the volume of services supplied to decrease. Consequently, an increase in the amount of services provided in response to a payment reduction would provide evidence of demand inducement (assuming any alternative explanations can be invalidated).

This conclusion is based on the assumption that physicians attempt to maximize their income (see Section 4.2.3, below). Most evidence indicates that this is not the case, however. Things that also matter to physicians include, perhaps most importantly, the availability of leisure time. Other commonly noted elements of a physician's utility function are professional ethics (e.g., having the patient's interest at heart or alternatively, distaste toward inducing services) and having an interesting caseload.

If a physician tries to maximize both income and leisure jointly, his or her supply curve may exhibit a "backward-bending" shape. At low levels of fees—for example, point A in Figure 4.3—higher payment rates will induce more work. At some level, such as point B, unit payment rates are so high that the physician may decide to enjoy more leisure as fees climb even higher. Thus, a reduction in payment rates would lead to an *increase* in the quantity supplied. Note that this is the same result as under demand inducement—but without there being any inducement whatsoever. As Hurley and Labelle (1995) note, "one cannot empirically distinguish the inducement and no-inducement models based on predicted utilization effects" (p. 424).

More recently, some U.S.-based studies have been conducted that explicitly take into account the fact that physicians treat patients in more than one market—for example, Medicare and private insurance patients.

Figure 4.3: Backward-Bending Supply Curve

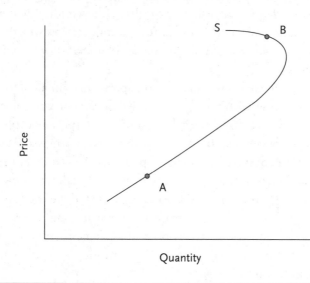

In a theoretical piece upon which several subsequent empirical investigations have been based, McGuire and Pauly (1991) show that how physicians respond to fee changes depends on the relative importance of the *substitution effect* and the *income effect*. The substitution effect predicts that if one insurer reduces fees, physicians will treat fewer of its patients, substituting more lucrative patients from the other insurers. The income effect, in contrast, predicts that physicians will also treat more patients of the insurer whose fee declined, to compensate for the loss of income. This latter effect is consistent with the notion of demand inducement.

Like the previous literature discussed, studies testing this model have also been ambiguous. Yip (1998) examined the provision of coronary artery bypass grafting surgeries by physicians in two states. This study's findings tend to be supportive of demand inducement, in that physicians who were most affected by cuts in Medicare fees were the ones who increased the volume of services the most—even the volume of Medicare services. Other studies (Tai-Seale, Rice, and Stearns 1998; Mitchell, Hadley, and Gaskin 2000), however, found more ambiguous results, with the results varying according to specialty and type of service.

Perhaps a good summary of the state of the art is provided by Jeremiah Hurley and Roberta Labelle (1995), who conclude,

It appears that, in response to economic considerations . . . physicians *can* induce demand for their services, they *sometimes do* induce demand, but that such responses are neither automatic nor unconstrained. Further, physicians do not always respond in ways that can be predicted. (p. 420)

Other Methods of Testing Demand Inducement

Partly as a result of the difficulty in using the above strategies for analyzing demand inducement, some analysts have employed other means.[11] One novel approach has been to see whether physicians and their families use more or fewer medical services than other people, the theory being that if physicians induce demand among their patients, they and their families are likely to avail themselves to fewer (unnecessary) services than others.

Two studies that have examined this have found that physicians and their families use *more* services than others, thus contradicting the notion of demand inducement (Bunker and Brown 1974; Hay and Leahy 1982).[12] One problem with studies like these, however, is the difficulty of controlling for the fact that physicians, other medical providers, and their families often get care at much cheaper prices. In addition, it is hard to account for other differences between medically oriented and other families.[13]

A final approach is to ask physicians how much money they would like to make and compare this to their actual income. It is then possible to determine whether this differential is correlated with their practice behavior. One such study found that the further physicians were below their targeted income, the more they charged their patients—evidence of demand inducement (Rizzo and Blumenthal 1996).[14]

---

11. For a thorough list of different approaches, see Labelle, Stoddart, and Rice (1994).

12. The Bunker and Brown study was not about demand inducement, per se, because it was written before the debate started to rage.

13. One possible difference is that health professionals are less tolerant than others of uncertainty with regard to their own health, and therefore demand more services when they are patients in an effort to minimize this uncertainty (Harold Luft, personal communication, 1997).

14. For critiques of this research, see the commentaries by Thomas McGuire and Uwe Reinhardt, along with the authors' reply, in the same issue of *Medical Care Research and Review* (volume 53, number 3).

Summary Remarks

There will likely always be doubts about how much demand physicians induce among their patients. Part of this is a result of the inherent ambiguity in the tools available, as the above discussion implies. We simply do not have sufficient information available to answer the question definitively. Gavin Mooney (1994) has stated that, to understand whether patients are being *induced* to use more services than they really want, we need to know how many they would demand if they were as well-informed as the physician, but no such studies have ever been conducted. Reinhardt (1989) makes a similar point when he states,

> [H]ighly sophisticated econometric methods ultimately cannot define what proportion of observed utilization [is] simply *accepted* by sick patients (or their anxious relatives) and what proportion the latter would have *demanded* of their own free will, had they been as well-informed as their physicians. (p. 339)

Another, very different reason may explain why agreement is likely never to be reached, however. The issue of demand inducement seems to raise the hackles of followers of conventional economic theory. Reinhardt (1985) makes this point, writing that:

> [O]ne suspects that vested interest in neoclassical economic theory has added at least some fuel to the flames. Mastery of the neoclassical framework requires a heavy personal investment on the part of the analyst. Among the payoffs to that investment is entree into a fraternity whose power has derived in good part from the unity of thought forged by this shared analytic paradigm. One need not be an utter cynic to believe that, quite apart from our profession's yearning for truth, the defense of that unifying framework can take on a life of its own. (pp. 187–88)

Although there has been great disagreement over the subject, demand inducement is becoming less of a policy issue, at least in the United States. In the early 1990s, it garnered some national attention when the Department of Health and Human Services (DHHS) drafted Medicare payment rates, under the new Medicare fee schedule, that were 16 percent lower than the medical profession had anticipated, in large part because of the *anticipation of* physician-induced demand in the wake of lower payment rates. After an outcry by the medical profession, DHHS dropped the assumption that physicians would respond to lower payment rates through demand inducement.

With the increased penetration of HMOs in the United States, demand inducement has not been as pressing an issue. Even if physicians can induce demand, they do not have a financial incentive to do so when they are paid on a capitated or a salary basis. But with the "backlash" against managed care continuing, more HMOs may revert to fee-for-service payment, making the issue relevant again. In addition, demand inducement is still germane to discussions of the U.S. Medicare program, as well as for countries that continue to rely on fee-for-service medicine.

Finally, and perhaps most important of all, whether physicians can induce demand directly addresses the competitiveness of the marketplace for health services—which is what this book is mainly about. The existence of demand inducement would in and of itself *mean* that the market for medical services is radically different than most other goods and services, which further implies that a different set of public policies might be called for. Indeed, much of Chapter 6 focuses on the many supply-side policies that various developed countries have adopted to deal, in part, with the uniquely strong role of suppliers in this market.

4.2.2 Do Firms Have Monopoly Power?

Of the 15 assumptions about a competitive market that are discussed in this book, the issue of whether firms have monopoly power has perhaps received the most attention from economists. Monopolies exist when only one firm sells a particular product in a market, but *monopoly power* means something a bit more subtle. A firm has monopoly power if it can raise prices without losing its entire market. When a firm has monopoly power, it can charge more than can a firm in a competitive market. Because conventional theory assumes that suppliers cannot influence demand, these higher prices will mean that the amount of output demanded will be lower than in a competitive market.

Figure 4.4 shows the conventional analysis of how monopolists and competitive firms compare with regard to pricing and output. To understand the drawing, one needs to know that monopolists maximize their profits by producing up to the point where the marginal revenue derived from providing an additional service equals the marginal cost of providing that service. They then set price at the highest level the market will bear, which is the point on the demand curve that corresponds to (i.e., is

Figure 4.4: Pricing and Output Decisions by Competitive Firms and Monopolists

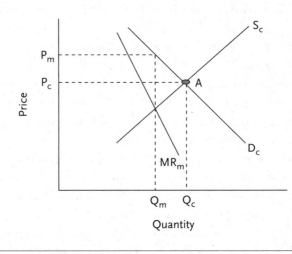

directly above) the profit-maximizing quantity of output. In the figure, S_c and D_c are the supply and demand curves, respectively, in a competitive market, and MR_m is the monopolist's marginal revenue curve.[15] The output produced by competitive firms is indicated by point A, where the supply and demand curves intersect, as well as the corresponding output levels P_c and Q_c. The monopolist, however, produces less (Q_m) and charges more (P_m).

Because monopoly power has been studied so thoroughly, we will deal with it only briefly in this section. In the area of health services, firms clearly have monopoly power. A hospital that raises its charges for a room may possibly lose some business, but will not lose all of its business. This is true for a number of reasons: hospitals differ with respect to quality,

15. If all output is sold at only one price, the marginal revenue curve must be below the demand curve for a monopolist. This is because if the firm wishes to increase output by one unit, its marginal revenue increases by an amount less than the market price at which the output sells. This is true, in turn, because the firm must lower the price it receives on all of the goods sold, not just the last one. If, in contrast, a monopolist can charge a different price to all customers (or different classes of customers), then it can reap even higher profits. Such monopolists are called *price discriminators* because of their ability to charge different prices to different buyers.

Figure 4.5: Pricing and Output Decisions by Competitive Firms and Monopolists with Demand Inducement

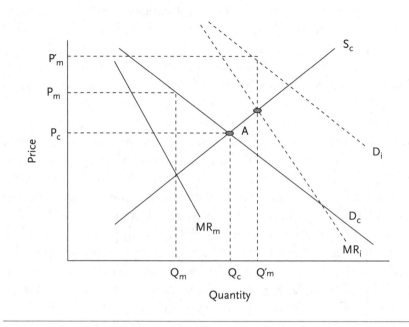

amenities, and location; patients may wish to be treated by a physician who prefers one hospital over another; and patients tend to pay out-of-pocket only a small fraction—about 3 percent—of the total hospital bill (U.S. DHHS 2001).

Similarly, as indicated in the previous section, physicians also appear to have some degree of monopoly power, demonstrated by their ability to induce demand for their services, which in turn allows them to derive even greater profits. This is because suppliers can shift the demand and marginal revenue curves in Figure 4.5 to the slashed curves D_i and MR_i. This would result in the (monopolist) physician producing more than would be predicted by the conventional monopoly model (Q'_m), and charging more as well (P'_m).

In the United States, over the past two decades there has been a strong movement toward more monopoly power in two other key components of the health services market: hospitals and health plans. One of the earliest examples of a very competitive market in the United States was Minneapolis–St. Paul. During the 1980s, health plans began to concentrate their purchasing power through a series of mergers, up until the point that two large HMOs controlled 90 percent of the HMO market (Christianson et al. 1995). In response, hospital systems and multispecialty group practices began their own consolidation to retain bargaining power, until only three hospital networks controlled the bulk of hospital beds (National Health Policy Forum 1995).

More recently, several communities being tracked by the Center for Studying Health System Change have shown increased consolidation, particularly in the hospital market. In Cleveland, for example, after the closure of several for-profit and inner-city hospitals, two hospital systems had garnered two-thirds of the market. As a result, health plans had reduced ability to successfully bargain to keep their hospital payments down (Christianson et al. 2000). In a somewhat smaller community, Lansing, Michigan, a single hospital system controlled 60 percent of the market, and a single health plan, 70 percent (Devers et al. 2001).[16]

The ultimate effect of such consolidations is difficult to predict; it depends in large part not only on the relative bargaining power of different market participants, but also on the importance consumers put on issues such as health plan premiums and quality of care. Thus far, it appears that increased HMO penetration has resulted in lower premiums, although these savings decline when there are few competing provider groups (Zwanziger and Melnick 1996; Bamezai et al. 1999). In addition, a recent upsurge in U.S. health insurance premiums raises doubt as to whether the savings generated by HMOs can be sustained. The effect on quality is less clear and is discussed in Section 4.3.1.

4.2.3 Do Firms Maximize Profits?

In otherwise competitive economies, the health services area is often an exception, in that many of the providers operate on a nonprofit basis. This is particularly true in the hospital sector, where for-profit status is the exception rather than the rule in the vast majority of countries. Even in the United States, only about 13 percent of community hospital beds are in for-profit facilities (U.S. DHHS 2001).

We will not focus on this issue here, however, since it has already been dealt with extensively in the literature. Rather, we briefly raise a different

---

16. The Center is studying 12 U.S. communities over time in depth. Reports can be obtained from http://www.hschange.com.

reason to doubt the profit-maximization assumption: managers in the health services sector, like their counterparts elsewhere in the economy, may seek to fulfill objectives other than maximizing their firms' overall profits. Because a vast literature on this subject exists (e.g., the study of total quality management), no attempt will be made to review the literature. Nevertheless, a few points about this assumption should be made.

In the 1960s, economist Harvey Leibenstein (1966) coined the term *x efficiency*. The use of this term signified his belief that factors other than those that economists usually considered—in sum, the "x" factor—had potentially very substantial effects on efficiency in the economy. To substantiate his argument, Leibenstein reviewed previous work on the social cost of traditional economic inefficiency, such as monopolies and trade barriers, and showed that these inefficiencies tended to have only minuscule effects on welfare. He then showed that, in contrast, the x factor often tended to have a significant effect on efficiency. What, then, is the x factor? It is essentially the idea that motivational factors affect how firms translate their inputs into outputs. Leibenstein (1966) wrote, "Neither individuals nor firms work as hard, nor do they search for information as effectively, as they could. The search arises because the relation between inputs and outputs is *not* a determinate one" (p. 407).

Standard economic theory assumes that firms maximize profits. Although most owners of firms (often the shareholders in publicly traded companies) certainly *want* to maximize profits, they do not run the companies by themselves. Rather, they hire managers and other employees to carry out the day-to-day business. In economic lingo, the owners of the firm are the principals, and the hired employees are the agents. Agents, however, may pursue some very different goals than profit maximization in carrying out their jobs. For instance, they may prefer not to work as hard as they could, they may be too cautious, or they may even plot against other employees to work their way up the hierarchy.[17, 18]

---

17. The extent to which managers and employees can deviate from profit maximization depends, to some degree, on how easy it is for other firms to enter the market. If entry costs are high, then an existing firm will be able to tolerate a larger degree of inefficiency without being subjected to competition from new entrants.

18. Even if employees do strive to maximize profits, another theory, the "Peter Principle," posits that such employees will eventually rise through the hierarchy until they reach their "level of incompetence," where they will remain (see Peter and Hull 1969). Although written in a humorous style, the book's theme would appear to contain more than a grain of truth.

One especially relevant application of this theory concerns independent practice association (IPA)–type HMOs. In IPAS, the owners of the HMO and its principal agents, the physicians with whom the IPA contracts, are physically separated and may have quite different goals. As a result, IPAS must come up with motivational factors to get physicians to act in the company's interest, but this is difficult to do and could reduce the quality of care provided. This issue will be further considered in Section 4.3.1, on capitation and incentive reimbursement.

4.2.4 Do Increasing Returns to Scale Exist?

Generally, economic markets observe constant or decreasing returns to scale in production. That is, when a firm expands the use of all inputs by a certain proportion, the corresponding increase in output is the same (constant) or less than (decreasing) the increase in input usage.

One important implication of constant or decreasing returns to scale is that there is no advantage for society in having a monopoly. This can be understood by supposing the opposite for a moment: imagine increasing returns to scale. In such a case, the average cost of production would decline as we move from many firms that each supply a fraction of the total output, to one firm that supplies all of the output. A society might therefore be better off in encouraging the monopolization of such an industry, along with the subsequent regulation of that monopoly to ensure that it did not take advantage of its monopoly status to charge too much, produce too little, or both. In contrast, without increasing returns to scale, there would seem to be little advantage to encouraging monopolies.

In the United States, a possible case can be made for the existence of increasing returns to scale in the hospital sector, particularly with regard to the provision of particular services. Stephen Finkler (1979) conducted the classic study of this type, examining economies of scale in the provision of open-heart surgery in California in the 1970s. Using a methodology called component enumeration, he essentially observed exactly what hospital resources were necessary for performing additional open-heart surgical procedures. He found that the average costs of such procedures did not bottom out until a hospital had provided about 500 per year, but that only 3 percent of California hospitals provided that many services. Finkler calculated that, in 1975 dollars, the United States could have saved $400 million by *regionalizing* open-heart surgery—that is, by providing such surgery in a select few regional facilities. He further calculated that the resulting incremental travel and other inconvenience costs would have absorbed only 6 to 9 percent of the savings. He also noted that "[h]eart surgery is only the tip of the iceberg" (p. 270). A much more recent study was carried out by Menke and Wray (1999), who examined the effect on costs of closing open-heart surgery units in selected U.S. Veterans Affairs hospitals. Even after accounting for the associated costs of transferring patients between hospitals and transportation expenses, they found that closing one of four underused facilities would reduce costs by 18 percent.

One must be cautious in interpreting the above results because they apply only to hospitals. Less information is available on increasing returns to scale in other parts of the health system, although one certainly suspects that such increasing returns would be less common since hospitals are the main area in which fixed costs are high.

Another aspect of increasing returns to scale in the hospital sector that is perhaps more often overlooked concerns health outcomes from surgery. One area of agreement among most health services researchers is that hospitals and physicians that have more experience in providing surgical services tend to obtain better health outcomes for their patients—the so-called "practice makes perfect" hypothesis. One of the earliest studies of this type found that hospitals that performed more than 200 operations per year of a particular type had mortality rates 25 percent to 41 percent lower than lower-volume hospitals, after controlling for case-mix differences (Luft, Bunker, and Enthoven 1979). A more recent study found that, when coronary artery bypass operations were done by high-volume surgeons in high-volume hospitals, mortality rates were 38 percent lower (Hannan et al. 1991). These results are also an indication of increasing returns to scale, in that quality is one of the chief outcomes in the hospital market.

4.2.5 Is Production Independent of the Distribution of Wealth?

A final assumption of the conventional economic model noted here is considered only rarely by economists, but is very important—the assumption that production is not related to the distribution of wealth.[19] Typically, firms are assumed to face *production functions* that look like Equation 4.2:

$$Q = f(L, K) \qquad (4.2)$$

---

19. For a succinct discussion of this assumption, see Graaff (1971).

where Q is the quantity of output over some period of time, and L and K are the quantities of labor and capital inputs over that same period. The term f indicates the state-of-the-art technology that is used to transform these inputs into output. What the conventional model assumes is that this function f is unaffected by the way in which Q is distributed among the population.

Alternatively, what if this is not the case, and the distribution of output affects productivity? This would seem to be plausible. If people are poorly fed, then they are less likely to be productive workers. In developed economies, where malnutrition is less widespread, the dependence of productivity on distribution would still hold in the following way. On average, poor people tend to be less educated and also tend to have more problematic health behaviors, which in turn reduces their health status and subsequent productivity. In a set of studies on the subject, Harold Luft (1973, 1978) found a causal relationship in which low socioeconomic status resulted in lower health status, which in turn led to lower productivity, particularly among people with chronic conditions. Some health implications of this relationship are discussed in Section 4.3.4 as well as in Section 5.3.3, where the concept of "social capital" is presented.

4.3 IMPLICATIONS FOR HEALTH POLICY

This chapter has attempted to show that the typical, passive role generally attributed to suppliers in competitive markets does not appear to apply very well to the field of health services. We questioned the validity of five assumptions of the competitive market, perhaps the most important of which, for our purposes, is that supply and demand are independently determined. In this section we discuss several ways in which relaxation of these assumptions results in a number of important implications concerning how suppliers' behavior can be influenced.

4.3.1 Capitation and Incentive Reimbursement

One of the key implications of the demand-inducement literature is that physicians can and do influence patients' decisions in a way that results in the provision of too many, and/or more complex, services. But physicians' ability to induce patient demand does not, by itself, mean that more services will be provided. A necessary corollary is that physicians are also paid more for providing more services—which is what happens when they are reimbursed on a fee-for-service basis. To see this, suppose that physicians had the ability to induce demand but were not paid more for each service they provided. In such a case, they would have no financial incentive to provide more services, even if they had the ability to do so.

This interaction between payment method and demand inducement provides one of the key motivations for capitated payment systems. Under a fully capitated system, providers receive a fixed payment over a set period of time regardless of how many services they provide. Thus, they have no direct economic incentive to provide additional services. In fact, the incentive is the opposite; if they provide fewer services, profits will be higher, since the capitation rate is unrelated to the number of services provided. Of course, if caregivers provide too few services, quality will be inhibited, providers may face possible lawsuits, and patients will likely become dissatisfied and move elsewhere.

The issues surrounding capitation and other forms of incentive reimbursement are fairly extensive, and they are complicated by the fact that these payment methods may apply to both health plans (e.g., insurers, HMOs) and providers. The following two subsections focus on these two groups separately.

Other supply-side measures that have been adopted to control costs are not reviewed here because they do not add any additional insights to the arguments being made. Some references are given to those wishing to pursue these topics: DRGs,[20] utilization review,[21] and practice guidelines.[22] A few broader supply-side measures used outside of the United States, such as technology controls and global budgeting, are presented in Chapter 6.

Paying Health Plans

In the United States, working-age individuals who have health insurance coverage usually obtain it through an employer. Typically, the employer contracts with several *health plans* to provide care to enrollees, although

---

20. For a review of the results of many DRG studies, see Coulam and Gaumer (1991).

21. For a review of the literature on second-opinion surgery, see Lindsey and Newhouse (1990). Useful studies on preadmission certification requirements for hospital stays include Wickizer, Wheeler, and Feldstein (1989); Scheffler, Sullivan, and Ko (1991); and Wickizer and Lessler (1998).

22. At the time of writing, little research had been published that evaluated the effect of practice guidelines on health costs. Detailed information on U.S. efforts to develop and disseminate practice guidelines can be found at: http://www.ahrq.gov/clinic/cpgonline.htm.

some employers choose a single plan for all employees. Health plans include *indemnity*[23] *insurers* such as nonprofit Blue Cross and Blue Shield plans or for-profit commercial insurers, HMOs, and PPOs. In recent years, however, organizational innovation has blurred the lines between these health plans. For example, conventional insurers now often offer both indemnity insurance and HMO coverage, and HMOs often offer "point-of-service" benefits that allow members to go to out-of-network providers and still receive some reimbursement of the costs, as would be the case in fee-for-service coverage.

HMOs are almost always paid by employers on a capitation basis—a fixed amount of money per person per time period. One of the most important policy questions in the field of health economics is, "How much money do HMOs save over fee-for-service medicine?" One would expect some savings because, by being paid on a capitation basis, HMOs have a strong financial incentive to spend less. Although it is generally agreed that money is saved, a great deal of controversy is voiced about exactly how much. Estimates vary from as low as 4 percent to as much as 25 percent.[24] The true savings certainly lie somewhere in between and probably depend on several factors, such as the type of HMO (group versus individual physician practice) and geographic area. The concern, of course, is whether these cost savings come at the expense of unacceptable reductions in the quality of care provided.

One should not underestimate the tremendous power of the incentives that underlie capitation. To understand the stark differences between fee-for-service and capitation, it is useful to use an analogy. Being paid by fee-for-service is like getting a signed check from someone where the amount of the check has not been filled in; the incentive is to do more to get more. Capitation, however, is like getting a signed check

---

23. Strictly speaking, these companies rarely sell true indemnity insurance. Under a true indemnity scheme, the insurer pays a fixed dollar amount per covered illness event (e.g., $50 for a visit to a doctor). Because such policies put the policyholder at much financial risk, insurers long ago found that *service benefits*, in which the policy pays a portion or all of the costs of a particular service, are more popular. Nevertheless, the term "indemnity insurance" is often used to distinguish conventional fee-for-service insurance from HMOs and PPOs.

24. The low-end estimates are from reviews of the literature conducted by the Congressional Budget Office (1994). The high-end numbers are from the RAND Health Insurance Experiment (Manning et al. 1984).

where the amount has already been filled in. Since the recipient already has the money and is not going to get any more by performing more services, the incentive is to do less to profit more.

The concern about quality under capitation is heightened with additional competition among HMOs. As HMOs compete against each other for employers to offer their products and consumers to choose them, they need to cut their costs to keep their premiums competitive—and, by and large, they have done so (Zwanziger and Melnick 1996; Christianson et al. 1995; Buchmueller 1998). But if consumers do not have sufficient knowledge to determine which plans offer the best quality, as was argued in Chapter 3, the cuts that HMOs make are more likely to reduce the quality of care provided.

Much research is being conducted on quality of care in HMOs versus fee-for-service medicine, the results of which are still far from certain. Most of the research to date has concerned patient satisfaction, one component of quality but perhaps not as convincing as looking at health outcomes.[25] In general, HMOs appear to perform better than fee-for-service in terms of satisfaction with keeping costs down and in coordinating care among different physicians, but do worse with regard to continuity of care (e.g., seeing the same doctors), providing access to care (e.g., waiting times, or providing care at off hours or on short notice), and perceptions about both the technical and personal sides of care (Safran, Tarlov, and Rogers 1994; Rubin et al. 1993; Miller and Luft 1997).

To most analysts, the more important issue is how HMOs have affected patients' medical outcomes. A review of the literature through the mid 1990s reported that most studies up until that time had found comparable quality between HMOs and fee-for-service medicine for various process and outcome measures of quality (Miller and Luft 1997), although some evidence raises particular concern about how well the poor and elderly fare in HMOs (Ware et al. 1996).

Research on health outcomes in HMOs, other types of managed care systems, and fee-for-service continues to be conducted. The results of future studies will be of particular interest as they demonstrate the effect of more competition in the HMO market. It is difficult to predict just

---

25. This issue—whether a health system should be judged based on improving patients' health or on increasing their utility or satisfaction—is discussed at greater length in Chapter 5.

how increased competition may alter the quality findings. On the one hand, more competition could improve quality if quality is the primary basis on which health plans compete, and if consumers are perceived as savvy judges of the quality of care provided. On the other hand, health plans, which are under extreme competitive pressures to control premiums, might cut resource use enough to result in reduced quality of care.

The material in this subsection might strike the reader as rather unsurprising. This is because nearly all health economists agree on the different incentives of capitation versus fee-for-service payment. What may generate more disagreement is exactly *why* these are important issues. What we posit here is that the reason we even consider capitation is that the marketplace for health services deviates so far from the competitive model that traditional, demand-side policy tools are largely inadequate. This issue is further pursued in Section 4.3.2, where we consider the issue of patient cost-sharing, the primary demand-side policy lever.

Paying Providers of Care

The previous subsection discussed how health plans tend to respond to payment incentives, but health plans do not respond alone. A health plan does not provide care, rather, doctors and other providers do. A health plan that is paid on a capitation basis must find ways to get doctors to act to conserve resources, and to keep plan premiums competitive.

Section 4.2.3 introduced the term "x efficiency" to indicate that other factors besides those usually considered in microeconomics—most notably, ways in which a firm motivates its employees—are necessary for firms to be successful. In the HMO arena, this issue becomes especially important. The problem typically is not as great for group-model and staff-model HMOs, which either employ their own physicians or contract with a medical staff as a whole. These HMOs tend to pay physicians a salary, which means that the physicians do not have a personal financial incentive to provide additional, marginally useful services. Nevertheless, such HMOs often also include incentive clauses to help ensure that the physicians consider the HMO's finances when making clinical decisions (Gold et al. 1995; Medicare Payment Advisory Commission 2000).

Compared to IPAS, group-model and staff-model HMOs have a big advantage in this regard: physicians work in a common setting with a *corporate culture*. Such HMOs have any number of levers to help ensure that the medical staff acts in a manner that is in the company's overall interest. Besides salary and capitation, such levers would include promotion within the organization, scheduling issues, and a variety of disciplinary actions, to name a few.

The problem faced by the HMO in influencing physicians' behavior is much greater in IPAS. Because physicians work in their own offices, and because they treat the patients from many HMOs as well as fee-for-service patients—not just from a single IPA—instilling in these physicians any sense of corporate culture is difficult, if not impossible. In addition, because they practice away from the HMO setting, the physicians have no direct oversight.

The IPA has an enormous problem. Obviously, physicians are needed to treat enrollees, but the IPA has almost no control over these physicians. How can the IPA motivate physicians to act in a way to conserve resources, so that the IPA can keep its cost below its capitation payments? Early IPAS were unsuccessful in this regard, and analysts expressed skepticism that such IPAS were able to control costs.[26] More recently, as IPAS and *network-model* HMOs (essentially, a network of several local IPAS) have become the dominant HMO model, some of this skepticism has eased.

Calculating just how much IPAS save compared to other HMOs or fee-for-service providers is difficult because conducting such comparative studies is difficult. With the exception of the RAND Health Insurance Experiment in the 1970s and early 1980s, in which people were randomly assigned to a single, staff-model HMO, researchers are plagued by the problem of *selection bias.*[27] This means that some health plans end up enrolling members who are either healthier or sicker than the rest of the population. Thus, the fact that IPAS might have lower costs than fee-for-service medicine may be a result of true cost savings, or alternatively, it may be due to the fact that they tend to have healthier enrollees. Although statistical techniques exist to help correct for this problem, the data available are rarely sufficient to fully solve it.

Some of the more recent literature is beginning to show that IPAS may be able to achieve the same sort of savings as group-model and staff-model HMOs. For example, findings from the Medical Outcomes Study—which examined 20,000 patients in about 350 physician practices in 1986—found that prepaid multispecialty groups had hospitalization

---

26. For an analysis of HMOs before 1980, see Luft (1981).

27. A vast amount of literature has been published on the issue of selection bias. A good policy perspective appears in Newhouse (1994). For more recent evidence on the extent of selection bias in U.S. insurance markets, see Hellinger and Wong (2000).

rates and ancillary test expenses that were lower than those of traditional HMOs (Greenfield et al. 1992).

How, then, are IPAS overcoming some of their inherent disadvantages regarding cost control? The main way is through a strong physician motivational factor—incentive reimbursement. Early IPAS generally paid physicians on a fee-for-service basis, which gave them no incentive to control costs. More recently, IPAS have adopted payment methods to help ensure that member physicians feel financial incentives similar to the HMO as a whole.

A variety of payment incentives exist, as shown in Table 4.1 from a U.S. survey of health plans conducted in 1999 (Medicare Payment Advisory Commission 2000).[28] Physicians can be paid by salary, capitation, and fee-for-service, and within these, can earn bonuses or "withholds" for meeting or not meeting certain productivity or cost-containment goals. One common method is to withhold a certain amount of a primary physician's capitation fee, which is returned only if certain goals regarding low referral and hospitalization rates are met. Such incentives can also be tied to the ordering of diagnostic tests and radiological procedures. As shown in the table, most health plans (61 percent) capitate primary care providers, but a large majority (75 percent) base specialist payment on fee-for-service. More than 40 percent of plans use bonuses or withholds for primary care physicians, and about 30 percent, for specialists (Medicare Payment Advisory Commission 2000).

The Medicare Payment Advisory Commission published other findings as well. When physicians are paid on a capitation basis, the capitation payment always includes primary care office visits and usually (more than 80 percent of the time) includes other services provided in their offices as well as inpatient visits. It also includes ancillary care provided by others and referrals for specialist care 46 percent of the time. Finally, the study examined the types of performance measures used by health plans to adjust payments to primary care physicians. It found that quality measures were used most often (68 percent of the time), followed by consumer surveys (48 percent of the time), utilization and cost measures (46 percent of the time), patient complaints (42 percent of the time), and

---

28. For a further discussion of these methods, see: Hillman, Pauly, and Kerstein (1989); Hillman, Welch, and Pauly (1992); Welch, Hillman, and Pauly (1990); and Medicare Payment Advisory Commission (2000).

Table 4.1: Predominant Methods Used by Health Plans to Pay Primary Care and Specialist Physicians, 1999

	Primary Care Physicians (%)	Specialist Physicians (%)
Fee-for-Service (Total)	24.7	75.3
Without withholding or bonuses	15.1	52.2
With withholding or bonuses	9.7	23.1
Capitation (Total)	61.2	13.3
Without withholding or bonuses	29.2	7.1
With withholding or bonuses	32.0	6.2
Salary (Total)	14.1	11.4
Without withholding or bonuses	13.3	11.4
With withhoulding or bonuses	0.8	0.0

Source: Medicare Payment Advisory Commission. 2000. "Health Plans' Selection and Payment of Health Care Providers, 1999." (Medicare Payment Advisory Commission, Washington, DC), Table B.5.

enrollee turnover rates (23 percent of the time). On average, between 6 percent and 10 percent of compensation was affected by the physician's performance on these measures (Medicare Payment Advisory Commission 2000).

Some limited evidence indicates that the prevalence of physician capitation may have peaked in the United States. A study by Robinson and Casalino (2001) examined changes in physician compensation arrangements between six health plans and a single insurer. The study found a reduction in the scope of services included in capitation contracts. Although it is too early to say that a retreat is in progress, such a trend is a possibility for several reasons: more physician practices finding themselves in financial stress; the specter of malpractice liability resulting from compensation methods; and a continuing consumer backlash against managed care and the tools of the trade.[29]

---

29. The October 1999 issue of the *Journal of Health Politics, Policy, and Law* was devoted to various researchers' views about the consumer "backlash" against managed care in the United

Although research on the effect of these incentives has been limited, most studies find the incentives to be at least somewhat effective, and sometimes very effective, in controlling HMO utilization and expenditures. In one study of Wisconsin employees enrolled in an IPA, a change from fee-for-service to capitation payment (with physicians sharing in the financial risk of hospitalization and specialty costs) resulted in an 18 percent increase in primary care visits, along with a 45 percent decline in referrals to specialists outside of the IPA. In addition, hospital admissions decreased 16 percent, and length of stay dropped 12 percent (Stearns, Wolfe, and Kindig 1992).

Similarly, in a study of an Illinois IPA, physicians were switched from fee-for-service payment with a 15 percent withhold (returned at end of year if utilization is kept below a target) to capitation payment with bonuses for reduced hospitalization and shared financial risk for specialty referral costs. Specialist costs increased 2 percent in the year after the change, after rising by 12 percent the previous year. Hospital outpatient service costs declined 7 percent, after increasing 12 percent in the previous year. But inpatient hospital utilization demonstrated little change (Ogden, Carlson, and Bernstein 1990).

On the international front, Mooney (1994) relates an interesting study on the power of incentive reimbursement. He reports on a study from Denmark in which physician payment methods were altered rather dramatically (see also Krasnik et al. 1990). In October 1987, general practitioners in Copenhagen changed from fully capitated payment to payment based partly on capitation and partly on fee-for-service, to conform with physicians in the rest of the country. This new system resulted in the ability of general practitioners (GPs) to make extra money for consultations, prescriptions, certain procedures and tests, and some other procedures. As a result, the provision of services that provided extra fees increased substantially and referrals to specialists and hospitals decreased significantly. From this, Mooney (1994) concludes that "[t]here clearly is considerable discretion on the part of GPs in how they act and remuneration systems can push them to go one way or another in how they treat their patients and whether they treat them themselves or refer them on in the system" (p. 127).

States. Since then, managed care plans have shown some tangible signs that they are responding to consumer concerns. Perhaps most prominent is that some HMOs no longer require referrals from primary care gatekeeping physicians before seeing a specialist.

No studies currently exist that specifically examine how changing physician payment methods, per se, affects the quality of care provided. Without such studies, addressing the overall question of whether patients and society are better off in a managed care environment is extremely difficult. The concern, however, is that if physicians are given a financial incentive to cut back services, a plausible effect of that incentive is deteriorating quality.[30] In this regard, Marc Rodwin (1993) has written:

> Society makes a statement about the role of physicians when it provides incentives for them to help government or health care organizations reduce their costs. This is especially so if there are no equivalent financial incentives for physicians to improve quality of care. By using financial incentives to change the clinical practice of physicians, society calls forth self-interested behavior. In asking physicians to consider their own interest in deciding how to act, we alter the attitude we want physicians ideally to have. For if physicians act intuitively to promote their patients' interests, we will worry less that they will behave inappropriately. But if their motivation is primarily self-interest, we will want their behavior to be monitored more carefully. (p. 153)

Much interest has been expressed in developing "mixed" payment systems, ones that are neither fee-for-service nor capitation, but rather include aspects of each. In this regard, James Robinson (2001) has written:

> There are many mechanisms for paying physicians; some are good and some are bad. The three worst are fee-for-service, capitation, and salary. Fee-for-service rewards the provision of inappropriate services, the fraudulent upcoding of visits and procedures, and the churning of "ping-pong" referrals among specialists. Capitation rewards the denial of appropriate services, the dumping of the chronically ill, and a narrow scope of practice that refers out every time-consuming patient. Salary undermines productivity, condones on-the-job leisure, and fosters a bureaucratic mentality in which every procedure is someone else's problem. (p. 149)

---

30. Keep in mind, however, that the fee-for-service system that is being replaced in the United States had its own problems—the main one being the provision of services that were unnecessary, or in some cases, harmful.

Robinson discusses various innovative methods that are being developed to pay physicians in the United States. Some examples include:

- Paying a monthly capitation rate to primary care providers, but supplementing this with fee-for-service payments for services that the payer wants to encourage, such as vaccinations, preventive care, as well as services in which it is more economical to provide primary rather than specialty care such as nursing home visits or fairly straightforward procedures.
- Paying "case rates" for particular episodes of care (e.g., cardiology) that cover all services provided by specialists during a particular window of time. This makes physicians cost conscious for services over which they have control, but does not penalize them for other care for which they have little control.

4.3.2 Issues Surrounding Patient Cost-Sharing

As noted several times in this book, the traditional economic method of trying to improve efficiency in the marketplace is to make patients pay more out-of-pocket for services. As may be recalled from Section 3.3.1, health insurance results in a societal "welfare loss" under the conventional model because people purchase services with a marginal benefit far below the cost of those services. Health economists therefore often are keen on increasing patient cost-sharing as a way of reducing this welfare loss (see Figure 3.6). This viewpoint was critiqued in Section 3.3.2.

In the United States, most employer-sponsored health insurance that is based on fee-for-service payments requires annual deductibles that averaged about $530 for a family in 2001, as well as a 20 percent coinsurance rate (Jensen et al. 1997; Gabel et al. 1994).[31] In addition, most HMOs require cost-sharing in the form of a copayment for each patient visit and prescription drug (the latter of which varies depending on whether or not generic or brand-name drugs are used). Chapter 6 discusses the extent of cost-sharing in several other countries.

---

31. There is nearly always an annual maximum amount for out-of-pocket costs, after which the insurer pays 100 percent of covered expenses. Recent surveys, however, do not report this information. In 1989, this typically ranged from $500 to $2,000 per year (Gabel et al. 1990).

In this section, we examine two issues associated with patient cost-sharing. The first part addresses problems in determining the effect of patient cost-sharing on controlling utilization and costs, while the second addresses equity. A further discussion of equity is included in Chapter 5.

The Effect of Patient Cost-Sharing on Utilization and Costs

The major study of patient cost-sharing, the RAND Health Insurance Experiment (Newhouse et al. 1993), concluded that patient cost-sharing was an effective method of reducing utilization and expenditures. People who had to pay 95 percent of charges had annual expenditures that were 28 percent lower than those who paid nothing, and those with a 20 percent coinsurance rate had expenditures that were 18 percent lower than those with free care (Manning et al. 1987). (See Table 3.1, in the previous chapter, for a summary of the results.) In addition, because the study also found little improvement in health outcomes among those with free care, study researchers concluded that comprehensive (i.e., first-dollar) national health insurance would be a wasteful way to spend a nation's resources (Newhouse 1993).

Because the RAND study was the only major one that has used a true experimental design (i.e., random assignment of different types of insurance), it is the one that is normally used when making projections of the effect of patient copayments. Nevertheless, the use of an experimental design jeopardizes the extent to which the results can be generalized to many health policy applications.

Two major classifications designate the *validity* of research studies: internal validity and external validity. Internal validity refers to how well study results accurately represent what actually occurred in the specific setting being examined. For example, suppose a researcher studied 50 IPAS and found that they resulted in a 15 percent reduction in expenditures. The extent to which this study is internally valid is measured by how accurate this result is compared to the true reduction in expenditures among that sample of IPAS. For a moment, let us say that this study was a good one, and that the findings appear to be reasonably accurate. But further suppose that the IPAS chosen were not representative of all IPAS because they were located on the west coast of the United States. External validity refers to how well the results from a particular study can be generalized to other settings and/or populations.

It is generally agreed among the health services research community that the RAND Health Insurance Experiment was very strong in terms of its internal validity.[32] External validity is more of a concern, however. Some issues include the fact that the elderly were excluded and that the sample included only six sites in four states. Another such concern is whether the study, which was conducted from 1974 to 1982, is still timely. For example, during the 1980s and 1990s, hospital days per capita in the United States fell by 55 percent (U.S. DHHS 2001). If the study were conducted today, the results concerning the price responsiveness of hospital care might be much lower. Even if people had free care, they might not want or might be prevented from obtaining hospital care. Other concerns include whether the findings with regard to health status would still hold, but such concerns are not directly relevant to the point being made here.

An even greater threat to the external validity of the RAND study's utilization and cost findings exists. To understand the issue, consider the experimental design in the RAND experiment. A random sample of individuals in six areas of the United States was chosen. Each site had an average of only about 1,000 study participants, many of whom were assigned to insurance plans that were equally generous as or more generous than those they had previously owned. Participants who were required to pay for care did indeed use fewer services. However, because only a small fraction of the population in each site participated—at most, 2 percent (Newhouse 1993)—almost no effect was felt on an individual physician's practice. Most doctors would have had, at most, only a handful of patients assigned to the high-coinsurance cells, so any reductions in service usage by those patients would not have markedly affected physician practice revenues. If everyone in an area had faced changing copayments—as might have occurred under various national health insurance proposals— the results could have been very different. Suppose that the plan called for coinsurance rates higher than the standard 20 percent level. Physicians might respond to the initial fall in business by inducing patient demand for services. This response could take the form of providing more follow-up services, more complex services, or even more surgery. The

---

32. Not everyone agrees with this, however. For some criticisms of the study, see Welch et al. (1987); and Hay and Olsen (1984). For responses to these criticisms by those who carried out the RAND study, see Newhouse et al. (1987); and Duan et al. (1984).

experiment examined only patient responses, not physician responses, to cost-sharing.

The converse may also be true. Suppose that a national health insurance plan removes all coinsurance. Subsequent demand may not rise as much as the RAND study would lead one to believe, for two reasons: (1) physicians may have less of a financial need than before to induce demand; and (2) governmental and private payers are likely to introduce other measures (e.g., tighter utilization review, expenditure targets, global budgeting) to quell the initial increase in patient demand.

The inability to deal with provider (and policymakers' regulatory) response in the RAND study has raised criticism since the inception of the experiment. In a discussion of these issues in 1974, when the experiment began, James Hester and Irving Leveson (1974) wrote,

> The utilization of health services is the result of a complex balancing between demand for health care and the supply system that provides it. While the changing needs of one individual or small group will not affect this overall balance, the large-scale shifts in quantity and source of medical care that would result from a major national change in the financing of health care certainly would. Large changes in aggregate demand can be expected to produce substantial changes whose exact form is strongly influenced by specific administrative and financial regulations. . . . These changes will, in turn, feed back into the overall use patterns and costs, and influence again the users of the system. (pp. 53–54)

In response, Joseph Newhouse noted that the study was not "designed to replicate what would happen if various health insurance proposals were enacted into law," and furthermore, the study "deliberately selected sites that vary considerably with respect to the amount of stress on the delivery system" (Newhouse 1974, pp. 236–37). That is, the six sites varied with respect to provider-to-population ratios.

A number of economists, although notably mostly from outside the United States, have provided similar criticisms of the generalizability of the RAND findings.[33] The ability to test the issue directly has been slight,

---

33. See, for example, Evans (1984) and Mooney (1994). One U.S. economist who has made the same point is Alain Enthoven (1988), who wrote, "There are . . . problems in applying

however.[34] Thus, the RAND study results are more safely used to indicate the effect of cost-sharing on patients' demand for services (independent of any resulting provider response), rather than indicating ways in which overall utilization of services will change in response to large-scale policy initiatives concerning changes in patient cost-sharing.

Is Patient Cost-Sharing Equitable?

No matter how one defines equity—and several possible definitions will be discussed in Chapter 5—a strong case can be made that patient cost-sharing is inequitable. This is because of two interrelated issues: cost-sharing payments account for a greater proportion of income for those with lower income; and those with lower income tend to be sicker and to require more services. Families with lower incomes who do seek medical care will spend a greater proportion of their income to meet these cost-sharing requirements. Differences in wage and salary rates abound among all countries. In the United States, the average wage of people with managerial and professional jobs, for example, is more than double that for those with service-related jobs. In 1998, median household income for Whites was a about $41,000, compared to $25,000 for Blacks and $28,000 for Hispanics (U.S. Census Bureau 2000).

---

the results of the RAND experiment to national policy. RAND studied the behavior of about 7,700 people in six different cities. Thus, the proportion of the population affected by the experiment in any city was too small to have a noticeable effect on doctors' incomes, but the effects might be very different if everyone in a city were changed from a coverage with little co-insurance to one with a great deal. Initially, visits to the doctor would drop, but as the doctors found more time on their hands, all our experience suggests they would find other ways to make themselves useful: extra visits and consultations for hospitalized patients, more frequently advising patients who telephone that they should come in to be seen, and the like. What applies to a small sample might not apply to the whole community" (p. 17).

34. The only U.S. study that addresses this issue was from a small natural experiment that was analyzed by Marianne Fahs (1992), on the experience of one multispecialty group practice located in Appalachia in 1977. Fahs compared utilization in the year before the institution of cost-sharing with that during the two years following its institution, for two groups: mine workers who faced increasing cost-sharing requirements, and steel workers who did not. The study found that physicians responded to the imposition of cost-sharing on their mine worker patients by changing their practice behavior for their steel worker patients. Fahs concludes that "when the economic effects of cost-sharing on physician service use are analyzed for all patients within a physician practice, the findings are remarkably different from those of an analysis limited to those patients directly affected by cost-sharing" (pp. 25–26).

This problem is accentuated when health status is taken into consideration. To illustrate, in 1999, 23 percent of Americans classified as poor rated their health as "fair" or "poor," compared to only 6 percent who are nonpoor (U.S. DHHS 1999). Eight percent of Whites rated their health as fair or poor, compared to 15 percent of Blacks and 12 percent of Hispanics (U.S. DHHS 2001). Age-adjusted hypertension rates are about 50 percent higher among Blacks than Whites. Both Blacks and Hispanics have about twice the rate of untreated dental caries as Whites (U.S. DHHS 2000). Among Medicare beneficiaries, 42 percent of Black beneficiaries and 44 percent of Hispanics rated their health as fair or poor, compared to 25 percent of Whites. Similarly, members of both minority groups are twice as likely to have diabetes. Two-thirds of Black Medicare beneficiaries have hypertension, compared to half of Whites (Gornick 2000).

Although the RAND Health Insurance Experiment did not find too many instances in which reduced patient cost-sharing improved health status, there was evidence of such an effect for those with lower income. Some examples:

- Low-income families at elevated risk benefited the most from free care. The reduction in diastolic blood pressure among lower-income persons who were judged to be at an elevated risk for hypertension was 3.3 mm Hg, compared to only 0.4 mm Hg for similar people with higher incomes (Brook et al. 1983).
- Low-income persons in poor health who were given free care had the largest reduction in serious symptoms (Shapiro, Ware, and Sherbourne 1986).
- Among children of poor families who were at the highest risk, those with free care were less likely to have anemia than those in the cost-sharing plans (Valdez 1986).

Additional evidence also comes from looking at how coinsurance affected the receipt of general medical examinations. Low-income adults in the cost-sharing groups received 46 percent fewer exams than their counterparts with free care, compared to only a 29 percent reduction for other groups. For the children of those with cost-sharing, the figures were 32 percent and 21 percent fewer exams, respectively (Lohr et al. 1986). Finally, the RAND study examined the influence of coinsurance on the probability of obtaining medical care that was judged to be highly effective at treating a particular episode of illness. Among nonpoor children, those who had to pay coinsurance were 85 percent as likely to obtain care as the nonpoor with free care. For poor children, however, cost-sharing was a much bigger deterrent to obtaining medical care judged to be highly effective for a particular illness episode. Compared to those with free care, poor children whose families faced coinsurance were only 56 percent as likely to receive services. A similar pattern, although not as marked, was found for adults (Lohr et al. 1986).

To only a limited extent does U.S. health policy deal explicitly with the equity problems arising from the burden of patient cost-sharing. The primary way is through the Medicaid program, which does not require patient copayments. However, Medicaid only actually covers 41 percent of the poor (U.S. Census Bureau 2000).

Summary Remarks

Some of the problems with relying on patient cost-sharing have been summarized by Canadian economists Greg Stoddart and colleagues (1993, p. 57), who found four overriding reasons to eschew the implementation of cost-sharing in their own national health system:

1. Charges do not lead to selective reductions in utilization of only unnecessary or less necessary services, but affect the utilization of needed services as well (while much ineffective care continues to be delivered);
2. The distribution effects—both financial and health effects—of charges are potentially quite serious for certain groups in the population, especially as healthcare use becomes more concentrated within small and very ill segments of the population;
3. Analyses of the effects of user charges must take into account the significant, offsetting response of suppliers to reductions in patient-initiated utilization; and
4. Charges are neither a necessary nor a sufficient condition for overall cost control in healthcare systems.

The equity problems can possibly be ameliorated in a few ways. The present author, for example, was involved in formulating a proposal for U.S. health reform in which cost-sharing requirements were explicitly tied to patient income (Rice and Thorpe 1993). Such proposals would probably be difficult to enact, however, for both political and administrative reasons.[35]

Other countries have focused their efforts on alternative means of controlling expenditures, as described next.

4.3.3 Allowing Only Selected Hospitals to Provide Particular Services

In a free market, any firm wishing to compete can do so. Generally, increased competition can only benefit consumers by providing a wider variety of choices at a lower price. But as discussed throughout this book, the health field deviates from a free market in many ways. One implication is that more competitors may not necessarily be desirable. An example of this concerns whether all hospitals should be permitted to provide any service that they wish.

As discussed above in Section 4.2.4, returns to scale appear to increase for the provision of certain specialized hospital services such as open-heart surgery. This implies that if services are concentrated in fewer hospitals, costs will be lower. In addition, evidence was presented that quality (as measured by lower surgical mortality) tends to be higher in hospitals that provide a greater volume of services.

One approach, of course, is simply to provide this information to consumers and let them decide whether or not to use low-volume hospitals. A problem with this approach, however, was discussed in detail in Chapter 3: consumers often do not have access to the relevant information, or when they have access, do not use it. As a result, almost all studies have found that a large percentage of patients seek care from hospitals with lower volumes than are considered necessary to provide the highest quality care.

An interesting example of consumers' lack of ability or willingness to use such information comes from the United States, which has taken a lead in developing and disseminating information about quality of care to consumers. Between 1984 and 1992, the federal government collected and disseminated information on risk-adjusted hospital mortality rates in all of the nation's hospitals, documenting which hospitals

---

35. Perhaps the largest impediment is that the proposal relies on the income tax system to determine patient liabilities. This likely would result in people viewing cost-sharing as a tax, and taxes tend to be very unpopular.

had poorer outcomes than would be predicted given their case-mix. Furthermore, instances in which particular hospitals performed poorly were well-publicized in the local media. In spite of this, the publication of these reports had almost no effect on subsequent admission rates (Mennemeyer, Morrisey, and Howard 1997). Consumers continued—at nearly the same frequency—to seek care from hospitals that provided lower quality.

The alternative is for government to determine which hospitals would be allowed to perform which procedures. This approach—which has been used in various Canadian provinces and other developed countries—has the advantage of ensuring that hospitals that are chosen to provide particular services have sufficient experience for providing high-quality care. (Costs may be lower as well due to higher volume.) Of course, this approach has some potential disadvantages: the lack of competition could result in monopoly profits; hospitals might have fewer incentives to strive to provide the best care possible; and patients would have to travel longer distances. Nevertheless, these advantages and disadvantages could be weighed to determine whether such a policy would, in net, be beneficial.

4.3.4 Improving Productivity by Providing Insurance

Despite their belief that additional health insurance results in a welfare loss to society, many if not most health economists believe that everyone should be provided at least some health insurance coverage. The basis of such a belief typically is from the viewpoint of equity or fairness; that is, for ethical reasons people should receive at least some level of coverage. Less often will health economists argue for universal, comprehensive health insurance coverage from an *efficiency* standpoint.

One can also make a strong argument for providing health insurance coverage from an efficiency as well as an equity standpoint—especially for the poor. As alluded to in Section 4.2.5, a competitive market may underprovide health insurance coverage if poor income distribution results in the inability of some people to be as productive in the workplace as they might otherwise.[36]

---

36. An even greater improvement in health might possibly occur if income distribution itself were more nearly equal, but as argued in Chapter 5, much stronger support exists for in-kind rather than in-cash transfer payments to the poor.

This argument rests on three assumptions: (1) health insurance increases utilization; (2) greater utilization increases health status; and (3) better health status improves worker productivity. Health economists are in general agreement about the validity of propositions 1 and 3, but some doubt 2.

Much of this doubt about proposition 2 comes from the RAND Health Insurance Experiment, where it was found that, among the nonelderly, care provided free of coinsurance and deductibles did little to improve health status among the nonelderly population (Brook et al. 1983; Keeler 1987).[37] But as discussed earlier in Section 4.3.2, other findings from the study indicated that poorer people did indeed benefit from free care.

The fact that programs such as Medicaid exist in the United States indicates a belief that poor people should be provided with health insurance so that they may be able to achieve up to their capabilities. Nevertheless, the lack of coverage for more than 15 percent of the nonelderly population indicates that far more can be done in this regard.

---

37. The study did not examine the elderly mainly because they already had Medicare coverage.

Chapter 5

Equity and Redistribution

IT IS PERHAPS misleading to discuss issues about equity and redistribution so far into the book because this masks their importance. Although economists often focus on what is efficient, most people would appear to be more concerned about what is fair. In this regard, Daniel Hausman and Michael McPherson (1993) write, "Notions of fairness, opportunity, freedom, and rights are arguably of more importance in policy making than are concerns about moving individuals up their given preference rankings" (p. 676). Despite the importance of these issues, they have not received sufficient attention from health economists.

Section 5.1 provides a brief summary of ways in which traditional economic theory deals with the subject of the redistribution of wealth. Section 5.2 provides a critique of this theory, focusing on problems with "ordinal utilitarianism," the philosophy on which most policy conclusions are based. Section 5.3 then provides several applications of this critique to health policy.

5.1 THE TRADITIONAL ECONOMIC MODEL

Although many economists have given considerable thought to the issues of equity and the redistribution of wealth, such issues play little part in the traditional microeconomic model. Rather than concerning itself with how people come into possession of their initial stock of wealth, the traditional model devotes nearly all of its attention to how they allocate the resources over which they have already been assigned property rights (Young 1994).

To recap, we will reproduce the Edgeworth Box shown in Figure 2.7 with a few modifications to make Figure 5.1. For simplicity, we assume

Figure 5.1: Edgeworth Box, Modified

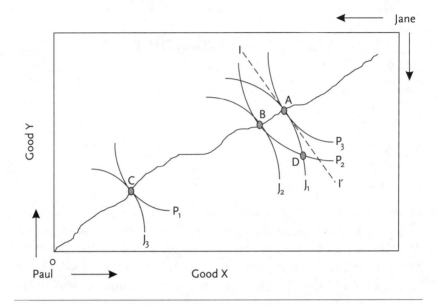

that society produces only two goods (this time, called X and Y) and that only two people, Paul and Jane, consume these goods. We saw in Chapter 2 that any allocation of the two goods that falls along the contract curve $o–A$ is defined to be economically efficient because no reallocations will make one of the consumers better off without making the other worse off. (Unlike in Chapter 2, we will ignore the issue of envy here.)

With the Edgeworth Box, we can see how any initial allocation of resources will be transformed, through trading, to a final equilibrium. To illustrate, suppose that Paul is initially endowed with about three-quarters of good X and just less than half of good Y (with Jane getting the remainder of each), which is depicted at point D. This is not a Pareto-optimal point because it is possible to make one or both of the consumers better off. Paul and Jane will therefore engage in trading, and afterward, the final allocation will fall along the contract curve somewhere between points A and B. The exact point depends on the relative bargaining skills of the two people.

However, only one point on the contract curve will also maximize *social* welfare. (See Section 2.1.4 for a discussion of social welfare functions.)

To reach that point, the economic model assumes that society will engage in redistribution of the initial endowments of wealth so that this particular point on the contract curve will be reached after the market has reached an equilibrium through trading.

Thus, under the traditional model, competition is used to ensure that resources are being used efficiently. Wealth is redistributed, through money transfer payments (since in the real world there are numerous goods, not just two), to ensure that the final competitive equilibrium results in a distribution of resources that is in accordance with society's desires. (The issue of how to carry out such a redistribution through taxation, without marring the efficiency brought about by competition, is a major problem, but one that was already addressed in Sections 2.2.2 and 2.3.2.)

5.2 PROBLEMS WITH THE TRADITIONAL MODEL

A number of criticisms have been leveled against the traditional model in terms of how it deals (or, perhaps more appropriately, does not deal) with equity and fairness as well as with the distribution of resources. These objections share one common element: they dispute the notion of ordinal utilitarianism, on which the traditional model is based.

This section critiques two of the assumptions listed in Table 1.1:

Assumption 9.   Social welfare is based solely on individual utilities, which in turn are based solely on the goods and services consumed.

Assumption 15.   The distribution of wealth is approved of by society.

5.2.1 Overview of Utilitarianism

Utilitarianism is the philosophy that assumes that social welfare is simply the sum or aggregate of all individuals' welfare. Under this philosophy, utility is a personal psychological perception, and, to the economist, is based on the goods a person possesses.

As discussed in Section 3.1.1, early advocates of "classical utilitarianism" such as Jeremy Bentham believed that these utilities not only could be quantified, but could also be added across individuals. Modern economics rebelled against such a concept, relying instead on the notion of *ordinal* rather than *cardinal utility*. Under ordinal utility, individuals choose which bundle of goods they prefer to any other instead of quantifying how much utility is derived from one bundle versus another.[1]

One needs to be careful in discussing utilitarianism because the term encompasses a number of seemingly distinct beliefs.[2] As noted, under classical utilitarianism, individual utilities can be quantified using a metric that is consistent across individuals. Ordinal utilitarianism, on which modern theory is based, requires only that individuals be able to rank alternative bundles of goods (which allows economists to employ indifference curves). But there are other utilitarian concepts as well. Under incremental utilitarianism, goods should be put in the hands of those who accrue the most gain from them. One hybrid form of utilitarianism allows intensity of preference to come into play (e.g., one good brings three times as much utility as another to a person), but does not permit utilities to be added across individuals.[3]

We have noted that economic theory is based on the concept of ordinal utilitarianism. In support of this concept, Kenneth Arrow (1983), a strong advocate of the use of ordinal utility in evaluating social welfare, has stated that,

> [T]he implicit ethical basis of economic policy judgment is some version of utilitarianism. At the same time, descriptive economics has relied heavily on a utilitarian psychology in explaining the choices made by consumers and other economic agents. The basic theorem of welfare economics—that under certain conditions the competitive economic system yields an outcome that is optimal or efficient—depends on the identification of the utility structures that motivate the choices made by economic agents with the utility structures used in judging the optimality of the outcome of the competitive system. As a result, the utility concepts which, in one form or another, underlie welfare judgments in economics as well as elsewhere . . . have been subjected to an intensive scrutiny by economists. (p. 97)

---

1. Some critics, however, believe that modern economists have gone too far in eschewing interpersonal comparisons of utility. Little (1957), for example, claims that most people are able to make valid judgments about whether one person is happier than another, or gets a greater amount of utility than another person from a particular good.

2. For a discussion of the different types of utilitarianism, see Elster (1992).

3. Elster (1992) has coined this as "Neumann-Morgenstern utility," after the founders of game theory.

What Arrow is saying is that the belief that competition results in socially desirable outcomes hinges on:

- Individuals making choices that maximize their well-being; and
- Society evaluating its own well-being solely on the basis of the utility enjoyed by its individuals.

Chapter 3 was devoted, in large part, to examining the first bulleted point. Much of the present critique will focus on the second.

5.2.2 Problems with Ordinal Utilitarianism

This section explores three problems with the concept of utilitarianism employed by modern economics, each of which has important implications concerning equity and the distribution of wealth. The first problem concerns lack of breadth; the concept ignores issues of social justice and fairness. The second problem concerns lack of depth; utilitarianism is defined solely in terms of a single, goods-based, psychological metric, ignoring other potentially important conceptions of what drives individual and social welfare. The third problem is perhaps more practical; utilitarianism mistakenly assumes that the socially optimal redistribution of wealth should take the form of cash grants rather than transfers of the goods and services themselves.

Social Justice and Fairness

Modern economics in general, and utilitarianism in particular, does not concern itself with what is right or fair. Rather, the possession of goods brings utility to individuals and therefore to society, which is conceived of as simply the aggregate of all individuals.

No concern is given to whether the overall distribution of wealth is *justified.* This is not to say that issues of income distribution are ignored. In fact, the people in a society may indeed be concerned about distributional issues and may choose to tax the rich to provide for the poor. But in such a situation, the distribution is the result of social choice (as exemplified by the social welfare function) and not necessarily based on social justice.

To understand this distinction—a crucial one—consider the difference between altruism and equity. The former is based on preferences, for example, I want the poor to have more so I provide donations or vote to increase taxes. Thus, providing for the poor makes *me* better off because their welfare enters my utility function. In contrast, according to Adam Wagstaff and Eddy van Doorslaer (1993),

> Social justice (or equity), on the other hand, is not a matter of pref-
> erence. As [Anthony] Culyer puts it: "the source of value for making
> judgments about equity lies outside, or is extrinsic to, preferences. . . .
> The whole point of making a judgment about justice is so to frame
> it . . . independently of interests of the individual making it." Social
> justice thus derives from a set of principles concerning what a person
> ought to have *as a right.* (p. 8)

The issue of what people should have as a right is obviously a controversial one, and one that has held the attention of philosophers and
economists alike. As noted, traditional economic theory, based on an ordinal view of utilitarianism, sidesteps this issue; rights do not come into
play, except insofar as society has defined property rights. But how property rights are assigned is not part of the purview of economics; rather, it
is a societal decision based, presumably, on other considerations.

The best-known modern exposition of social justice and rights is the
book by John Rawls (1971), *A Theory of Justice.* The next two subsections
will describe and critique Rawls's viewpoint.

Rawls's Theory

Rawls's theory, which he calls "justice as fairness," provides an alternative
to utilitarian philosophy. To determine what is fair, he invokes a concept
called the "original position," in which people choose the principles of a
just society from a position where "no one knows his place in society, his
class position or social status, nor does anyone know his fortune in the
distribution of natural assets and abilities, his intelligence, strength, and
the like" (Rawls 1971, p. 12).

In addition, one does not know the sort of society in which he or she
will be placed; it may be a democracy or, alternatively, a dictatorship in
which there is a small ruling class, with the rest of the population assigned
to slavery. Rawls calls this lack of information about one's talents and
standing, a "veil of ignorance." His goal is to determine the system of
justice that rational, self-oriented people would choose when placed in
the original position.

The other term that needs definition is "primary goods," which are
defined as "rights and liberties, powers and opportunities, income and
wealth" (p. 62). Self-respect turns out to be another key primary good.

Rawls posits that people in the original position would accept the proposition that primary goods should "be distributed equally unless an unequal distribution of any, or all, of these values is to everyone's advantage. Injustice, then, is simply inequalities that are not to the benefit of everyone" (p. 62).

The upshot—the system of justice that Rawls believes would be adopted by a society whose members consider these issues under the veil of ignorance in the original position—is what he calls the "difference principle." Under the difference principle, society is better off only when it makes its least well-off people better off. In other words, society's resources should be devoted to increasing the primary goods possessed by the most disadvantaged people. The only time that resources will go to the group that does not occupy the bottom rung is when by doing so, benefits will trickle down to the most disadvantaged group.

This result—that in the original position, people will adopt the above method of allocating primary goods—is called "maximin."[4] In essence, people will choose to maximize the lot of those who have the minimum. The unusual nature (at least to an economist) of this philosophy can be seen from Figure 5.2, which shows a set of L-shaped social indifference curves under the theory. Let the x axis be the primary goods enjoyed by person X, and the y axis those enjoyed by person Y. Each curve shows distributions that are, from society's viewpoint, equally desirable. Higher curves (i.e., those farther from the origin) represent higher levels of social welfare. The 45-degree line shows equal distributions of primary goods.

The indifference curves are L shaped; society is no better off when Y has more primary goods if those possessed by X do not increase. The only way to increase social welfare—that is, to get on a higher indifference curve—is to provide more to the person who has the least.

Why would people, placed in the original position, come up with such a conception of justice? Rawls has a simple answer:

> Since it is not reasonable for [a person] to expect more than an equal share in the division of social goods, and since it is not rational for him to agree to less, the sensible thing for him to do is to acknowledge as the first principle of justice one requiring an equal distribution. Indeed, this principle is so obvious that we would expect it to occur to anyone immediately. (pp. 150–51)

---

4. This stands for *maximum minimorum.*

Figure 5.2: Social Welfare Under Rawls's Theory

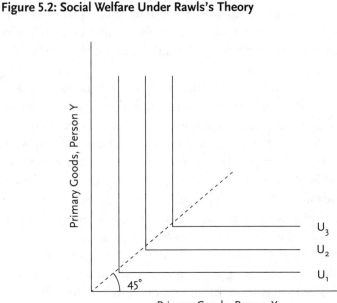

Source: Reprinted by permission of the publisher from *A Theory of Justice* by John Rawls, p. 5, Cambridge, MA: The Belknap Press of Harvard University Press, Copyright © 1971 by the President and Fellows of Harvard College.

Before moving on to a critique of Rawls's theory, note its policy implications. Although the theory is abstract and cannot be applied directly to many problems,[5] one implication overrides all others: society should engage in far more redistribution than it currently does. This is because many, if not most, redistributive programs are not targeted solely at those who are worst off in society. In fact, one could argue that relatively little goes to this group. In this regard, Gordon Tullock (1979) has written,

> So far as I know there is absolutely no reason to believe that majority voting or any of the variants of democratic government transfer an "optimal" amount. Indeed, I would argue that they do very badly, since the bulk of the transfers they generate are transferred back and

---

5. See Elster (1992) for a more thorough discussion of this criticism.

forth within the middle class; and, so far as I know, there are no arguments that would indicate that these transfers are desirable. (p. 172)

Although Rawls did not list health as one of the primary goods, some analysts have disagreed with this decision. According to Ronald Green (1976), "Access to health care is not only a social primary good, but possibly one of the most important such goods [because] disease and ill health interfere with our happiness and undermine our self-confidence and self-respect" (p. 120). The types of services that would be included as part of a universal health plan would include such things as "basic preventive and therapeutic services" (Green 1976, p. 120).[6] Norman Daniels (1985), in particular, has explored the extension of Rawls's theory to health.

Critique of Rawls's Theory
Although Rawls's theory is usually praised even by its critics, a number of objections have been leveled against it. Here we discuss some of them.

People Would Not Choose Maximin. Rawls assumes that rational people would choose the maximin principle to distribute primary goods. Many analysts, particularly economists, disagree, claiming that to reach this conclusion, one must assume a huge amount of risk aversion among the population. To illustrate, suppose that people were asked to choose between two alternative societies, one in which 95 percent of the people were endowed with $10,000 in resources and the other 5 percent with $1,000; and another society in which everyone was endowed with $1,500. It seems unlikely that most people would choose the latter—but that is what Rawls predicts. Indeed, survey research on how people claim they would behave under the original position indicates that they would prefer the first scenario, so long as they did not view the $1,000 as too low for subsistence. In general, when asked, people seem to choose to maximize average income subject to some minimum constraint or floor, rather than the maximin solution (Miller 1992).

In fairness to Rawls, however, there are two responses to the above argument. First, Rawls makes it clear that under the original position, one does not know the kind of society in which one would be placed. It may be dictatorial, with almost all wealth lavished on a few and the

---

6. For more views on this topic, see Daniels (1985).

rest of the populace living in poverty. Given that uncertainty, one might more easily come up with maximin—rather than risk being a member of the (subjugated) masses, why not choose a system of justice in which resources are equally distributed? In surveys that have been conducted, people likely imagined themselves placed within a democratic society like the one they were used to.

Second, although one could argue that Rawls's theory will result in unreasonable choices "on paper," such odd results might be unlikely under real-world circumstances. In the above example, the implication is that, somehow, the subjugation of 5 percent of the population will allow the other 95 percent to accrue far more wealth. In this regard, Rawls (1971) states, "it seems extraordinary that the justice of increasing the expectations of the better placed by a billion dollars, say, should turn on whether the prospects of the least favored increase or decrease by a penny" (p. 157). This is indeed unlikely; testing the validity of the theory using these kinds of numbers might in itself be unfair. Nevertheless, Rawls's theory might sacrifice too much efficiency to gain a small amount of equity.

More Groups Should Receive Favorable Treatment. Under Rawls's theory, the only group that receives a greater portion of primary goods is the one that is worst off. This is not necessarily desirable—why not help the nearly worst off at the same time you are helping the worst off; might not that be what people would choose in the original position (Sen 1982)? In addition, some people might not fully enjoy or use the primary goods that they are transferred and that others might need more to enjoy life. These issues, which are explored in the next section, are not dealt with through the application of Rawls's theory (Sen 1982).

This raises a related issue: how do we know who is worst off? In the theory, Rawls uses a "representative person" within each subgroup of society. The problem is that some of these representative people may be better off in some characteristics and worse off in others. If that is the case, who would be assigned the first primary goods to be redistributed? Furthermore, the way in which decisions are made in society clearly demonstrates that all aspects of a person's background are not considered in distributing scarce resources. To give one example in the literature, the fact that you do not get a scarce kidney for transplantation (and therefore must remain on dialysis) will not typically increase your chances of being admitted to a university over other qualified candidates (Young 1994). Societal decision making is typically done on a "local" rather than "global" basis (Elster

1992; Young 1994). In the above example, those who decide on college admissions do not also decide on kidney allocation, nor do they usually consider such factors.

Other Factors Should Form the Basis of Reallocation. This argument will be mentioned only briefly to avoid repeating what is in the next section, which examines other conceptions of welfare (besides utilitarianism). Just as utilitarianism is limited in its conception of ways in which resources should be distributed, so, it can be argued, is Rawls's theory.

In the theory, the only basis for redistribution is where a person stands in society with respect to his or her possession of primary goods. This viewpoint would appear to be rather limited for a number of reasons, two of which are listed here:

1. Under the theory, people are entitled to an equal share of resources irrespective of their work effort, motivation, and so on. This is because what a person is born with is, according to Rawls, really just the result of a "natural lottery," which "is arbitrary from a moral perspective." As a result, he believes that "[e]ven the willingness to make an effort, to try, and so to be deserving in the ordinary sense is itself dependent on happy family and social circumstances" (Rawls 1971, p. 74). Thus, if people exhibit a lack of motivation, it is not clear that they should be endowed with less of a share of primary goods because, in essence, it really is not their fault. Needless to say, relying on such criteria to carry out policy could result in a very large sacrifice of efficiency.
2. Equalizing resources does not necessarily solve people's problems because they still might not be born with the wherewithal to use these resources in a manner that will be of benefit to them. In fact, some people might need more resources than others (e.g., the disabled).

Nozick's Libertarian Critique of Rawls. As might be imagined, different philosophers (and economists) have reached different conclusions about what things people should have as a right. Robert Nozick (1974) has proposed an "entitlement theory," which is a libertarian philosophy in which the distribution of wealth is just if: (1) the original assignment of wealth was arrived at fairly, and (2) the current distribution was arrived at through voluntary exchange.

Nozick begins by developing a conception of a *just* role of government, concluding that this would be a "minimalist state" in which government's role is limited to such things as mutual protection and enforcement of contracts; "any state more extensive violates people's rights" (Nozick 1974, p. 149). He concludes that:

> The minimalist state treats us an inviolate individuals, who may not be used in certain ways by others as means of tools or instruments or resources; it treats us as persons having individual rights with the dignity this constitutes. Treating us with respect by respecting our rights, it allows us . . . to choose our life and to realize our ends and our conception of ourselves, insofar as we can, aided by the voluntary cooperation of other individuals possessing the same dignity. How *dare* any state or group of individuals do more. Or less. (pp. 334–35)

Nozick's entitlement theory contains two main aspects pertinent to justice. The first is the "principle of justice in acquisition of holdings," which pertains to how a person originally attained a resource, and the second is the "principle of justice in transfer of holdings," which concerns resources that they subsequently obtain from others. Essentially, what Nozick says is that if a person originally obtained a resource without violating anyone else's rights, or from another person voluntarily, then he or she is entitled to it.

Unlike Rawls, Nozick believes that people should be able to enjoy the full fruits of any natural advantage they possess. If, say, a person is born smart, and, as a result, becomes rich, that individual should keep all of his or her wealth if the person violated nobody else's rights. Rawls, however, would likely contend that being born smart is a lucky advantage that does not make the person deserving of additional primary resources. Nozick interprets Rawls's view as saying that "everyone has some entitlement or claim on the totality of natural assets . . . with no one having differential claims. The distribution of natural abilities is viewed as a 'collective asset'" (Nozick 1974, p. 228).

At one point in his book, Nozick uses health as an example. He presents and then refutes an argument made by Bernard Williams (1962), who claimed that societal resources should be redistributed to those in poor health who cannot afford necessary medical care. Nozick (1974) counters that Williams, ignores the question of where the things or actions to be allocated and distributed come from. Consequently, he does not consider whether they come already tied to people who have entitlements over them (surely the case for service activities, which are people's *actions*), people who therefore may decide for themselves to whom they will give the thing and on what grounds. (p. 235)

Many objections can be raised about Nozick's conception of justice. From a philosophical standpoint, the major objection is that people who start at a disadvantage are likely to remain at one. Recall that Nozick says that holdings that were acquired fairly must not be taken involuntarily from an individual. Who is to say what is a fair way of acquiring resources? And how can it be called fair if some people are born in such a disadvantaged position that they effectively have no way to overcome it? Even Nozick (1974) admits that he is "as well aware as anyone of how sketchy [his] discussion of the entitlement conception of justice in holdings has been" (p. 230). A less charitable view is that it is a philosophy espousing the rule of "finders keepers" (Elster 1992; Stone 1996).

Other Conceptions of Welfare

One reason that *A Theory of Justice* was such an important book is that it allowed others who may not have completely agreed with Rawls to formulate their own bases for thinking about alternative conceptions of social welfare. Rawls poked a number of holes in the utilitarian philosophy; since then, others have enlarged them. A few key ideas will be presented here. Those interested in pursuing the topic may wish to consult the references for additional reading.[7]

The Role of Equality. Readers often have difficulty understanding why philosophers might not believe that people should be granted full property rights over the resources that they have inherited and/or earned. Rawls (1971) states that "[n]o one deserves his greater natural capacity nor merits a more favorable starting place in society" (p. 102), and interestingly, most philosophers and even many economists agree. Arrow (1983), in writing about Rawls's books, notes that under the theory,

---

7. Some especially useful books about this topic have been written by Amartya Sen (1987, 1992).

Even natural advantages, superiorities of intelligence or strength, do not in themselves create any claims to greater rewards. . . . Personally, I share fully with this value judgment. . . . But a contradictory position—that an individual is entitled to what he creates—is widely and unreflectively held; when teaching elementary economics, I have had considerable difficulty in persuading the students that this *productivity principle* is not completely self-evident. (pp. 98–99)

The literature on moral philosophy is very clear that in creating a fair society, something must be equalized. Amartya Sen (1992) provides a reason:

It may be useful to ask *why* it is that so many altogether different substantive theories of the ethics of social arrangements have the common feature of demanding equality of *something*—something important. It is, I believe, arguable that to have any kind of plausibility, ethical reasoning on social matters must involve elementary equal consideration for all at *some* level that is seen as critical. The absence of such equality would make a theory arbitrarily discriminating and hard to defend. A theory must accept—indeed demand—inequality in terms of many variables, but in defending those inequalities it would be hard to duck the need to relate them, ultimately, to equal consideration for all in some adequately substantial way. (p. 17)

Sen notes that even Nozick's (1974) libertarian philosophy (described above) calls for the equalization of something—libertarian rights.

Unfortunately, deciding that something ought to be equalized does not solve most of our problems. Rather, it seems to raise more questions than it answers. The main problem, of course, is that such a decision does not tell us *what* should be equalized. Before confronting this, it is important to distinguish between two similar-sounding, but quite different, concepts: "equality" and "equity." The former implies equal shares of something; the latter, a "fair" or "just" distribution, which may or may not result in equal shares.

In economics, the difference between the two terms can be seen by examining the two common forms of equity: horizontal equity and vertical equity. Horizontal equity implies that similar people are treated the same with respect to some characteristic (the choice of which is a major issue in itself)—what we are referring to here as equality. But vertical equity is much different; it is, according to Gavin Mooney (1996a), "the unequal but equitable treatment of unequals" (p. 99). For example, we might, in the name of equity, establish a lower tax rate for the poor than for the rich.

The distinction among all of these terms is illustrated by Deborah Stone (1996), who discusses how to divide up and distribute "a delicious bittersweet chocolate cake" among students in her public policy class. One way, of course, is to give equal slices to all, but that seemingly fair method may lead to protests that "equality" does not result in an "equitable" distribution. Some possible objections to equal slices noted by Stone, each of which results in a different distribution of cake, include:

- Everyone in the university should get a slice, not just class members.
- Higher-ranked persons deserve bigger slices (or more frosting).
- Because males traditionally have had less access to homemade cake, each sex should get half the cake to divide among their members.
- Those who were given smaller main courses should get more cake.
- People who can't appreciate the cake should get less (or none).
- *Access* to the cake, not the cake itself, should be equalized by giving everyone a fork; competition for the cake would then ensue.
- The cake should be distributed by lottery.
- The allocation should be decided on by voting.

It is not hard to come up with close analogies to each of these arguments when allocating scarce medical goods and services.

As noted above, persuasiveness in issues involving resource allocation requires advocating the equalization of something. What is being equalized under utilitarianism? The answer is not as straightforward as it might seem because, as noted earlier, the concept embraces several different formulations. In general, though, utilitarianism is not about equalizing something so much as maximizing something else (Sen 1992). Under classical utilitarianism, the sum of all individuals' utility is being maximized. Under ordinal utilitarianism, society is best off when each individual succeeds in maximizing his own utility, although some income redistribution is likely to be necessary to maximize the social welfare function.

We are most concerned with ordinal utilitarianism because it forms the basis of modern economics. What is being equalized under ordinal utilitarianism? One possibility is that each individual's interests are being treated equally; my utility counts as much as yours.[8] Another possibility might be that people have equal rights to produce and trade to maximize their utility. This is not to say that they have equal ability or opportunity to do so. Rather, in a competitive market, no explicit restrictions prevent participation in the marketplace. It is not hard to see why moral philosophers, in considering the vagaries of social advantage in the real world, would view this concept as wanting.

What, then, should be equalized? As before, no attempt will be made to review this literature; those seeking additional information should consult some of the references listed in the footnotes.[9] One line of thought, advocated by Ronald Dworkin (1981), is that people's "resources" should be equalized—a philosophy that would appear to be not terribly different from Rawls's equalization of primary goods.[10]

Another line of thought, by John Roemer (1995), is that people's "opportunity" should be equalized. The idea is that people should be responsible for their own actions once a "level playing field" is established. To operationalize this, Roemer distinguishes between factors that are beyond a person's control and factors that are within a person's control. He gives the following example. Suppose we want to compensate people when they contract lung cancer (so that, perhaps, they can afford their medical care). We first come up with a list of factors over which people have little control; examples Roemer uses are age, ethnicity, gender, and occupation. We then look at smoking behavior within these subgroups. Suppose that the average 60-year-old, male, Black steel worker has smoked for 30 years, and the average 60-year-old, female, White college professor has smoked for eight years. Using these figures provides a way to gauge the behaviors of others who fall into these subgroups. If we then have a Black steel worker and a White professor contracting lung cancer, and they have smoked for 20 years and 15 years, respectively, the steel worker would receive more compensation—because his behavior was more responsible *given the circumstances over which he had little or no control.*

---

8. Gavin Mooney, personal communication, 1997.

9. Two goods sources that contain a thorough set of references are Sen (1992) and Hausman and McPherson (1993).

10. Dworkin (1981) devotes several pages to explaining the difference between his theory and Rawls's theory. One difference is that Dworkin claims that his theory is tailored to the individual, whereas Rawls focuses on one representative person in a social class. Individuals are apparently more responsible for their actions (how they spend their resources) under Dworkin than under Rawls.

A final candidate for equalization, advocated by Sen (1992), will be particularly relevant in Section 5.3.2, under health applications. This is the equalization of capabilities, which "reflect a person's freedom to choose between alternative lives" (Sen 1992, p. 83). The idea here is to give people the wherewithal to be able to achieve the things they want. Capabilities focus not on resources themselves, but on what resources can do for a person.

Equalizing capabilities is different than the other systems of equalization discussed earlier. It differs from Rawls's theory, and from equalizing resources, because under those systems people are given physical resources but not necessarily the ability to use them to achieve what they want. And it differs from equality of opportunity because giving people an opportunity does not necessarily mean that they will be able to use it effectively to their own advantage. Equality of capabilities might mean that more resources would be given to a disabled person because that person could need more to be capable of achieving his or her goals. Or it might mean actually giving unskilled laborers the skills to achieve more—rather than simply plying them with cash grants.

Alternative Concepts of Utility

Economists do not typically inquire into why people derive utility from particular goods. Modern theory is interested simply in which bundle of goods a person prefers; the preference need not be justified. An economic system that is best able to satisfy such preferences is desirable because the preferences themselves are beyond questioning. Sen (1992) has deemed this a "welfarist" viewpoint: the only thing that matters in evaluating an economic system is how well it satisfies these preferences.

Many objections to this viewpoint can be raised; a few were mentioned in Chapter 3:

- It essentially sanctions preferences that we might view as immoral; for example, equal favor is given to those preferences that may involve harming others as compared to those that we might find to be more lofty. In this regard, Mark Sagoff (1986) writes, "It cannot be argued that the satisfaction of preferences is a good thing in itself, for many preferences are sadistic, envious, racist, or unjust" (p. 302).
- It also sanctions preferences that might be, in some sense, faulty (e.g., behaviors that are self-destructive). One example is shortsightedness. Sagoff (1986) writes, "Literary and empirical studies amply

confirm what every mature adult discovers: happiness and well-being come from overcoming or outgrowing many of our desires more than from satisfying them" (p. 304).

• It focuses on goods rather than other values such as freedom. This leads to the seemingly faulty prediction that people will be equally happy with a particular bundle of goods that is assigned to them, versus the same bundle that they freely choose (Hahnel and Albert 1990).

This conception of utility also does a poor job in predicting other aspects of people's behavior. One concerns why people even bother to vote. Given the infinitesimally small chance that your vote would decide an election, why go to all the effort? Another example is income taxes. Why be honest when it is so easy to cheat and so hard to be caught (Aaron 1994)? As a final illustration, a summarization of Howard Margolis's (1982) discussion of people's contributions to charity is useful.

Suppose that a public radio station embarks on a fundraising campaign, and you decide to contribute $10 (but not $11); that is, you maximize your utility by spending $10 for this charity in the place of spending it on other goods and services you could purchase. But just as you are about to call in your pledge, the station announces that someone else has just given $10. Under the conventional model, this new information will make you will forgo your contribution—the station is already $10 richer; you can now keep the $10 and be that much better off than before. Not contributing allows you to have your (bittersweet chocolate) cake and eat it too.

If people really behaved this way, then there would be no way public radio (or for that matter, almost any charity) could exist. Once a single, large donor announced his or her intention to contribute, getting anyone else to contribute would be nearly impossible. Everyone else would "free ride" on this donation. The outcome would be economically inefficient because far less would be contributed to charity than is desired by the public.

Fortunately, something still drives people to contribute to charities. To explain paradoxes such as these a broader definition of utility is necessary. An example from Chapter 2 was Sen's use of people's recycling behavior as an example of commitment—a behavior that people engage in, even though it does not seem to be in their self-interest. Another formulation is from Margolis (1982), who explains people's behavior by positing that they have two distinct altruistic motivations. One, which he calls *goods altruism*, is the one we normally conceive; people receive utility when other, less-well-off people have more goods to consume. The other is *participation altruism*, a very different concept. Under it, people receive utility from the act of giving resources away (including their time) because it makes them feel good about themselves. This dual form of altruism, according to Margolis, can explain the paradoxes discussed earlier (why a person would vote, give to charity, not cheat on taxes).

More recently, Henry Aaron (1994) has provided a critique of utility theory, calling for "a new economics of human behavior." Although spelling out the details was beyond the scope of his work, he believes that,

> [E]ach person [has] more than one, possibly many, utility functions. In one or more of these sub-functions the arguments, as in standard theory, are particular goods and services. In others the arguments are intangible objectives such as adherence to duty, altruism, or spite, characteristics necessary for reputation or self-respect. Particular economic commodities may enter more than one function. In contrast to standard theory, however, the marginal utility of a given object may vary widely in different utility functions and may even have different signs. (pp. 15–16)

Cash Versus In-Kind Transfers

One of the most common applications of ordinal utility theory is the supposed superiority of cash over in-kind transfers. The argument is as follows. Suppose that society wishes to transfer wealth from wealthier to poorer individuals, and there are two choices: giving people money or giving them goods or services directly. The former would always be superior because, by letting people choose exactly how to spend their money, they are able to maximize their utility (i.e., reach their highest affordable indifference curve). In contrast, if goods or services are provided, maximizing utility would be almost impossible. We could never do better than through transferring cash, and could only do as well if the goods transferred were *exactly* what would have been purchased had the grant been in the form of cash.

The issue, to most economists, is one of consumer sovereignty. Should people be allowed to make their own choices, or alternatively, should society act paternalistically by telling people how they should spend the resources that are redistributed to them? As was made clear in Chapter 3 and earlier in this chapter, ordinal utilitarianism has a clear preference for cash transfers because it assumes that people will make choices that are in their best interest.

One obvious issue that arises is whether people will really spend money in a way that is best for them. For example, suppose that a person is ill; society feels sympathy and gives that person $5,000. If the person takes the money and spends it on frills, alcohol, or the like, can we really say that the person is better off than having the care that the money would have purchased? Although this is certainly an important question, it will not be dealt with here, since issues like it were discussed at some length in Chapter 3. Rather, in this section we will assume that however the person spends the money will indeed maximize his or her utility.

Three other reasons contribute to the belief that providing goods and services may indeed be superior to providing cash; each will be addressed briefly in the following subsections.

The Desires of Donors. The first, and probably the most important, reason to provide goods over cash is that the superiority of cash over in-kind subsidies is based on the following propositions being true:

• We do not care about the utility of the people who make the donations (or pay the taxes); or
• We do care about the donors, but they do not care about how the money is spent.

Because these two issues are related, we will deal with them together.

Why should we ignore the wishes of the donors? One possibility is that how the recipients spend the money is none of the donors' business. But this belief contradicts a tenet of economic theory—that preferences simply exist and do not have to be justified. If donors do indeed care about how the money is being spent, then this element must be taken into account in determining what is in society's best interest. And if total welfare is simply the sum of all individuals' welfare, it is incumbent on the analyst to consider everyone's preferences, including those of the donors.

What, then, do donors care about? In considering this problem, George Daly and Fred Giertz (1972) posit that two kinds of (positive consumptive) externalities are to be considered in providing transfer payments to those who are less well off. One, which they call a "goods externality," exists when the donor obtains utility from a recipient having specific goods such as housing, food, education, or health services. The other, labeled a "utility externality," is when the donor cares only about the recipient's utility, not the goods via which this utility is obtained.

The question that Daly and Giertz pose is this: "Do people, individually or collectively, extend aid to others in hopes of improving the real welfare of the recipients or in order to alter their consumption pattern?" (p. 135). To answer it, they observe people's preferences in private charity, where donations are purely voluntary, and they find that private charities "almost invariably redistribute it in the form of particular commodities" (p. 135). Furthermore, when one looks at the support for public redistribution programs (e.g., housing support), the justification is often explicitly to alter recipients' consumption patterns. In this regard, the authors add,

> [A] majority of voters might approve of public housing for slum areas but be strongly opposed to the transfer of money to people living in those slums. . . . For donors the crucial issue may be not the level of well-being achieved by the recipient but rather *how* he achieves it. (p. 136)

Although some people may claim that they are only interested in the utility of the recipient, such an attitude seems a bit farfetched, as suggested in the following quotation by David Collard (1978):

> The overwhelming weight of impressionistic evidence is that people are concerned less with other people's incomes or utilities than with their consumption of specific commodities. Any reader who believes himself to be entirely non-paternalistic in his concern is asked to perform the following mental experiment. I notice that my neighbour is badly fed and badly clothed so I give him some money which he then spends on beer and tobacco. Do I feel entirely happy about this or do I somehow feel that my intentions have been thwarted? (p. 122)

Ensuring Sufficient Donations. As was shown in Section 2.2.2, the presence of positive externalities of consumption necessitates a transfer of income to ensure an economically efficient, Pareto-optimal outcome. But now suppose that donors, fearing that recipients will squander their donations, decide not to give (or vote to reduce taxes). This reduces donations to a level that is less than economically efficient. By allowing for in-kind rather than cash subsidies (and very illiquid ones at that), more money is likely to be donated, resulting in a more efficient outcome (Daly and Giertz 1972).

Improving Productivity. Another topic raised in Chapter 2 is the fact that few, if any, "neutral" transfer payments exist. In general, taxes and subsidies result in a work disincentive that will result in a less-than-optimal amount of production. Readers are well aware of the fact that welfare payments may reduce the incentive to work because, as earned income rises, welfare payments decline.

A. C. Pigou (1932), in his classic book, *The Economics of Welfare,* raises an important reason why in-kind transfers might be superior to cash:

> [T]ransference of objects not capable of being sold or pawned, and designed to satisfy needs, which, apart from the transference, a recipient would have left unsatisfied, have a different effect. The last unit of money which a man earns for himself in industry will be required to satisfy the same needs, and will, therefore, be desired with the same intensity as it would have been if no transference had been made. Hence no contraction will occur in the contribution which, by work and waiting, he makes to the national dividend. (pp. 725–26)

This point has apparently been overlooked by most analysts: provision of a good or service that would not have been purchased otherwise by the recipient provides no work disincentive. (An example would be medical care services that a poor person could not otherwise have afforded.) Some important health applications arising from the issues raised in this section are dealt with next.

5.3 IMPLICATIONS FOR HEALTH POLICY

This chapter has focused on problems with the concept of ordinal utilitarianism, the key tool in the economics of social welfare. By relying on it, the field has been able to sidestep issues of great importance to societies, such as determining what is a fair and equitable allocation of resources. In addition, the concept was shown to be flawed because of its inability to predict such basic things as reasons why people contribute to charitable causes, and the nature of these contributions. Based on the above critique, this section provides three implications for redistributive policy in the health services area.

5.3.1 Providing Health Services Rather than Cash

The last part of Section 5.2.2 showed several reasons to believe that it is better to implement redistributive policies by providing services rather than cash. This is, of course, in sharp contrast to the predictions of the conventional economic model, which posits that cash contributions will always be superior.

Needless to say, most health policy makers have eschewed the conventional model. What they have tended to do, instead, is promote insurance coverage or reimbursement for services. No countries rely on giving low-income people money and leaving them the choice of purchasing or not purchasing health coverage.

Further evidence is provided by examining how redistribution policy is carried out in the one industrialized country that has not adopted national health insurance: the United States. In 1998, $290 billion in cash and noncash benefits were provided to persons with low income in the United States. Of this amount, only 24 percent was cash aid. The remaining 76 percent was for the direct provision of goods and services such as medical care, food, and housing. In fact, more than twice as much was spent on providing just one in-kind service—medical care—than was spent on cash subsidies (U.S. Census Bureau 2001, p. 343).

The provision of health insurance coverage is not exactly the same as providing services directly, however. Unlike the latter, where the recipient is given no choice, when a person has health insurance he or she can choose the types of services to be received—so long as they are among the menu of services covered by the insurance program. In that respect, insurance coverage bears some resemblance to cash. But these choices are limited to a specified set of health-related goods. As discussed earlier in the chapter, donors (private charity) and taxpayers (public programs) would be unlikely to tolerate having recipients spend these resources on non–health-related items.

Thus, we see that social policy, worldwide, is conducted in a manner that is not consistent with what is predicted by the conventional economic model. And, except in the United States, countries have gone the extra step of providing guaranteed health insurance coverage for the entire population, an issue considered in Section 5.3.3, national health insurance.

5.3.2 Focusing on People's Health, Not Utility

Under the conventional economic model, society strives to allow people to maximize their utility. This is because, under utilitarianism, social welfare is simply the aggregate of individual utilities. Because utility is purely subjective, not directly measurable, and not comparable across different people, public intervention is typically not advised. Rather, people should choose to spend their resources in whatever manner they think will maximize their welfare.

But as argued above, utilitarianism suffers from various shortcomings, one of which is that it is silent on a basic issue of social justice: people should not be penalized for things over which they have little or no control. It was argued that, for a theory to have any moral sway, something very important needs to be equalized. This "something" has to do with people's opportunities, or alternatively, their capabilities to achieve their life goals.

For decades, health economists have debated whether health is "different."[11] Much of this literature has focused on informational problems —certainly an important issue, but not terribly convincing because other sectors of the economy also have major (although perhaps not quite as severe) information problems. Other literature has focused on the fact that health is perhaps associated with stronger positive externalities. Arrow (1963b), for example, has stated, "The taste for improving the health of others appears to be stronger than for improving other aspects of their welfare" (p. 954). Although this provides a somewhat stronger case that health is special, one can still imagine other needs—food, education, housing—that are equally compelling.

What would appear to be truly different about health concerns opportunities and capabilities: good health provides people with the opportunity and/or capability to achieve other desired things. As A. J. Culyer (1993) has written, "One reason for such beliefs may be to do with the important role [things like health] have in enabling people to fulfill their potential as persons" (p. 300). He also states that, "If it is felt that all residents of a political jurisdiction ought to have equal opportunities for their lives to flourish, then it follows that *health care* is one of the goods and services whose right distribution must be ensured" (Culyer 2001, p. 276). Such a viewpoint is consistent with the reason given by Lester Thurow (1977): "[S]ociety's interest in the distribution of medical care springs, not from unspecified externalities that affect private-personal utility, but

---

11. See, for example, Pauly (1978) and Sloan and Feldman (1978), as well as the following comment by Reinhardt (1978).

from our individual-societal preferences that 'human rights' include an *equal* 'right' to health care" (p. 93).

The idea that society should consider other, nonutility aspects of welfare has been coined the "extra-welfarist" approach. (Under a welfarist approach, only individual levels of utility matter to society.) In health, these nonutility aspects have to do with access to health services, good health itself, or both.[12] Some researchers, such as Lu Ann Aday, Ronald Andersen, and Gretchen Fleming (1980), have advocated that access to health services is the key dimension of equity, whereby "[t]he greatest 'equity' of access is said to exist when need, rather than structural or individual factors, determine[s] who gains entry to the health care system" (p. 26). More recent work by Mooney et al. (1991) appears consistent with this viewpoint. They advocate "equal access for equal need," because this "provides individuals with the *opportunity* to use needed health services" (p. 479).

Other analysts, notably Culyer (1989), have advocated that health status rather than access to care be considered the key outcome,[13] and the determinants of health the key research issue.[14] If one considers health rather than utility as an outcome, the meaning of economic efficiency is very different from the one typically used in economics. Under this conception, Culyer (1993) states that efficiency is achieved "by prioritizing the more 'urgent' and so distributing health between A and B [such] that, at the margin, the cost of A's and B's additional health is equal to the social value attached to the health of each" (p. 312).[15]

---

12. For a good discussion of the pros and cons of equalizing health, utilization, or access, see Chapter 5 of Mooney (1994).

13. Some of Culyer's more recent writing has begun to move away from this position. In 1993, he writes: "I now think that it is more helpful in studies of distribution to focus on the need for health care than on the need for health. . . . [Adam] Wagstaff and I have also come to a stipulative definition of need as 'the minimum resources required to exhaust an individual's capacity to benefit from health care'" (p. 318).

14. For a thorough model of the determinants of health, see Evans and Stoddart (1990).

15. A perhaps similar view is advocated by Alan Williams (1997), called the "fair innings" argument. He writes that this "reflects the feeling that everyone is entitled to some 'normal' span of health. . . . The implication is that anyone failing to achieve this has in some sense been cheated, whilst anyone getting more than this is 'living on borrowed time'" (p. 119). One implication is that more medical resources should be devoted to the young, who have not yet had their fair innings, with correspondingly less spent on the elderly.

Under this sort of allocation rule, society is interested not so much in what people demand as in how much of an improvement in health can be purchased with a given amount of money—a very nonwelfarist viewpoint. Both this view and the one centered on access to care seem to dictate health policy worldwide much more so than the conventional economic model. The view that centers on access as the key outcome is consistent with the fact that most government-sponsored programs seek to equalize people's ability to obtain needed medical care. The view that focuses on health itself as the key outcome forms the basis of the growing reliance on cost-effectiveness analyses in health-related studies, and on the relatively new focus on clinical outcomes and effectiveness in the field of health services research.

In contrast, what is worrisome about some of the recent developments, not only in the United States but in other countries as well, is a renewed interest in rationing the use of services by higher out-of-pocket price. (Medical savings accounts, discussed in Section 3.3.4, are one obvious example.) Such policies may indeed turn out to be effective in quelling the use of services; according to conventional theory, these policies will lead to more efficient economic outcomes if people choose to forgo services that they do not find very useful. But if one views access to health services, or health itself, as the outcome society is trying to maximize (per dollar of expenditures), then the results could be very different. By inhibiting economic access, policies aimed at reducing demand may, at the same time, lead to reductions in access, health status, or both, to levels below those that society deems optimal. These issues are discussed in detail in Chapter 6.

5.3.3 National Health Insurance

Section 3.3.1 demonstrated that comprehensive national health insurance is not necessarily economically inefficient. Here, we consider some equity rather than efficiency issues. This section focuses only on equity and is quite brief because Chapter 6 contains a detailed discussion of various issues surrounding the national health insurance systems that have been developed and implemented by a number of developed countries.

If, as was just argued, societies believe that either equal access to health services or equal access to good health is necessary in the name of social justice, then a clear-cut justification for national health insurance exists. Research on views about equity in several developed countries, conducted by Wagstaff and van Doorslaer (1993), show that such programs are consistent with the prevailing ethical viewpoints in nearly all developed countries.[16]

The one country without a national health insurance program is the United States; *why* this is the case has been debated for decades and will only be briefly touched on here. One possible reason is that the United States may indeed hold a somewhat different ethic than other countries. A survey reported on by Robert Blendon and his colleagues (1995b) found that only 23 percent of Americans agreed with the statement, "It is the responsibility of the government to take care of the very poor people who can't take care of themselves." The numbers for other countries were considerably higher: 50 percent of Germans agreed with the statement, as did 56 percent of Poles, 62 percent of British and French, 66 percent of Italians, and 71 percent of Spaniards (Blendon et al. 1995b).

This corresponds with the findings of Wagstaff and van Doorslaer (1992) on the actual amount of equity in different countries. With regard to finance, the United States, which relies on private insurance, was the least equitable of ten countries studied; the results with regard to the equity of service delivery are less easy to generalize. Thus, an (albeit somewhat simplistic) argument can be made that, in eschewing universal health insurance coverage, the United States is accurately reflecting an ethic of its citizenry.

Suppose that most of the U.S. public does not favor universal coverage, given its cost. This raises a most interesting question: should policymakers respect these wishes, or alternatively, still attempt to achieve universal coverage? In a discussion of these issues between Mark Pauly and Uwe Reinhardt, Pauly (1996) suggests that voters could probably be convinced that the value of certain reforms aimed at reducing the rate of uninsurance is worth the costs. However, he asserts that, "If we cannot convince the decisive voters of the value of what we value, then I think we need to accept the verdict of democracy" (p. 14). Reinhardt (1996) takes a very different view. Citing a number of instances in which the policy elites prevailed over the citizenry to abolish unjust laws, he states,

> I, for one, believe that, if this nation is ever to have truly universal health insurance coverage and a truly humane safety net all around,

---

16. For a summary of research on this topic, see van Doorslaer, Wagstaff, and Rutten (1993).

an elite espousing those goals would have to impose that state of affairs on a generally confused plebs that has quite unstable, often logically inconsistent and utterly malleable preferences on this matter. (p. 24)[17]

National health insurance makes a great deal of sense when one considers the alternative conceptions of social welfare that were discussed previously. If, as Margolis (1982) and Aaron (1994) argue, people have more than one element in their utility functions—if, in addition to regular "goods-based" utility, they also derive satisfaction from helping others—then they derive utility from being part of a society that helps those who do not have access to health services or good health.

In this regard, Mooney (1996a) writes that,

> Individuals recognise that they are members of a society and that they get some form of utility or increased well-being from being in a society, being able to make a contribution to that society, and being an active participant in that society. The source of this form of utility seems much more to be non-individualistic or at least stemming from a recognition on the part of the individual that he or she is a member of a society and that such membership does convey certain benefits but also perhaps certain responsibilities. (p. 100)

This attitude has been denoted by the term "communitarianism," where, as applied to health, there is a "desire on part of the members of that society to create a just health care service as part of a wider just society" (Mooney 1996a, p. 101).[18] A key element in enacting the appropriate type of health system for a particular country is determining the extent to which the country's population holds such an ethic—a fruitful area for future research.[19]

---

17. Support for this viewpoint is provided from survey data (Blendon et al. 1994), which shows that Americans' support for national health reform is quite volatile, depending in large part on the specific messages they receive from special interest advertisements.

18. A related area of inquiry is how people's sense of community affects their attitudes. In a study conducted among 1,200 Florida residents, Ahern, Hendryx, and Siddharthan (1996) found that a person's positive or negative feelings about his or her community were the best predictor of that person's perceived experiences with the health system.

19. In 1996, Gavin Mooney presented an extensive discussion of these issues in "A Communitarian Critique of Health (Care) Economics" at the inaugural meetings of the International Health Economics Association in Vancouver, British Columbia (Mooney 1996b). Mooney is currently at Curtin University in Perth, Australia.

In recent years, researchers worldwide have investigated these issues, often under the area of "social capital" theory. Although many definitions of social capital exist (see Macinko and Starfield [2001] for a summary), most involve the empowerment of individuals through their membership in a group that shares like characteristics. Similarly, many different pathways have been hypothesized between social capital and health. One is social cohesion, the idea being that a more socially disparate society with large gulfs between the well and poorly off, or between the races, results in numerous adverse consequences, including individual ones like additional psychological stress, as well as group ones such as unresponsive government (Kawachi and Kennedy 1999). Another is social relationships, where some researchers have found that the quantity and quality of human interactions have a causal effect on health status (House, Landis, and Umberson 1999). The existence of a national health insurance program could be argued to improve social cohesion, although it would be more challenging to find a link to social relationships.

In summary, the case for a national health insurance program that guarantees universal coverage is very strong. Universal coverage is consistent with prevailing notions of fairness; people should not be penalized for circumstances—such as their sociodemographic background or their current state of health—over which they may have little control. (The case for providing coverage to all children is especially compelling, since they are *clearly* not responsible for the circumstances in which they find themselves.) In addition, unlike other characteristics, good health is instrumental in allowing people to have the capabilities to achieve their personal goals. Consequently, financial barriers to obtaining care are doubly unfair because they not only result in poorer health, but they also frustrate people's ability to attain the other things that they value. Furthermore, most people would appear to be endowed with a communitarian spirit in which they draw pride in being part of a society in which the well-being of others is an important part of their own welfare. That nearly every developed nation is committed to providing health insurance to its population, regardless of the individual's ability to pay, is not surprising.[20]

---

20. The Appendix contains brief descriptions of the health insurance systems in ten developed countries.

Chapter 6

The Role of Government

THE PREVIOUS CHAPTERS have focused on limitations of markets. The first five chapters concluded that economic theory has been misused to support the viewpoint that markets should be relied on more in the health services sector. The alternative to relying on markets is varying degrees of government involvement in the financing and delivery of these products and services. Although nearly all health economists agree that government must play a role in the market, the nature and magnitude of such involvement is controversial.

As indicated in the previous chapters, markets are problematic not only with respect to providing services equitably, but also providing them efficiently. This begs the key policy question: would government do any better? Economist Henry Sidgwick (1887) once stated that, "It does not follow that whenever laissez-faire falls short government interference is expedient; since the inevitable drawbacks of the latter may, in any particular case, be worse than the shortcomings of private enterprise" (p. 414).[1] More than 100 years later, Mark Pauly (1997) seems to express a similar view when noting that "a government staffed by angels could undoubtedly do a better job than markets run by humans" (p. 470); he is less sure when humans run the government. Charles Wolf (1993) adds:

> The actual choice is among imperfect markets, imperfect governments, and various combinations of the two. The cardinal economic choice concerns the degree to which markets or governments—each

---

1. This quote was obtained from Wolf (1993), p. 17.

with their respective flaws—should determine the allocation, use, and distribution of resources in the economy. (p. 7)

Indeed, all countries use both markets and government, in varying degrees, to determine the allocation of goods and services in the health services area. The choice is not "either/or"; markets and government can and do complement each other. Markets help improve on government by helping ensure that consumer demands are met and resources are not squandered. Governments help improve on markets in ensuring that poor and sick individuals have access to care and that providers and insurers do not reap unreasonable profits from selecting healthier patients (Morone 2000; Rice et al. 2000). All countries must decide on how much government involvement to employ and just where it should intervene in markets.

Because this chapter—unlike the previous ones—does not focus on providing a critique of conventional economic theory as applied to health, it is organized differently. Section 6.1 presents alternative views on the role of government, discussing both reasons that government should intervene in markets, as well as problems that government intervention may have in allocating (and even distributing) resources in a socially desirable manner. Section 6.2 applies this to health services issues, addressing various ways different countries have used government in the health services sector. Section 6.3 provides cross-national data on access, utilization, expenditures, quality/satisfaction, and equity to help assess the success of different policy approaches. Section 6.4 then furnishes ten "lessons" on the role of government in health systems.

6.1 ALTERNATIVE VIEWS ON THE ROLE OF GOVERNMENT

This section explores different viewpoints on the appropriate role of government, focusing on the issue generically and leaving the most of the specific application to health to the remainder of the chapter. Section 6.1.1 presents reasons that markets might fail, and Section 6.1.2, why government might fail.

6.1.1 Market Failure

Traditional economic theory provides two main sets of reasons for government involvement in a market: to overcome market failures that result in inefficient outcomes, and to change the distribution of resources among the population.[2] Because Chapter 5 focused on issues of equity and distribution, for now we focus largely on efficiency. Equity will be considered again in Sections 6.2 through 6.4.

Traditional economic theory provides a number of ways to classify the various types of market failure that can occur in an economy. One way of classification follows:

- Structural deficiencies exist in the market; in particular, either consumer information is poor or there is an insufficient number of competing firms or barriers to entry.
- The product in question is a "public good."
- There are externalities associated with the product.
- The product is characterized by increasing returns to scale.

If any of these occurs, government intervention could possibly— although not necessarily—result in greater efficiency than relying on markets alone. In this instance efficiency is usually defined in terms of technical efficiency—producing a greater output for a given expenditure of resources.

Almost all of these situations have been discussed earlier in the book.[3] The only one not previously mentioned explicitly is public goods. A public good is one in which the consumption by one person does not diminish its consumption by another; a second characteristic is that it is nearly impossible to exclude someone from using the good. Radio waves and national defense are two commonly cited nonhealth examples. In the area of health, clean air is a good example; some would also include investments in medical knowledge such as provided through the U.S. National Institutes of Health. Although more controversial (although perhaps not as much in European countries with a history of universal coverage), another possibility might be the social solidarity that is gained by knowing that the entire population of a country has access to good care.

---

2. Another reason that is sometimes mentioned for government involvement is *economic stabilization*. In the United States, for example, the Federal Reserve System is responsible (in part) for maintaining the stability of the U.S. financial system. To do so it engages in a number of activities including regulation of monetary supply and key interest rates.

3. Consumer information was discussed in Chapter 3; lack of competition (monopoly) and increasing returns to scale in Chapter 4; and externalities in Chapter 2.

Public goods are underproduced, or not produced at all, by markets. If a good can be enjoyed by all and excluding someone from consuming it is difficult, a firm cannot easily recover its costs. Government provision, financed through tax revenues, is the only alternative. Nevertheless, just because something is a public good is not enough reason for government to embark on its production. The overall gain to society in its production first needs to be determined to exceed the associated costs.

The above discussion focuses on the traditional economic formulation of market failure. This book has contended that a number of other assumptions exist (i.e., many of those listed in Table 1.1) that, if not met, could also cause markets to fail. To give a single example, Chapter 2 noted that one such assumption is that consumer tastes are predetermined and not influenced by the consumer's experience in the marketplace. If, as was argued, this assumption is not met, this would provide additional reasons for the possibility of market failure.

Even if one ignores these additional assumptions, an argument can be made that a market environment creates more reasons for government intervention (either through regulation or direct provision) than those typically considered by economic theory. For example, poor consumer information is one reason that markets can fail. Proponents of markets often believe this is not a justification for government intervention beyond ensuring the quality and quantity of information and its wide dissemination. Advocates of more aggressive government intervention, however, often believe that this will be ineffective, either because the information cannot be made understandable to most people or because they may not use the information in the way considered desirable by experts or policymakers.

To illustrate, one issue facing countries is to decide whether all hospitals should be allowed to provide the services they wish, or alternatively, if government should act more paternalistically and *regionalize* care, which means that specific hospitals are assigned to provide particular (often, but not always, "high-tech") services. In this case, those leaning toward markets might choose the former option, with government ensuring the provision of information on health outcomes at alternative facilities. Those favoring government are more likely to believe that consumers do not understand and/or use such information, and therefore the provision of services should be provided only by certain (government-selected) institutions that have demonstrated their ability to provide high-quality care. Needless to say, government should not make such decisions lightly. It needs to convince itself that consumers would not use or misuse availability information, and in addition, it must weigh not only the quality of care provided by alternative hospitals, but also such things as patient proximity to local facilities from which they might want to seek care.

6.1.2 Government Failure

Just as markets may fail, so might government. Although the field of economics has devoted considerable effort to studying the topic of market failure, much less effort has been expended on developing a comparable theory of government failure. This is not terribly surprising. For such analyses to be tractable, simplifying assumptions are necessary. Economists have been successful in analyzing consumers by assuming that they focus on maximizing utility, and in studying firms by assuming that they seek to maximize profits. Providing a convincing theory of government behavior is much more difficult, and can hardly be captured by employing a few simplifying assumptions.

Some of the pioneering work in the area of government failure was conducted by Charles Wolf (1979, 1993). Wolf contends that just as a market may fail in the ways mentioned above, government intervention in a market may fail for similar (although not precisely the same) reasons. Government, according to Wolf, faces a number of challenges, including: the difficulty of defining and measuring outputs (e.g., the quality of education); by nature, government is monopolistic and doesn't have to adhere to a "bottom line" of profits or losses; and government is overseen by politicians who tend to prefer quick fixes rather than long-term solutions. As a result, one often sees government operate inefficiently and, in addition, inequitably, since it is often beholden to special interests who contribute in one way or another to the politicians and political parties.[4]

Some of these criticisms could also be applied to markets. In particular, when markets are used to carry out activities that traditionally are part of government's role (e.g., primary education), they have an equally difficult time defining outcomes. And just as government workers are not subject to profit-and-loss statements, evidence indicates that employees

---

4. Wolf's analysis has been critiqued by Julian Le Grand (1992). He posits that government failure is better considered separately with regard to different types of government intervention in a market (e.g., provision, taxation/subsidy, regulation), and goes on to consider such failure in each of these contexts.

and managers in private industry often serve their own goals rather than those of the shareholders.

Other economists have contributed a great deal to one aspect of understanding the potential for government failure, an area called the "economic theory of regulation." George Stigler (1971) is usually credited as pioneering this field, although there were various antecedents to it, both within and outside of the economics literature.[5] Previously (and still today), many researchers and laypersons alike took what Stigler calls a more idealistic view of regulation: that it is designed to serve the public interest. Regulation, it was believed, served the public interest by improving efficiency (e.g., correcting externalities, controlling the behavior of monopolists) as well as equity (e.g., redistributing income from the wealthy to the poor) (Feldstein 1996)—or by protecting health or enhancing safety.

Stigler found this "public interest theory" unsatisfactory and proposed instead what is sometimes called "capture theory"—which is quite the opposite of the public interest theory. Rather than serving the public, regulation serves those that it is designed to regulate. Viewed this way, regulation is, by its nature, anticompetitive and anticonsumer.

How can regulated industries capture the regulators whose role, purportedly, is to keep them in check? To answer this, Stigler brought in the political process to his analysis. Just as firms attempt to maximize profits and individuals, utility, so politicians also attempt to maximize their self-interest. Politicians, he believed, are interested in being re-elected so they can retain their power, and for that to occur they need votes and money. Special interest groups can provide this but will do so only if the politician can offer them something in return. That "something" is regulations that, through various means, make members of the group better off. Examples include regulations that keep out competitors or make entry into a market difficult, price supports or subsidies, or actions that harm competitors that sell substitute goods.

Interestingly, small interest groups, not large ones, are most effective in this regard. So long as members of these groups share a common interest, they can concentrate their resources (say, to influence legislation) and

---

5. In the economics literature, see Mancur Olson's book, *The Logic of Collective Action* (1965). To cite one noneconomic example, in the 1960s, historian Gabriel Kolko observed that, "The dominant fact of American political life at the beginning of this century was that big business led the struggle for the federal regulation of the economy." This quote is from High (1991), p. 1.

avoid the "free-rider" problem, which occurs when those who benefit do not contribute to the effort because of their belief that others will instead. But why would consumers allow this to happen? Stigler hypothesized that their interests were too disparate; consumers could not possibly be expert enough to keep up with all industries, and even if they could, they would not bother because cost-increasing regulations for a single product would have little overall effect on their disposable incomes.

The theory can be extended to regulatory agencies as well as elected officials. Legislators do not have time to directly oversee all aspects of government, nor do they and their staffs have the necessary expertise. These tasks are delegated to administrative agencies. The employees of these agencies, it is argued, are motivated "by job security and higher salaries [which] . . . are more likely to occur when an agency's budget is expanding" (Feldstein 1996, p. 30). This, in turn, will happen only if the agency's behavior is in accordance with the desires of the legislature.

Over the years various economists have further honed the economic theory of regulation. The major contribution was made by Sam Peltzman (1976), who formalized the theory and worked out some of the kinks. Just as the public interest theory ignored the interests of special interest groups, Stigler's theory seemed to put all of the power in the hands of special interests. Under his formulation, this was a single special interest group, essentially the one that was the highest bidder for the favors of the regulator.

Peltzman theorized that regulators would not necessarily serve a single special interest group. Rather, they would consider all competing interests, although not equally.[6] By trying to serve a variety of interests, a self-interested politician or regulator would gain more—in a sense, by trying to make everyone happy. But this does not mean that consumers would have as much clout as producers. As noted, those groups that are best able to concentrate their resources toward a particular goal will tend to be most influential in the regulatory process.

---

6. Regulators, like consumers and firms, are assumed to reach an equilibrium in which the ratio of marginal benefits to marginal costs is equalized—here, across competing interest groups. Marginal benefits can be viewed as the extra political support or contributions received by helping a particular interest group, and marginal costs, the loss of support or contributions. If certain groups, such as producers, can do a better job at marshaling their resources than consumer groups, under the theory politicians and regulators would focus more of their attention on aiding such groups.

An extensive literature related to the economic theory of regulation, but more wide ranging in scope, is a school of thought called "public choice" or "rational choice"—not to be confused with the "public interest" literature discussed above that assumed that regulation benefits society by improving efficiency and the distribution of resources. Public choice theory studies (among other things) how public organizations make decisions (Stanbury 1986). This theory has been characterized "as the economic study of nonmarket decision making, or simply the application of economics to political science" using the assumption "that man is an egoistic, rational, utility maximizer" (Mueller 1989, pp. 1–2). Its proponents have examined such issues as why people vote, the implications of rulemaking by majorities and alternatives to it, the formation of coalitions and political parties, and theories of government and bureaucratic behavior.[7]

The basis of public choice theory is that individuals act in their own interest. Politicians seek to become and stay elected to retain power, prestige, and sometimes wealth. Government workers seek job security, pleasant working conditions, and higher pay; one way to achieve the latter is to increase the size of their agency or the number of people whom they supervise. Interest groups form to obtain favors from government. In return, they provide campaign contributions, attempt to sway the public in favor of certain positions or candidates, and perhaps provide useful information about the preferences of voters.

A number of criticisms have been leveled at public choice theory as well. On the theoretical side, it is unclear that public officials act in a solely self-interested manner. The theory, for example, predicts that political parties and individual candidates will focus almost entirely on enticing voters by espousing centerist positions, but oftentimes this is not the case. Similarly, the theory leaves little room for ideology in politics; rather, politicians are assumed to choose their positions to get elected rather than seeking election so as to implement their vision,[8] and civil servants also are driven by factors devoid of ideology. This is not to say that the theory

---

7. For a detailed review of the public choice literature, see Mueller (1989), and for a critique, Green and Shapiro (1994).

8. Some public choice theorists have tried to incorporate ideology into models of competition among political candidates, but one problem in doing so is that it makes it hard to distinguish the theory from more traditional ones used in political science (Green and Shapiro 1994).

is always wrong—it surely describes many actors in the political scene—but it may be viewed as unusually cynical. In addition, public choice theory has been criticized as not being consistent with empirical evidence of actual behavior in a number of areas (Green and Shapiro 1994). One area that has been most criticized is understanding citizen involvement in public affairs. Public choice theory does a poor job explaining why people vote in elections (when their chance of influencing an election is almost nil) or vote to raise their own taxes (Mueller 1989).

One final point in appreciation of the economic theory of government, government failure, and public choice theory should be noted, however. These theories have helped make society far more aware of the *potential* for self-serving behavior on the part of participants in governments. This is enormously helpful in that it alerts the public to areas in which government failure is most likely to be manifested, and consequently, assists the public in averting its manifestations. As noted by Dennis Mueller (1989):

> [F]rom a knowledge of past mistakes we can design institutions that will avoid similar mistakes in the future. Public choice does provide us with this knowledge. Because of this, I remain optimistic . . . even about the possibility that this research may someday help to improve the democratic institutions by which we govern ourselves. (p. 465)

6.2 DIFFERENT APPROACHES TO THE ROLE OF GOVERNMENT IN THE HEALTH SERVICES SECTOR

Every country formulates its own way of involving government in the financing and delivery of health services. These methods, of course, are not fixed in stone. Most nations continually tinker with their systems, and occasionally they enact major changes—for example, the movement toward more competition through "internal markets" in the United Kingdom (described in more detail in the Appendix), which began during the Thatcher administration but has been quelled somewhat since the Labour Party came into power in 1997.

Different observers have different views on the proper role of government in the health services sector. Nevertheless, some agreement holds on where government should have a very strong role, and where it should have little. One area that nearly everyone would agree is government's responsibility is monitoring the health services sector and making policy. Most would also agree that the production of medical supplies such as latex gloves should be left to markets. For example, Robert Evans (1983), a critic of market-based systems, has written that:

> Where commodities are concerned—pharmaceuticals, optometric goods, and health appliances—there is both analysis and empirical experience to suggest that an open, competitive market combined with product inspection and certification (but not licensure of providers) might significantly enhance efficiency and lower costs. (p. 37)

In such cases, the potential for a great deal of competition among producers exists, and information is not much of a problem because it is reasonably straightforward to measure outputs (Preker, Harding, and Travis 2000).

Most societal choices in the health services area, however, fall between these two extreme cases. Consequently, the optimal degree of government involvement is not obvious. This section explores the different ways in which government is involved in the health services sector, illustrating some of the different choices made with examples from selected developed countries.

Every country is presented with thousands of choices related to whether and how government should be involved in the organization, financing, delivery, and monitoring of health-related goods and services. Table 6.1 lists some of the major roles the government can play involving five overall areas: the structure of the system; the nature of coverage and delivery; regulation of prices and expenditures; regulation of volume; and control of input supply. The remainder of the section elaborates on the roles.

A basic understanding of the health systems in various developed countries is useful to fully understand the remaining sections of this chapter. The Appendix[9] contains a short description of the organization, financing, and delivery of services in ten selected countries: Australia, Canada, France, Germany, the Netherlands, Japan, Sweden, Switzerland, the United Kingdom, and the United States. These countries were chosen because they are among the largest in the developed world and/or have health systems that are often discussed in policy circles.

---

9. The Appendix was coauthored by Miriam J. Laugesen and Thomas Rice.

Table 6.1: Alternative Roles for Government in the Health Sector

Structure of the System
 Universality of coverage
 Publicly vs. privately administered coverage
 Coordination of payers
 Locus of administrative authority

Nature of Coverage and Delivery
 Role of private insurance
 Benefits in publicly mandated systems
 Cost-sharing requirements
 How providers are paid
 Choice of providers

Regulation of Prices and Expenditures
 Hospital prices and expenditures
 Physician prices and expenditures

Regulation of Volume

Control of Input Supply
 Hospital
 Physician
 Capital and medical technology

The following discussion is, by necessity, fairly general. Fifteen different societal decisions are discussed, so it is not possible to go into detail about how each of several countries has dealt with each of these decisions. Rather, the text discusses the issue in general, provides examples of selected countries that have used different approaches, and provides an overview of the advantages and disadvantages of alternative policy choices.

6.2.1 Structure of the System
Universality of Coverage
Nearly all developed countries except the United States provide guaranteed health coverage to almost all of their citizens. In most cases, such coverage is the cornerstone on which the system is based. Germany, for

example, has a history of solidarity through a social code, *Sozialgeset-zbuch*, which "holds that medical care should be provided solely according to an individual's needs, whereas the financing of care should be based solely on the individual's ability to pay" (Pfaff and Wassener 2000, p. 907). The federal government in Canada will contribute to provincial health plans only if care is provided to all citizens with minimal financial impediments. The United Kingdom's National Health Service was established more than 50 years ago to provide comprehensive universal coverage with no financial access barriers (Roemer 1991; Smee 2000). In fact, this sort of ethic is common among almost all European countries (Wagstaff et al. 1992).

Coverage is not completely universal in several of these countries; people do fall through the cracks. In some instances individuals have to sign up for coverage but do not. In others, some are allowed to opt out of public coverage and may fail to procure private insurance. Germany provides a notable example; the 10 percent or so of the population with the highest incomes are not required to enroll in sickness funds. Most instead choose private insurance, which tends to pay providers more and, as a result, may make these patients more financially attractive to providers. The Netherlands also allows some of the population to opt out of joining sickness funds.

The United States provides universal coverage only to a subgroup of the population—those age 65 and over and individuals with disabilities—through the Medicare program. Although many low-income individuals also receive coverage through the Medicaid program, such coverage is hardly universal for this group. States have much discretion in setting income thresholds, and furthermore, individuals often must be "categorically eligible"—for example, be a dependent child or the mother of dependent children. As a result, in 1997 just 39 percent of Americans below the poverty level had Medicaid, and 34 percent were uninsured (U.S. DHHS 2000, pp. 339–41).

The many advantages of universal coverage include potential to (Rice 1998):

- Improve the health and productivity of the population by making health services financially accessible to all
- Obviate the need to provide for a large array of safety-net facilities for uninsured sick people who cannot afford care

- Generate cheaper administrative costs because processes such as verifying eligibility for the program will not be necessary
- Provide government with more clout in keeping provider payments in check
- Reduce problems of adverse selection into health insurance plans[10]
- Enhance fairness in society

A possible argument against universal coverage is that it forces those who do not want coverage to pay for it, either through higher taxes or lower take-home wages. This situation was discussed in some detail in Chapter 3. As argued by Mark Pauly (1968), universal coverage, coupled with first-dollar coverage, could result in a reduction in social welfare if the benefits resulting from the extra utilization are exceeded by their costs. A counter-argument, however, is that providing coverage for preventive care could actually lower future expenditures for care—although little evidence is available to demonstrate whether this is the case.

Publicly vs. Privately Administered Coverage

Generally speaking, countries with near-universal coverage administer their health systems in two ways (Saltman and Figueras 1998). One system is sometimes referred to as "Beveridge style," after British academician William Beveridge, who is often credited with masterminding the post-war welfare state in the United Kingdom that included the National Health Service. Under such systems, which are also characteristic of Scandinavian countries such as Sweden, government is the provider of most services. Canada's system, although different in that it relies more on private providers, is similar to the extent that nearly all payments to providers are from government—a system known as "single payer." These systems tend to obtain the bulk of their funding through tax revenues.

The other type is sometimes referred to as "Bismarck style," after nineteenth-century German Chancellor Otto von Bismarck, who (in part, as a way of staving off political support for socialism) enacted the modern world's first system of social welfare, including health and old-age insurance. Under this kind of system, government does not provide

---

10. Universal coverage does not eliminate adverse selection because different people may be covered by different plans. It does ensure, however, that sicker individuals are not excluded from obtaining coverage.

most health services directly. Rather, it oversees healthcare's provision by private nonprofit organizations such as sickness funds, which are often although not exclusively operated by occupational consortia. Examples of countries that use such a system include France, Germany, and the Netherlands. Rather than being financed largely through taxes, these systems rely more on contributions by employers and employees (van Doorslaer et al. 1999).

One of the main advantages of publicly administered coverage concerns its method of financing. Tax systems usually do more to enhance equity than those that rely on employer and employee contributions—although both are generally considered more equitable than systems that rely on private insurance, as do the United States and Switzerland. Tax systems also may be less disruptive to the economy. For example, mandatory payroll taxes may make it difficult for small employers to compete. In contrast, others tout privately administered systems as more removed from the political process, perhaps enhancing the systems' stability (White 1995).

Coordination of Payers

In countries that rely on sickness funds or private insurers to administer health coverage, an issue arises concerning the extent to which these entities coordinate provider payment. The United States has no statutory requirement for coordination, nor any formal system of coordinating payment. Each insurer establishes its own provider payment mechanism. Even when two insurers use similar systems (e.g., fee-for-service with withholds), the actual amount they pay usually differs.

In contrast, under an "all-payer" system, all insurers pay providers the same amount. Japan has what some consider to be the purest type of all-payer system in which fees paid are the same regardless of the provider from whom treatment is sought or place of treatment (Ikegami 1991; Ikegami and Campbell 1999). In some cases (e.g., hospital payment in France and the Netherlands), government regulators establish these fees. In Germany, government is less involved; a consortium of sickness funds negotiate joint rates with hospitals (Glaser 1991). In such countries, all-payer rates are the norm for physician payment as well.

Although all-payer rates are typical in many of these countries, some exceptions exist. Perhaps the most notable exception is Germany: wealthier Germans can purchase private insurance rather than going through sickness funds. In addition, rather than joining the sickness fund associated with their occupational category or region, Germans can instead enroll in a "substitute fund," which is advantageous in that they sometimes provide more benefits and tend to pay providers more. Although these substitute funds used to be an option only for Germans above a certain income threshold, currently anyone can join.

All-payer rate setting has two main potential advantages. First, providers have much less of an economic incentive to favor one type of patient over another. This contrasts with the situation in the United States, where, for example, some physicians avoid treating Medicaid patients because historically program payment rates have been so much lower than those paid by Medicare and by private insurers. The second advantage is the inability of providers to "cost shift," that is, increase charges to one payer to compensate for lower payments from another. Among other things, cost shifting makes it difficult to control overall costs because providers can charge the patients of one payer more if another payer provides less.

The main potential disadvantage of all-payer rates is that all providers tend to receive the same payment, irrespective of their skills or the quality of care they deliver. Thus, to provide financial incentives to enhance quality, a country needs to find other ways to reward providers. (Of course, with an abundance of physicians, better ones presumably will be rewarded with more business.) Some would also argue that individuals should be allowed to make themselves desirable to the best providers. This can occur in countries that allow individuals to enroll in substitute funds or opt out of the public system entirely—but is not possible under a pure all-payer system.

Locus of Administrative Authority

All countries administer their health systems at both a national level as well as subnational levels. Some countries, however, rely on one type more than the other. Most European countries administer at the regional level (Jonsson 1989); the main exception is the United Kingdom, but in recent years it has also moved more toward regional involvement by having some budgeting carried out by district health authorities (Le Grand 1999). Most significant health-related decision making in Sweden and Switzerland is done at the regional level, in part because regional government is vested with strong powers (Jonsson 1989; Zweifel 2000). In Canada, provinces have the vast majority of power over the operations of their systems as well.

In the United States, the Medicare program is administered at the federal level. Day-to-day administrative tasks, however, are carried out by regional (often, statewide) intermediaries and carriers—usually insurers. In contrast, whereas the Medicaid program receives considerable federal funding, states run these programs—although they often must obtain federal "waivers" if they want to innovate.

Focusing government effort more at the national rather than the regional level affords two main advantages. First, national government tends to have more resources available to help ensure that a sufficient level of expertise is available to conduct its activities. To illustrate, in the United States, personnel in the Agency for Healthcare Research and Quality collectively would tend to have more expertise in ways of measuring quality of care than would personnel in the Medicaid agency of a single state. Second, administration and enforcement at the national level tends to lead to more uniformity and has the potential for ensuring equity across different regions.

Nevertheless, there are advantages for most government activity to be carried out at a subnational or regional level. The main one, of course, is that personnel at the regional level are more likely to understand the particular problems of their own populations and providers. Unlike central government, which often has a "one-size-fits-all" mentality, regional government may be able to craft solutions that better meet local needs.

6.2.2 Nature of Coverage and Delivery
Role of Private Insurance
Generalization of the role of private insurance across countries is difficult; each country has its own unique system. Among countries with universal coverage, two basic differences predominate. The first concerns the role of private insurers over and above what is provided under government-mandated coverage. The second is whether insurers can compete against each other.

Canada is unusual in that it effectively prohibits private health insurers to sell coverage for services already included in a particular provincial health plan. In Canada, private insurance does exist for services not covered under provincial health plans (as is the case with other countries),[11]

---

11. Nearly all countries allow for the sale of "supplemental insurance." Such coverage is sometimes provided through employment (Canada, France) and other times purchased

but little private insurance exists for provincially covered hospital and physician services. Although coverage for hospital and physician services is allowed in some Canadian provinces, hospitals and physicians seeing private patients cannot receive any payments from public sources—effectively eliminating a market for private insurance covering hospital and physician care.

Most other countries allow private insurance to compete against government-mandated coverage. About 10 percent of higher-income Germans have private health insurance. One of the attractions of private coverage is that it tends to pay providers more. In countries with long waits for elective procedures, this can be a very attractive feature. That, in fact, is undoubtedly the major attraction of private insurance in the United Kingdom; such insurance is possessed by 11 percent of the population. Other advantages include choice of specialist and more comfortable accommodations for hospital care (Smee 2000).

Letting people opt out or supplement public coverage provides two possible advantages. First, it allows them to use their own resources to purchase the coverage and services that they wish to have. People are allowed to purchase fancy homes and cars, advocates argue, why should they be precluded from purchasing the best health coverage available? A counter-argument, however, is that if those opting out are not required to purchase private coverage, they could re-enter the public system when they become ill, raising overall costs. Second, letting people opt out offers a way of reducing government expenditures. A person who has private coverage does not need to use as many public resources. In fact, this argument has been compelling to some governments. Australia, for example, has been aggressive in providing subsidies that encourage individuals to purchase such coverage (Hall 1999). In 2000, 45 percent of the Australian population had private insurance (Willcox 2001). Whether public expenditures are indeed reduced depends, however, on the extent to which private coverage is supplemented by the public sector. Australians, for example, receive a 30 percent premium rebate from the government when they purchase private insurance. In Ireland, an estimated

---

individually (Australia). It tends to cover services that are excluded from the public plan (e.g., dentistry, private hospital rooms) or that are part of patient cost-sharing requirements. There are differences across countries, however. Because of the ubiquity of this coverage across developed countries, it is not listed here as an explicit societal choice.

50 percent of the costs of private care in public hospitals is subsidized by government.[12]

Allowing a large role for private insurance produces two major disadvantages, however. First, as the percentage of the population with private coverage grows, those with public coverage may no longer have access to adequate care. When well-funded private plans compete with strapped public ones, members of the former tend to get the better providers and facilities and shorter waits. (The U.S. Medicaid program offers a good example of this.) As a result, the quality of coverage can become related to income—quite contrary to the notion of solidarity in which care is dispensed according to need rather than ability to pay. Second, with multiple payers, selection bias becomes an issue; the particular worry is that sicker and poorer people will stay in the public system, while healthier and wealthier ones gravitate toward the private sector.

The second issue involves whether insurers can compete against each other. This is the main characteristic of a system of *managed competition*. Under managed competition—a system that has never been fully implemented in any country—insurers would compete with each other on the basis of price, benefit offerings, service, and quality. As envisioned by Alain Enthoven (1978, 1980), who is credited with developing the concept, insurers would offer the best product possible to attract enrollees. To keep premiums manageable, they would also pressure providers to keep their fees down.

Although not fully implemented anywhere, its major characteristic—competing insurance plans—is being tested in more and more countries. (Volumes have been written both in favor of and against the concept, so a comprehensive treatment will not be attempted here.) In the United States, competing (but unmanaged) insurers is the norm. In the employment-based sector—the major portion of the population with health insurance—65 percent have a choice of two or more health plans (Kaiser Family Foundation and Health Research and Educational Trust 2000).

Choice of insurers is a fairly new concept in Europe, however. Some countries—for example, Switzerland and Germany—have begun to experiment with this (Zweifel 2000; Pfaff and Wassener 2000), with

---

12. Miriam Wiley, personal communication, February 2002.

generally mixed or, as yet, indeterminate results. Most notable, perhaps, is the Netherlands. In the early 1990s, sickness funds were permitted to compete against each other (partly on the basis of premiums) to try to attract subscribers. Previously, individuals were required to join the fund in their particular region. Another important change was that rather than being paid retrospectively, sickness funds received a prospective, risk-adjusted capitation payment per enrollee, which might have provided them with a strong incentive to control costs. One of the major problems thus far has been coming up with an effective risk-adjustment payment formula so that plans compete on the basis of efficiency rather than trying to attract the healthiest enrollees. (For more details, see: van Doorslaer and Schut 2000; Schut 1995; Saltman and Figueras 1998; and Light 2001a).

One of the potential advantages to managed competition in general and competition among health plans in particular is that costs may be controlled if plans do compete on the basis of keeping premiums down. They can attempt to do this by choosing providers that have shown themselves to be efficient, paying them in a way that gives them an incentive to conserve resources, and implementing programs that control the use of unnecessary and costly services. Quality can be enhanced if competition is also based on this outcome. This may be possible if consumers are able to effectively use comparative information provided on plan quality, an issue discussed in detail in Chapter 3. Finally, access can also be ensured if generous subsidies are provided to low-income persons that allow them to "buy into" mainstream health plans.

However, a number of concerns also exist—the potential for:

- Plans to consolidate and monopolize certain markets, leading to higher prices and less incentive to provide a good product. This is especially a problem in nonurbanized and smaller urbanized areas (Kronick, Goodman, and Wennberg 1993).
- Comparative plan information about quality that is difficult for individuals to use.
- Difficulties involved in adequately risk adjusting plan premiums to help ensure that plans do not attempt to control costs by selecting healthier patients.
- Perceived inequities arising when some individuals and population groups have perceptibly worse coverage than others (Rice 2001).

Benefits in Publicly Mandated Systems

All countries provide hospital and physician services as part of the benefits that are included as part of their universal coverage programs. Countries vary, however, in the other services offered, services such as pharmaceuticals, dentistry, and long-term care (Glaser 1991). Long-term care is often financed through a system parallel to that of health services. Pharmaceuticals, although often covered to some extent and nearly always provided to the poor, are most likely to be subject to substantial patient cost-sharing as a way of controlling utilization. Dental coverage is commonly provided through supplemental insurance.

The two primary advantages of having a more extensive list of services covered by public programs are (1) enhanced equity in that ability to pay is less of a criterion for receiving services; and (2) easier cost control with government coverage because providers have more difficulty shifting costs to others (although some would debate this point). In Canada, for example, by far the largest growth in health expenditures has been for services not covered by provincial health plans (Evans 2000).

Such an extensive list of covered services is not without its disadvantages. The most obvious disadvantage is costs; covering more leads to more expenditures that need to be paid for through taxes or social insurance funds. Second, more comprehensive coverage leads to more service usage. When these services are more discretionary and perhaps less necessary than others, costs may outweigh the services' benefits (although this point is disputed in Chapter 3).

Cost-Sharing Requirements

Historically, most developed countries have not relied on heavy cost-sharing for hospital and physician services. In that respect the United States has been an exception, particularly in the area of physician services, where deductibles and 20 percent coinsurance rates have been standard in the fee-for-service sector. Over the past decades, however, the percentage of U.S. health expenditures paid out-of-pocket has declined: from 27 percent in 1980 to 18 percent in 1999, in part because of greater enrollment in HMOs which, until recently, tended to charge relatively low copayments (U.S. DHHS 2001, p. 333).

A country that has eschewed patient cost-sharing is Canada. The country has five overall requirements that provinces must meet to obtain full federal funding, one of which is "accessibility." Provinces must ensure "reasonable access to insured health care services . . . unprecluded or unimpeded, either directly or indirectly, by charges (user charges or extra billing) or other means . . ." (Canada Health Act Overview 2001). As a result, provinces are prohibited from levying any cost-sharing requirements for covered services (Deber 2000). Other countries with relatively low levels of patient cost-sharing include Germany and the United Kingdom.

Some countries, notably France, Switzerland, and Australia, do have significant cost-sharing requirements. In general, however, these do not apply to many services, or most of the population has supplemental insurance to provide protection. In France, for example, many procedures are exempt from the cost-sharing requirements, and 80 percent of the population has supplemental insurance that covers most of these costs (White 1995). In total, direct payments for health services exceed 20 percent of health-related financing in France, Switzerland, and the United States. In contrast, the figures for Germany, the United Kingdom, the Netherlands, and Sweden are 10 percent or less (Wagstaff et al. 1999).

We will forgo the discussion of the advantages and disadvantages of patient cost-sharing here since they have been covered extensively in other parts of the book.

How Physicians Are Paid

Through the 1980s the predominant method of paying physicians in most countries was fee-for-service. One exception was the British National Health Service, which provided its physicians an annual payment that covered all of their office visits for the year for each patient registered in their practice. Another exception was that many countries paid a salary to specialists who practiced exclusively in the hospital. Most countries that use fee-for-service employ fee schedules. In most cases, the fee schedules are negotiated between medical associations and sickness funds or insurers (Glaser 1991).

However, recent years have seen an increase in incentive-based payment systems, not just in the United States but in several European countries as well. Reforms in some countries such as the United Kingdom have aimed to integrate primary and hospital care through integrated budgets. The United Kingdom allowed primary care physicians to register as "fundholders." Under this system physicians received financing for each patient in their practice to cover all primary care services, and also a budget for pharmaceutical and surgery services. Physician fundholders could retain their surpluses and use them to improve their facilities (Le Grand 1999). Since the Labour Party came into power in 1997, fundholding was replaced by a somewhat similar system of Primary Care Trusts (PCTs) (Enthoven 2000), which comprised larger regional groups of primary care providers. PCTs commission services for their patients; exceptions to services covered include long-term care and some hospital services. If PCTs underspend their budget, they can spend funds on additional services or practice facilities (Koen 2000). Over time, these trusts "will absorb increasing amounts of financial risk and clinical responsibilities for managing not only primary care but also the specialty and public health care of their populations" (Bindman and Weiner 2000, pp. 121–22).

The United States probably exhibits the greatest variation in physician payment. Under the Medicare program, 85 percent of enrollees are in the traditional fee-for-service program, with the remaining 15 percent in Medicare HMOs. In contrast, the majority of working Americans with health insurance are in some form of managed care: either HMOs (23 percent in 2001), preferred provider organizations (PPOs, 48 percent), or point-of-service plans (POSs, 22 percent), with just 7 percent in conventional fee-for-service plans.[13]

Although most PPOs pay physicians on a fee-for-service basis, compensation methods are more diverse for HMO and POS plans—as shown in Chapter 4 (Table 4.1). In paying for primary care, these health plans use fee-for-service 25 percent of the time, capitation 61 percent of the time, and salary 14 percent of the time. To pay specialists, the figures are 75 percent of the time for fee-for-service, 13 percent of the time for capitation, and 11 percent of the time for salary (Medicare Payment Advisory Commission 2000).

The advantage of fee-for-service systems for physicians is that they may help ensure that care is not underprovided. They are very costly, however, and also can lead to the provision of too much care. In contrast,

---

13. The figures in the text are from Gabel et al. (2001). PPOs typically contract with provider groups to provide care to enrolled patients. PPO patients receive discounts if they go to these participating providers, but still may use nonparticipating providers as well. Unlike HMOs, PPOs do not normally pay providers with incentive-reimbursement systems such as DRGs and capitation. POS plans are similar to PPOs, but usually exhibit several differences: patients must first see a gatekeeping primary care physician before seeking specialist care; cost-sharing requirements are higher (often 40 percent) for care provided outside of the network of participating providers (but unlike HMOs, enrolls *can* receive care from out-of-network providers); and like HMOs, POS plans often employ incentive-reimbursement techniques.

capitation-type systems can save money but do have the potential for the underprovision of services unless some forms of mediating incentives are provided. For example, capitation payments can be adjusted based on quality or satisfaction scores, and they can be coupled with fees-for-service for the types of services society might want to encourage, such as immunizations or preventive care. No matter what system of physician compensation is used, monitoring and safeguards will still be required.

Choice of Providers

Free choice of a primary care physician is the norm in nearly all developed countries. Patients in countries that rely on competing health plans, like the United States, often are limited to primary care physicians in their plan—but are usually given free choice among any physician within the plan (unless, of course, a physician's practice is already full). In contrast, choice of specialist varies a great deal among countries. In a review of policies in 19 European countries, Richard Saltman and Josep Figueras (1998) state that, "There is no clear consensus among [European] countries as to whether patients should be allowed to refer themselves to specialist care or whether general practitioners should serve as gatekeepers to specialty care" (p. 89). In U.S. HMOs, normally a patient cannot see a specialist without a referral from his or her primary care physician—although this has begun to change as HMOs begin to move away from "heavy" managed care practices. In contrast, patients in Japan generally can see any specialist that they like (Ikegami and Campbell 1999).

It is difficult to see any advantages to not allowing free choice of primary care provider—not surprising, perhaps, given the fact that almost all countries do provide this choice. The issue of free choice of specialist is not quite as straightforward, however. Because individuals often have less experience in and understanding of the procedures that specialists perform, they often are not in as good a position to make these choices, and in fact might choose surgeons who have little experience in performing complicated procedures.

The advisability of offering free choice of hospital is even less clear. Such a choice is characteristic of the fee-for-service system in the United States, but is less true elsewhere. In Germany, for example, hospital referrals usually must be obtained from a primary care physician, and normally the patient must go to the closest hospital appropriate for the medical condition (Brenner and Rublee 2002). However, the case may be made that the choice of hospital has never been truly free even in the

United States. Some years ago Paul Ellwood stated, "Hospitals don't have patients; doctors have patients and hospitals have doctors" (Fuchs 1983, p. 58). Indeed, U.S. doctors treat, on average, 90 percent of their patients in a single hospital (Miller, Welch, and Englert 1995).

Offering consumers a choice of hospital places an individual in the best position to weigh the trade-offs between proximity, convenience, costs, and *perceived* quality. In addition, if the consumer does sufficient research on quality, he or she can (in theory at least) insist on going to a hospital with excellent medical outcomes. Presumably, this would apply only to elective admissions, where enough time is available to conduct sufficient research.

On the other hand, providing free choice of hospital would not be best for individuals and for society as a whole for three reasons. First, patients may choose hospitals that provide poor quality. Second, economies of scale may be associated with concentrating volumes of particular services in a single hospital (Finkler 1979). Third, if a particular service is concentrated in a single hospital, hospitals do not have to spend resources competing for patients and physicians. This has to be weighed against higher costs that may accrue from giving hospitals more monopoly power.

6.2.3 Regulation of Prices and Expenditures

A key decision that countries must make is the extent to which they intervene in the marketplace either by setting unit prices or overall health expenditures. These policies can apply to many different types of providers and services: hospitals, physicians, outpatient clinics, pharmaceuticals. After a brief overview, this section will focus on the hospital and physician sectors.

A common method of controlling expenditures is through the use of "global budgets," which "tend to be prospectively set caps on spending for some portion of the health care industry" (Wolfe and Moran 1993, p. 55). A study conducted in the early 1990s found ten European countries that had adopted some form of global budgeting (Wolfe and Moran 1993), mainly for the government portion of hospital and/or physician expenditures, but sometimes (e.g., in the United Kingdom) for total government health expenditures. Global budgets tend to be administered regionally in most countries that use them (Jonsson 1989) and are not used in isolation, but rather as one of several tools for controlling health expenditures.

Hospital Prices and Expenditures

Hospitals prices and expenditures can be regulated in various ways. Some time ago, hospitals in most countries received per diem payments for each day of a patient's hospital stay, but this method was ineffective in controlling overall expenditures because it provided an incentive to keep patients longer (Glaser 1991) and was not based on the resource requirements incurred by different types of patients.

The United States was the first country to pay hospitals a fixed amount for an entire patient stay, as part of the diagnosis-related group (DRG) system first employed by the Medicare program and later by a few other private and public insurers. This quickly shortened lengths of stay. Although concerns continue to be raised about quality because DRGs encourage early discharge, no systematic evidence indicates that this has occurred.[14] If quality has not be dampened, then the fact that DRGs shortened stays implies that on average, patients were probably staying in hospitals too long. Indeed, hospital lengths of stay in most developed countries have shortened in recent years. It is not clear whether or not this was due, to a significant degree, to evidence from the United States that shorter stays were indeed possible. Advances in certain medical techniques, for example, have also made shorter stays possible.

More common in other developed countries, however, is the use of global budgets for paying hospitals. In some countries, notably Canada, each hospital negotiates its own budget with provinces. If a hospital exceeds its budget, compensation is not guaranteed. In France, hospital budgets are assigned based on historic costs but adjusted for case-mix (Fielding and Lancry 1993; Saltman and Figueras 1998), a trend in a number of European countries. In countries with multiple payers, each must contribute to a hospital's global budget. This is usually done by negotiations between the hospital and either government or a consortium of sickness funds. Each of the funds then contributes a portion of the hospital's total budget based on how much its enrollees contribute to the hospital's overall utilization (Glaser 1991).

---

14. One study conducted on the effect of DRGs during their first three years found no overall diminution in quality (Kahn et al. 1990), although another component of the study found that more patients were being discharged in a clinically unstable condition (Kosecoff et al. 1990).

Each of the current payment methods—negotiated rates used by private health plans in the United States, DRGs, and global budgets—has its own advantages and disadvantages. The potential success of each system hinges, in part, on the ability of payers to adjust payments according to severity of illness so that hospitals are appropriately compensated. Nevertheless, some generalizations about each of the payment systems are possible. The use of competitive forces to set rates has the advantage of allowing the market to equilibrate supply and demand, potentially enhancing economic efficiency. Critics, however, believe that hospital costs are impossible to control when multiple sources of payment exist. In addition, hospitals may end up favoring the patients of the more generous payers.

DRGs have the advantage of encouraging hospitals to keep patients no longer than medically necessary. However, DRGs also have several potential problems: quality will suffer if stays become too short, so it must be continually monitored; hospitals may still favor the patients of one insurer over another if DRG payment rates vary; providers have an incentive to "upcode," that is, bill for more remunerative DRGs; similarly, providers have an incentive to move care to sectors that are not paid on a DRG basis (e.g., outpatient departments); and the potential remains for providers to shift costs from one payer to another. The effect of DRGs might have been expected to be known by now, since they were implemented in 1983. However, because the method was implemented nationally, isolating the effect from other changes in the health system over this period of time (particularly the growth of managed care) is nearly impossible.

Hospital global budgets are difficult to evaluate in isolation because they are typically used in conjunction with other policies such as controls on bed supply and medical technologies. The main advantage of paying hospitals a global budget is that it allows payers, be they government or private, to control overall hospital expenditures. In addition, it may enhance efficiency because hospitals are free to allocate their budgets as they wish. Disadvantages include the difficulty of coming up with the appropriate total budget for each hospital, since this entails calculating how much the hospital would be spending if it were operating efficiently; concerns that hospitals will stint on hiring appropriate staff, since they are given a fixed budget; the potential for keeping beds filled with patients who use fewer resources to keep budgets up but costs down (a problem that can be ameliorated if payments are adjusted according to patient severity); and the lack of incentives to innovate.

Physician Prices and Expenditures

As noted earlier, fee-for-service payments remain the most common method of compensating physicians in developed countries, although hospital-based physicians are sometimes salaried. The typical system is one in which physicians are paid based on a fee schedule, which is simply a list of procedures with a fee associated with each. In some countries (e.g., the U.S. Medicare program) fees are the product of a set of relative values and a "conversion factor." The relative values, which generally are determined by physician associations, indicate the ratio of payment rates between different procedures. A conversion factor then converts these relative values into actual fee-for-service payment rates. For example, if a follow-up office visit has a relative value of ten, and the conversion factor is eight dollars, then total payment for the service would be $80. In contrast to the relative values, which tend to be determined by the medical profession,[15] the conversion factors are usually established by government or sickness funds, sometimes in negotiations with physician organizations.

Fee-for-service has been criticized for its inability to control costs and for the incentives it provides for overutilization of services. Some countries, notably Germany, the United States through its Medicare program, and most of the Canadian provinces, have dealt with these criticisms by attempting to control total expenditures for physicians—that is, the product of unit prices and the volume of services provided.

In the early 1990s the U.S. Medicare program began use to volume performance standards (VPSS). This was later replaced by a similar system called the *sustainable growth rate* (SGR). Under the VPS system, each year the U.S. Congress set a target rate of increase in Medicare Part B physician expenditures. If actual spending exceeded the target, the next year's physician fee update was normally reduced by that amount (although Congress could do whatever it chose when the time came). Conversely, if the growth in spending was less than the target, physicians would get more. Suppose, for example, that the target for a particular year was a 10 percent increase in spending. If actual spending increased by 12 percent,

---

15. The procedure used to establish the relative values used by the Medicare program was somewhat different. The values were originally based on a research study conducted at Harvard University and then modified by a congressional agency. The American Medical Association and various specialty groups participated in and contributed to the findings. See Hsiao et al. (1988).

the target would have been exceeded. Most likely, this would be extracted the next time Congress updated Medicare physician fees. If physicians were due a 5 percent cost-of-living increase, they would likely be granted only 3 percent.

The main difference between the SGR system, implemented in 1998, and the VPS system was in setting the target expenditure rate of "sustainable growth." The rate was determined by four factors: (1) the percentage change in physician input prices; (2) the percentage change in Part B fee-for-service enrollment; (3) the projected change in real gross domestic product (GDP); and (4) the percentage change in spending for physicians' services resulting from other changes in law (Medicare Payment Advisory Commission 2000).

The VPS system (and by analogy, its successor, SGR) has been criticized as being too blunt of an instrument to affect individual physician behavior. Because the system applies nationally, individual physicians who increase the volume of the services they provide are not penalized by experiencing a decline in their fees. The latter would happen only if all physicians behave this way. If a physician does not increase his or her volume but other physicians do, then that physician would suffer. His or her volume is constant, but the fee paid will fall because of the behavior of other physicians. The systems may therefore contain a "perverse" incentive to increase the volume of services, which is exactly what it was supposed to prevent. One way to improve the incentives would be to target smaller groups of physicians by having separate targets for each specialty, state, or state-specialty combination (Rice and Bernstein 1990; Marquis and Kominski 1994).

Most of the Canadian provinces have also adopted expenditure caps or targets in response to difficult economic times experienced by both the federal and provincial governments beginning in the late 1980s (Barer, Lomas, and Sanmartin 1996). As of the mid 1990s, eight of the ten provinces had established "hard" caps in which fees were reduced in proportion to the extent to which the caps were exceeded. One of the more interesting side effects is that the medical profession sought to reduce the supply of physicians as a way of stabilizing fees—the idea being that more physicians would result in more billings, which in turn would reduce payment rates. These policies are described below, under "Control of Input Supply."

The U.S. Medicare targets and the Canadian provincial caps just mentioned apply at the aggregate level. In addition, as of the mid 1990s, five of the ten provinces had adopted some form of individual income cap as well. Typically, this entails reducing unit fees after a physician has exceeded a certain income threshold. In Ontario, for example, fees were reduced by 33 percent after annual income reached $404,000, and by 67 percent after it reached $454,000 (Canadian dollars) (Barer, Lomas, and Sanmartin 1996).

A final example comes from Germany. Ambulatory care physicians are paid on a fee-for-service basis according to a fee schedule that is based on a national relative value scale. (Physicians providing inpatient care are salaried.) A national commission determines what the total growth in health expenditures should be, but payer and provider organizations in each region negotiate their own expenditure ceilings within nationally set guidelines. Fixed pools of funds, based on a capitated payment for each insurance fund member, are allocated to each region. In most regions, the capitation pools are further divided into separate risk pools for physician consultation, laboratory testing, and "other" services. The number of relative value points billed by physicians is tallied quarterly, and the pool funds are divided by the number of points to determine a conversion factor that can be used to convert points to payments. The higher the volume of services, the lower the conversion factor (Kirkman-Liff 1990).

One novel and important aspect of the system is that conversion factors are determined and payments are made retrospectively. That is, physician fees are not established until it is known exactly how many services were provided. Consequently, if some physicians raise volume, other physicians will be paid less for services already provided. Because of this, a system has been established that allows boards composed of both physician and insurance representatives to monitor each physician's practice, and to even withhold payment when high volumes cannot be justified (Rice and Bernstein 1990). Physicians that provide 15 percent more services than the norm are audited, and those providing 25 percent more than the norm actually have to return money to the physicians' association (Henke, Murray, and Ade 1994). Thus, German physicians have an incentive to police each other; if one physician overprovides services, fees for the others will be less.

6.2.4 Regulation of Volume

Just as regulating unit prices is one method of trying to control expenditures, another is to regulate the volume of services provided. With the exception of the United States, which has a history of utilization controls, most countries do not focus so much on direct volume controls. Rather, they tend to focus on limiting expenditures, as discussed above, or on the supply of inputs, which is discussed next.

In contrast, there has been and continues to be much direct regulation of volume in the United States. Examples in the fee-for-service sector include requiring certification before insurers pay for hospital stays, second opinions before surgery is paid for, and the profiling of physician practices. Similar examples are in place in managed care plans that use other forms of reimbursement, although their purpose sometimes is to ensure that enough, rather than too much, care is provided.

One way to think about this is to distinguish between two kinds of regulation: "micro" and "macro." Microregulation can be thought of as direct control. Macroregulation, on the other hand, is more indirect: the setting of ground rules to meet particular goals. Other developed countries, much more so than the United States, rely on macroregulation. Global budgets provide a good example. Little direct oversight is given to the provision of care, but strict controls are placed on how much money is paid out in total. Another example of macro-based policies are tight controls over the diffusion of medical technologies.

In the United States, health plans compete largely on the basis of premiums; as a result, they need to find ways to control their costs. Broadly speaking, controls are exerted in three ways: over prices, quantities, or total expenditures. The last of these is difficult to achieve directly, since a health plan has no way to set a global budget, rather, a single payer—or a tightly coordinated all-payer system—is needed to control total expenditures. Consequently, the emphasis has been on the first two.

Beginning with quantity, managed care plans employ a variety of microregulatory quantity controls. One example is preadmission certification of hospital stays. This involves having the physician contact a health plan employee in order for the stay to be covered. If the plan disagrees with the physician's assessment, a cumbersome appeals process can ensue. Another example is requiring that patients see a primary care gatekeeper before going to a specialist. To enforce this, health plans must examine every case. If the claim is denied, the patient can appeal, resulting in further administrative costs. In general, microregulation means that someone is watching over a large percentage of physician and patient activities.

The main way that prices can be controlled is through incentive reimbursement schemes. These, however, tend to result in microregulation, since it is necessary to monitor whether providers are skimping. A new tool for addressing the problem of skimping is disseminating information through report cards (discussed in Chapter 3), which increasingly are being administered not only to health plans, but to provider groups as well. The idea is to provide consumers with appropriate measures of performance, such as consumer satisfaction, clinical quality performance, and service performance like waiting times.

The advantage of direct control of volume is that it can focus on reducing the waste in the system. For example, if a particular procedure is inappropriate for a patient with a given diagnosis, such procedures can, in theory, be identified. The major disadvantage, however, is that these strategies often are cumbersome from an administrative standpoint, involving much bureaucracy, paperwork, and undue oversight over the practice of medicine.

6.2.5 Control of Input Supply
The Hospital
Developed countries vary a great deal with respect to whether hospitals are publicly or privately owned. Among those that are privately owned, variation exists regarding whether they are for-profit or nonprofit institutions. In the United Kingdom, for example, about 90 percent of inpatient beds are in public facilities (Smee 2000). In contrast, the majority of acute care hospitals in the United States and Canada are private, not-for-profit facilities.

Controlling the supply of hospital beds is a strategy used by most developed countries, particularly in the public sector. The logic goes back to Roemer's Law, which states that in a well-insured population, "a bed built is a bed filled" (Shain and Roemer 1959). This "law" was consistent with empirical evidence for decades, until the advent of DRGs and movement away from fee-for-service medicine. Nevertheless, controlling hospital supply and beds generally is not the only major method by which most countries attempt to control hospital expenditures. Equally common is the use of global budgets and restrictions on medical technologies (Saltman and Figueras 1998).

The Physician
Most countries are active in controlling the supply of physicians—usually because of the supposition that more physicians will result in higher health expenditures (see Section 4.2.1 on physician-induced demand).

In more recent years an emphasis, particularly in the United States, has been placed on augmenting the supply of generalists at the expense of specialists. This is because of perceptions of a shortage of the former and glut of the latter (although research on whether this is indeed the case is inconclusive). One way of trying to change these distributions, at least in the long run, is to provide more of a financial incentive to physicians who choose to become general or family practitioners, internists, or OB-GYNs. In the United States, the Medicare fee schedule that was implemented in the early 1990s resulted in a substantial redistribution of fees away from specialists toward generalists (Ginsburg, LeRoy, and Hammons 1990). Nevertheless, income differences by specialty in the United States still remain large. In 1997, U.S. radiologists earned an average of $260,000 and surgeons $217,000, compared to $147,000 for internists and $132,000 for general and family practitioners (U.S. Department of Labor 2000).

Countries have used a variety of techniques to control physician supply over the years. Most common are limiting medical school enrollment and reducing the number of foreign-trained physicians allowed in a country (Schroeder 1984). Some of the Canadian provinces have been particularly active in this regard as the country and provinces faced financial difficulties that began in the late 1980s. Additional strategies used by one or more provinces include: paying new physicians only 50 percent of usual fees unless they practice in particular geographic areas; not providing billing numbers (which are needed to obtain payment); and allowing older physicians to "buy out" their billing numbers so as to encourage retirement (Barer, Lomas, and Sanmartin 1996). The restrictions in billing numbers have not been terribly successful. Barer and colleagues (1996) note, "Yet despite the best intentions of the ministers of health in declaring their commitment to a national physician resource strategy, in reality provinces have pretty much done their own thing to keep others' graduates from their borders" (p. 223).

Controlling the supply of physicians has been considered necessary by most countries in order to have some control over total health expenditures—as well as to help plan for the desired distribution of health personnel. The major disadvantage is that government planners may mistakenly perceive shortages or surpluses of physicians and therefore make inappropriate policy decisions. Given the lead time it takes to train physicians, it may take years to correct any such mistakes.

Table 6.2: Availability of Selected Medical Technologies* (Units per Million Persons)

	CT Scanners	MRIS	Radiation Therapy	Lithotriptors
Australia	20.8	4.7	4.9	1.0
Canada	7.3	2.5	7.0	0.5
France	9.7	2.5	7.8	0.8
Germany	17.1	6.2	4.6	1.7
Japan	84.4	23.2	NA	4.0
Netherlands	9.0	3.9	7.2	0.8
Sweden	13.8	6.8	0.8	0.3
Switzerland	19.0	13.2	11.7	3.0
United Kingdom	6.1	4.5	3.3	NA
United States	13.2	7.6	4.0	2.4

*Data are from the most recent year available between 1990 and 2000, which varies by country.
NA = data not available.
Source: OECD. 2001. "OECD Health Data 2001: A Comparative Analysis of 30 Countries." (OECD, Paris). Used with permission.

Capital and Medical Technology

With the notable exception of the United States, developed countries have been active in controlling the dissemination and use of expensive medical technologies.[16] Table 6.2 shows the availability of four medical technologies—CT scanners, MRIs, radiation therapy, and lithotriptors —across the ten countries in terms of number of units per million

16. The United States was once active in this area as well. Certificate-of-need (CON) programs, which were coordinated through state and local planning boards, provided a means of controlling the number of hospital beds as well as medical technologies that cost more than a threshold amount. These programs were common beginning in the late 1970s, but had mostly been phased out by the 1990s. Evaluations of the programs tended to show that they were unsuccessful in controlling hospital expenditures. Although CON did control bed supply somewhat, the amount of resources per bed increased to compensate for those reductions. The failure of CON was largely the result of putting power in the hands of local planning boards, whose members had little or no incentive to prevent local hospitals from obtaining the resources they desired (Salkever and Bice 1978; Rice 1992b).

population.[17] In general, Japan has by far the most technologies: four times as many CT scanners, almost twice as many MRIs, and 30 percent more lithotriptors than any of the other countries. The probable reason for the preponderance of medical technologies in Japan is summarized by Yoshikawa and Bhattacharya (2002):

> Under Japanese fee-for-service medicine with the uniform fee schedule, hospitals cannot engage in price competition; under such market conditions, hospitals tend to engage in nonprice competition to attract patients. With legal restrictions on advertising, a hospital's options are quite limited. Hence, many hospitals may purchase high-technology medical equipment to signal a level of medical sophistication that will attract more patients. Hospitals located in markets with a high level of local competition have an incentive to quickly acquire high-technology medical equipment to compete with their rivals. (pp. 259–60)

Other than Japan, few clear patterns are evident in Table 6.2, except that for most technologies Canada ranked near the bottom.

The methods by which different countries control these technologies vary. In Canada, provinces finance most capital equipment, and hospitals do not receive increases in their global budgets for the use of medical equipment that has not been approved by provincial governments. After studying the considerable differences in the utilization of cardiovascular procedures between Canada and the United States, Diana Verrilli and colleagues (1998) found that lower rates in Canada, particularly for older individuals,

> [Are] accomplished both by implicit, discretionary rationing by physicians and by more formal restriction on the availability of services

---

17. CT or "CAT" scans, short for computed tomography scanners, provide images of the human body based on computer syntheses of x-rays taken from different directions. MRIs, short for magnetic resonance imaging, provide three-dimensional body images through the use of magnets and radio waves, thereby avoiding the use of radiation. Radiation therapy uses high-energy rays to treat disease, especially cancer. Lithotriptors use intense sound waves to destroy kidney stones. These procedures were chosen because they constitute four of the five reported by the OECD (2001). The other measure, hemodialysis stations (for kidney dialysis), was not available for three of the ten countries.

through resource constraints. Canadian provincial governments strictly control both the number of hospitals performing cardiovascular procedures and the funding for these procedures. (p. 481)

Other countries with similarly stringent controls include Sweden and the United Kingdom (McClellan and Kessler 1999).

The advantages and disadvantages of explicit supply controls are similar, whether they apply to hospitals, physicians, or medical technology. The advantages, like those mentioned for budget controls, include the potential for cost control and greater ability for governments to successfully plan for the provision of necessary services to the population. The two main disadvantages are the inability of policymakers to determine the appropriate amount of inputs to produce, and concern that controls will stifle life-enhancing or efficiency-producing innovations. This is of particular concern for medical technologies where advances are occurring at a quick pace.

6.3 CROSS-NATIONAL DATA ON HEALTH SYSTEM PERFORMANCE

This section provides recent data on the performance of different countries' health systems. It is divided into five subsections, each of which examines a particular aspect of performance: access, utilization, expenditures, quality/satisfaction, and equity of financing. The focus is on the ten countries discussed earlier and described in the Appendix: Australia, Canada, France, Germany, Japan, the Netherlands, Sweden, Switzerland, the United Kingdom, and the United States. Because comparable data are scarce, in some instances only a subset of countries is compared. Short descriptions of each country's system appear in the Appendix.

Before presenting and discussing these data, it should be mentioned that the World Health Organization (WHO 2000) did attempt to assess the performance of the health systems of its 191 member states in 2000. Performance was based on five indicators: overall level of population health, health inequalities within the population, two measures of health system responsiveness, and the distribution of the health system's financial burden within the population. For the sake of completeness, the rankings are noted here: Australia (32nd), Canada (30th), France (1st), Germany (25th), Japan (10th), the Netherlands (17th), Sweden (23rd), Switzerland (20th), the United Kingdom (18th), and the United States (37th). Curiously, Italy was ranked second in the world, in spite of the fact that "only 20 percent of Italians rate their health care system as satisfactory" (Jamison and Sandbu 2001, p. 1595).

This chapter does not rely on the WHO rankings because they appear to be fraught with methodological problems. Some of these include not controlling for any confounding variables other than national education levels and health expenditures; assuming that all differences in outcomes are the result of health system performance; extreme sensitivity of the results to changes in specification of the statistical model; ignoring such measures as satisfaction and health promotion and preventive care in the ratings of performance; and assuming that every country has the same goals for its system (Jamison and Sanbu 2001; Robbins 2001; Mooney and Wiseman 2000). Until such an analysis can adequately deal with these issues, it is premature to rank different countries' health systems' performance.

6.3.1 Access

This section presents data on three different aspects of access to care: coverage rates, whether individuals believe they can obtain care when they need it, and waiting times for obtaining procedures. The first of these is a measure of potential access, whereas the second and third are gauges for realized access.

Unfortunately, comparable cross-national data are not available on coverage rates. Although most developed countries have systems with universal coverage, in some of these countries a subset of the population receives coverage through private rather than public sources. Table 6.3 shows eligibility for health benefits under *public programs*. In seven of the ten countries, more than 99 percent of the population is covered in this manner. The figures are lower in Germany (92.2 percent), the Netherlands (74.2 percent), and the United States (45.0 percent). In the case of Germany and the Netherlands, almost everyone who does not have public coverage has private insurance. This is not the case in the United States, however.

Table 6.4 show the prevalence of uninsurance in the United States. In 1999, 38.5 million were uninsured—approximately 16 percent of the under age-65 population. Rates are much higher for particular subgroups: 27 percent for those age 18 to 24, 34 percent for Hispanics, and about 35 percent for those below 150 percent of the poverty level.

One limitation of the data in Table 6.4 is that it does not address the availability of medical care irrespective of whether individuals have

Table 6.3: Eligibility for Health Benefits Under Public Programs* (% of Population)

	Percentage of Population Covered
Australia	100
Canada	100
France	99.5
Germany	92.2
Japan	100
Netherlands	74.2
Sweden	100
Switzerland	100
United Kindgom	100
United States	45.0

*Data are from the most recent year available between 1997 and 2000, which varies by country.
Source: OECD. 2001. "OECD Health Data 2001: A Comparative Analysis of 30 Countries." (OECD, Paris). Used with permission.

health insurance. Although access to care might be supposed to be related to health insurance coverage, this is not necessarily the case. Uninsured individuals can receive care by paying for it themselves, or alternatively, through a "safety net" of facilities and providers designed to serve the poor and uninsured. Similarly, insured individuals may still face access barriers if, for example, the supply of medical personnel, facilities, and technologies is insufficient to serve the population. However, uninsured Americans are far more likely than the insured to say that they are not able to get the medical care that they need (Donelan et al. 1999). Other studies indicate that compared to the insured, the uninsured are more likely to forgo recommended treatments because of costs, receive fewer preventive services, are more likely to be hospitalized for "avoidable conditions," and are more likely to be diagnosed for cancer when the disease has reached a more advanced stage (Hoffman and Schlobohm 2000).

Table 6.5, which is based on data collected from telephone surveys of individuals in Australia, Canada, the United Kingdom, and the United States, examines various indicators of realized (as opposed to potential) patient access to health services across these countries (Donelan et al. 1999). Somewhat more Americans—14 percent compared to 10 percent

Table 6.4: Number of Uninsured in the United States and Percentage Insured by Selected Characteristics, 1999

Total Number of Uninsured (Millions)	38.5
Percentage Uninsured by Characteristic	
Age	
Under 6 years	11.0
6–17 years	12.3
18–24 years	27.4
25–34 years	22.1
35–44 years	16.3
45–54 years	12.8
55–64 years	11.4
Sex	
Male	17.2
Female	15.0
Race	
White	14.7
Black	19.4
Asian or Pacific Islander	16.3
Hispanic Origin and Race	
All Hispanic	33.9
White, non-Hispanic	12.1
Black, non-Hispanic	19.3
Percent of Poverty Level	
Below 100	34.4
100–149	35.8
150–199	27.7
200 or more	7.7
Geographic Region	
Northeast	12.2
Midwest	11.5
South	19.8
West	18.6
Location of Residence	
Within MSA	15.3
Outside MSA	18.9

MSA = metropolitan statistical area.
Source: U.S. DHHS. 2001. "Health, United States, 2001, with Urban and Rural Chartbook," http://www.cdc.gov/nchs/products/pubs/pubd/hus/hus.htm.

Table 6.5: Consumers' Reports on Access to and Cost of Care, 1998 (%)

	Australia	Canada	United Kingdom	United States
There was a time in the past 12 months when they needed medical care but did not get it	8	10	10	14
Level of difficulty seeing specialists and consultants when they needed it				
Extremely difficult	5	6	3	9
Very difficult	9	10	7	6
Somewhat difficult	21	30	19	24
Not too difficult	25	22	30	24
Not at all difficult	29	25	25	32
Had problems paying medical bills in past year	10	5	3	18
They or a family member have not filled a presecription because they could not afford it	12	7	6	17

Source: Donelan, K., et al. 1999. "The Cost of Health System Change: Public Discontent in Five Nations." *Health Affairs* 18 (3): 206–16. Used with permission.

or less from the other countries—indicated that there was a time during the previous year that they needed medical care but did not receive it. The disparity between the United States and the other countries was greater with respect to two indicators of affordability: having problems paying medical bills in the last year (18 percent in the United States vs. 10 percent or less elsewhere), and not filling a prescription because of its costs (17 percent vs. 12 percent or less).

In contrast, respondents from all countries reported fairly similar amounts of difficulty in seeing specialists and consultants when they needed such care; however, residents of the United Kingdom reported the least difficulty in obtaining care from specialists. This is an interesting result given (as shown below in Table 6.9) that the United Kingdom spends less on health relative to other countries. Americans were more

Table 6.6: Consumers' Worries and Anxieties About Their Health Services, 1998 (%)

	Australia	Canada	United Kingdom	United States
How worried are you that if you become seriously ill, you will not be able to get the most advanced medical care, including medicines, tests, or treatment?				
Very worried	19	29	16	21
Somewhat worried	29	34	30	26
Not too worried	52	37	51	53
How worried are you that if you become seriously ill, you will not be able to get medical care you need because you cannot afford it?				
Very worried	25	22	14	23
Somewhat worried	26	23	23	24
Not too worried	48	54	60	52
How worried are you that you will wait too long to get nonemergency medical care?				
Very worried	25	20	12	14
Somewhat worried	28	32	30	22
Not too worried	46	47	55	64

Source: Donelan, K., et al. 1999. "The Cost of Health System Change: Public Discontent in Five Nations." *Health Affairs* 18 (3): 206–16. Used with permission.

likely to report extreme difficulty but also were more likely to report no difficulty at all. This is a result, in part, of differential access between the insured and uninsured populations in the United States, and perhaps because some enrollees in HMOs find that they have trouble getting referrals. Regarding the differential access, twice as many uninsured as insured Americans (67 percent vs. 34 percent) said that they had somewhat or more difficulty accessing specialists (not shown in table).

Table 6.7: Self-Reported Waiting Times, 1998 (%)

	Australia	Canada	United Kingdom	United States
Waiting times for non-emergency surgery for themselves or a family member				
None	5	16	7	10
Less than 1 month	46	28	23	60
1–3.9 months	32	43	36	28
4 months or more	17	12	33	1

Source: Donelan, K., et al. 1999. "The Cost of Health System Change: Public Discontent in Five Nations." *Health Affairs* 18 (3): 206–16. Used with permission.

The same study also examined consumer anxiety about accessing care in the future (Table 6.6). The main patterns are: residents of the United Kingdom are less worried about the affordability of care than are others; Canadians are most concerned about not obtaining the most advanced treatments, and, along with Australians, that they will wait too long for care.

One issue that has received a great deal of attention internationally is waiting lists, particularly for obtaining surgical care and tests. Unfortunately, compiling comparable cross-national data on waiting lists is nearly impossible. Countries rarely keep consolidated lists of patients who are waiting for treatment. The alternative of using hospital records is problematic because patients may be listed at more than one hospital.

Perhaps a better way to study the problem is to examine *waiting time* rather than waiting lists. This gets around the problem that people may be on several lists at once. Unfortunately, no objective data are available on waiting time. A reasonable alternative is to ask consumers about their experiences. This was asked as part of the Donelan et al. (1999) study. Table 6.7 shows the results. Americans had, by far, the shortest average waits for nonemergency surgery. Seventy percent reported waiting less than one month, and only 1 percent waited more than four months. Undoubtedly this is due, in part, to the surplus of hospital beds in the United States. Occupancy rates in the United States were approximately

65 percent in the late 1990s, compared to more than 80 percent in most of the other countries examined (OECD 2001). Residents of all three other countries reported considerably more waiting. One-third of United Kingdom residents reported waiting four or more months, compared to 12 percent of Canadians and 17 percent of Australians. Although data on waiting time are difficult to obtain, in most countries, those with higher incomes are able to avoid waiting times by obtaining services through private insurance or self-payment. Indeed, in some countries, physicians have an incentive to make public patients wait as an incentive for some to pay more lucrative fees through the private market.

Another survey examined a related question: how much patients needing elective cataract surgery in three countries (Canada, Spain, and Denmark) were willing to pay to reduce waiting time (Anderson et al. 1997). One finding was that few—12, 15, and 24 percent of respondents in Spain, Canada, and Denmark, respectively—were in favor of higher income taxes to eliminate waiting times. Furthermore, relatively few were willing to pay market prices to avoid waits in public facilities. The authors conclude that, "in spite of expressed public dissatisfaction with waiting lists in all three sites, a majority of the respondents did not support the actions that could have reduced their own wait" (Anderson et al. 1997, p. 181).

6.3.2 Utilization
Utilization is not a measure of a country's health system performance, rather, it is an input into the process of providing and delivering care. It is discussed here briefly, however, because utilization figures provide a glimpse into how different countries manage their resources.

Table 6.8 shows four measures of usage, regarding inpatient care (acute care bed days per capita), outpatient care (physician consultations or visits per capita), and cardiovascular care (coronary artery bypass and coronary angioplasty operations per 100,000 population). Most countries have comparable rates of inpatient utilization, with the United States having somewhat lower rates than the others. Two countries, Germany and Switzerland, have rates considerably higher than the rest. Physician consultation rates show more variation, with Sweden much lower than the others and Japan and Switzerland substantially higher. Japan's rate is well more than double that of all counties except Switzerland. This is attributable both to a very low fee schedule, which encourages physicians to see many patients for short visits, as well as historically high levels of prescription drug use; it is likely that a disproportionate number of physician

Table 6.8: Utilization of Select Services

	Acute Care Bed Days per Capita*	Physician Consultations per Capita**	Coronary Artery Bypass Operations per 100,000⁺	Coronary Angioplasty Operations per 100,000⁺⁺
Australia	1.0	6.3	83	91
Canada	1.0	6.4	65	70
France	1.1	6.5	35	73
Germany	1.9	6.5	38	86
Japan	NA	16.0	NA	NA
Netherlands	0.9	5.8	60	72
Sweden	0.8	2.8	54	NA
Switzerland	1.7	11.0	60	65
United Kingdom	1.0	5.4	41	35
United States	0.7	5.8	203	339

*Data are from the most recent year available between 1996 and 1999, which varies by country.
**Data are from the most recent year available between 1996 and 1999, which varies by country. Data for Switzerland are from 1992.
⁺Data are from the most recent year available between 1991 and 1998, which varies by country
⁺⁺Data are from the most recent year available between 1993 and 1998, which varies by country.
NA = data not available.
Source: OECD. 2001. "OECD Health Data 2001: A Comparative Analysis of 30 Countries." (OECD, Paris). Used with permission.

visits in Japan are specifically for obtaining prescriptions (Ikegami and Campbell 1999).

The other noteworthy pattern in the table is the extremely high rates of use of the two coronary procedures in the United States. The United States rate is almost four times the average of the other countries for bypass operations and almost five times as high for angioplasty, a finding confirmed by a more systematic cross-national research study on differences in heart-attack care around the world (TECH Research Network 2001). This high rate is in part a result of explicit "supply-side" rationing as well as the use of strict global budgets in several of the other countries

244   THE ECONOMICS OF HEALTH RECONSIDERED

(Saltman and Figueras 1998; McClellan and Kessler 1999; TECH Research Network 2001).

Another, perhaps more intriguing reason is that use of cardiovascular procedures appears to be especially high in the United States for the "oldest old." A study of data from the United States and Canada in 1992 found that the difference in usage between the two countries rose dramatically with age. For example, among coronary artery bypass procedures, the ratio between U.S. and Canadian usage was 1.4 for ages 65 to 69, 2.6 for ages 70 to 74, 4.2 for ages 75 to 79, and 7.2 for those over age 80. The pattern for angioplasty (1.9, 3.2, 4.9, and 7.7) was very similar (Verrilli, Berenson, and Katz 1998). The authors conclude that:

> As a result of both resource constraints and societal and physician attitudes towards care of the elderly, physicians in Canada appear to use age as a basis for limiting the provision of technologically oriented medical care. In contrast, since the threshold for providing cardiovascular services to the elderly is higher in the United States than it is in Canada, it appears that U.S. physicians consider age a less important factor in determining who receives cardiovascular services. In the general absence of budgetary constraints, whether this encourages profligate service use or whether it contributes to improved outcomes among elderly persons in the United States is uncertain. (p. 482)

These differences in usage rates do not appear to have much effect on mortality. In another study, Tu and colleagues (1997) found that angiography was five times as common among seniors in the United States as in Ontario, Canada, whereas angioplasty and coronary artery bypass surgery were seven times as common. In spite of this, 30-day mortality rates were only slightly lower in the United States (21.4 percent vs. 22.3 percent), and one-year mortality rates were nearly identical (34.3 percent in the United States vs. 34.4 percent in Ontario).

Part of the reason for these stark differences in utilization, especially among older patients, is undoubtedly related to the way in which costs are controlled in the two countries. In the U.S. Medicare program, cost control is mainly done through limited physician fees and DRG payments, as well as aggregate expenditure targets for all physician services. In contrast, Canadian cost controls center around hospital global budgets and controls on the diffusion of medical technology. As a result, most provinces

Table 6.9: Total Health Expenditures, 1998

	Per Capita Expenditures in U.S. Dollars	Ratio of Expenditures to the U.S. Level	Percentage of GDP Spent on Health
Australia	2,085	2.00	8.6
Canada	2,360	1.76	9.3
France	2,043	2.04	9.4
Germany	2,361	1.76	10.3
Japan	1,795	2.32	7.4
Netherlands	2,150	1.94	8.7
Sweden	1,732	2.40	7.9
Switzerland	2,853	1.46	10.4
United Kingdom	1,510	2.76	6.8
United States	4,165	1.00	12.9

Source: OECD. 2001. "OECD Health Data 2001: A Comparative Analysis of 30 Countries." (OECD, Paris). Used with permission.

lack the capacity to provide as many surgeries to older patients as does the United States.

6.3.3 Expenditures

The first column of Table 6.9 shows per capita expenditures on health in each of the ten countries during 1998. These figures have been adjusted by "purchasing power parities," which account for different price levels across countries so that a given amount of money will purchase the same market basket of goods and services (OECD 2001). To aid in viewing these numbers, the second column shows the ratio of expenditures in each other country to the United States. The 2.00 figure for Australia, for example, means that per capita expenditures were twice as high in the United States. The final column shows the percentage of gross domestic product (GDP) devoted to health in each country during 1998.

Among half of the countries, expenditures are fairly similar, falling in a narrow range from $2,043 to $2,361. The United States is far above all others at a figure of $4,165, with Switzerland a distant second at $2,853. The U.S. level is particularly noteworthy given that about 16 percent of the under-age-65 population is uninsured; these individuals spend less on health services. The United Kingdom spends the least on health at $1,510, with Sweden and Japan fairly close to that amount. The patterns are similar with respect to the percentage of GDP spent on health, although the range among countries is narrower.

Because wealthier countries can devote a larger share of national income to health, it is useful to control for this factor when comparing countries. Figure 6.1 shows the relationship between wealth and health expenditures for all Organization for Economic Cooperation and Development (OECD) countries in 1997. In almost all instances, a country's health spending can be predicted quite accurately by the level of per capita GDP; almost all fall on the diagonal line. The main exception is the United States, which spends far more on health than would be predicted based simply on its income.

Comparing these figures to the utilization patterns shown in Table 6.9 to those in Table 6.8, care in the United States is much more expensive given that its overall usage rates for hospital and physician services are low by international standards. One explanation is the higher usage rates for the two cardiac procedures shown, which likely is indicative of patterns for many other procedures as well. Another explanation, not shown in these tables, are differences in unit prices between countries. Some research has been conducted that compares unit prices for medical care in the United States versus Canada. One study, using data from the mid 1980s, found that the ratio of U.S. private insurance physician fees to those paid by the Canadian provinces averaged 2.4, with ratios exceeding 3.0 for surgery (Fuchs and Hahn 1990). Although Americans may be getting "more" for their fees, these considerable differences in fees may not reflect major differences in the quality of care delivered (an issue addressed below). Rather, differences in provider incomes are more likely. Physician incomes are far higher in the United States than elsewhere— almost twice as high as those of Canadian physicians, and more than twice as high as those in the other countries examined here (OECD 2001).

However, higher unit costs are not necessarily a reflection of waste; the services being priced might not be comparable in terms of quality. A day in the hospital in the United States, for example, might entail better quality or more desirable amenities than one in Canada. Similarly, U.S. physicians could produce more for their higher fees. This is why comparing quality and satisfaction across countries is so important; some comparative data on these outcomes are presented next.

Figure 6.1: Relationship Between National Wealth and Health Expenditures

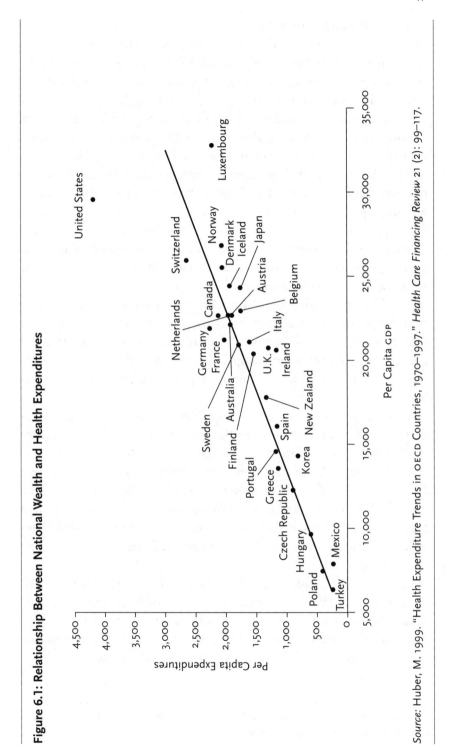

Source: Huber, M. 1999. "Health Expenditure Trends in OECD Countries, 1970–1997." *Health Care Financing Review* 21 (2): 99–117.

6.3.4 Quality and Satisfaction

In spite of the importance of quality to policy discussions on health system reform, very little cross-national information is available on the issue. The most common data that are available concern vital statistics such as life expectancy and infant mortality. Although extremely important, these figures are more reflective of sociodemographic conditions in a country rather than the quality of its medical care systems. Perhaps a better way of assessing quality across countries might be to *ask* individuals and physicians about their perceptions, although this obviously is subjective. Another flaw (as argued in Chapter 2) is that people's tastes are based on their experience, so perceptions are affected by what they are used to. Consequently, an even better way would be to conduct rigorous studies of important health outcomes across countries, controlling, as much as possible, for differences in population characteristics. Unfortunately, few such studies have been conducted.

Unlike quality, satisfaction is somewhat easier to evaluate across countries. Satisfaction is sometimes criticized, however, as being overly subjective and not targeted on aspects of quality that are of most interest to policymakers. Furthermore, compared to objective measures of quality, satisfaction measures based on survey responses are more prone to shift over time.

Beginning with the vital statistics, Table 6.10 shows average life expectancy and infant mortality rates for the ten countries. Life expectancy shows relatively little dispersion. Among the small differences, the averages are higher in Japan and lower in the United States than elsewhere.[18] A much greater difference, however, is found in infant mortality rates. Rates for Sweden (3.5) and Japan (3.6) are just half as high as the United States (7.2). The much higher infant mortality rates in the United States are due, in part, to lack of insurance and poorer living conditions among poorer residents.

Cross-national satisfaction surveys have been conducted among both individual residents and physicians. Tables 6.11 and 6.12 are from the same telephone survey of individuals in Australia, Canada, the United Kingdom, and the United States cited above in the section on access to care (Donelan et al. 1999). Table 6.11 focuses on overall satisfaction with the

---

18. The U.S. figures are also relatively low when one looks at life expectancy at age 40: it is tied for eighth among the ten countries for males, and ninth for females (OECD 2001).

Table 6.10: Life Expectancy and Infant Mortality Rates, 1998

	Life Expectancy at Birth (Years)	Infant Deaths per 1,000 Live Births
Australia	78.7	5.0
Canada*	78.6	5.5
France	78.4	4.6
Germany	77.5	4.7
Japan	80.6	3.6
Netherlands	78.0	5.2
Sweden	79.4	3.5
Switzerland	79.5	4.6
United Kingdom	77.3	5.8
United States	76.7	7.2

*Data for Canada are for 1997.
Source: OECD. 2001. "OECD Health Data 2001: A Comparative Analysis of 30 Countries." (OECD, Paris). Used with permission.

Table 6.11: Consumers' Views of their Health Services System, 1998*

	Australia	Canada	United Kingdom	United States
On the whole the system works pretty well, and only minor changes are necessary to make it work better	19	20	25	17
There are some good things in our healthcare system, but fundamental changes are needed to make it work better	49	56	58	46
Our healthcare system has so much wrong with it that we need to completely rebuild it	30	23	14	33

*Percentage of consumers that agree with the statements.
Source: Donelan, K., et al. 1999. "The Cost of Health System Change: Public Discontent in Five Nations." Health Affairs 18 (3): 206–16. Used with permission.

Table 6.12: Consumers' Views on Their Medical Care, 1998 (%)

	Australia	Canada	United Kingdom	United States
Medical care they and their family received in the past 12 months was				
Excellent	19	24	15	19
Very good	35	30	35	30
Good	31	30	31	33
Fair	11	11	12	12
Poor	2	2	2	3
Care received at last doctor visit was				
Excellent	36	37	19	29
Very good	32	30	37	30
Good	21	22	25	24
Fair	9	6	10	12
Poor	2	4	4	4
Length of most recent doctor visit was				
5 minutes or fewer	17	12	31	11
6–10 minutes	26	21	34	19
11–15 minutes	29	25	13	19
16–20 minutes	15	19	7	18
More than 20 minutes	12	20	5	30
Time their doctor spent with them was				
About right	84	82	78	74
Too short	13	15	14	23
Too long	2	2	2	1
Overall hospital experience was				
Excellent	27	28	28	26
Very good	30	26	34	28
Good	22	18	20	28
Fair	10	17	8	7
Poor	11	10	10	11
Length of their hospital stay was				
About right	73	72	77	78
Too short	17	19	11	12
Too long	9	8	12	10

Source: Donelan, K., et al. 1999. "The Cost of Health System Change: Public Discontent in Five Nations." *Health Affairs* 18 (3): 206–16. Used with permission.

system. In general, United Kingdom residents exhibit more satisfaction and less dissatisfaction than those in other countries, with Canada a clear second. The United States and Australia were the least satisfied, with almost one-third believing that the system needs to be completely rebuilt.

Table 6.12 focuses on consumers' views of the actual medical care that they receive. The first question concerns overall medical care, the next three, physician visits, and the last two, hospital stays. Consumers' views on overall medical care between the countries showed little difference. In all four countries, 49 percent to 54 percent rated care as excellent or very good, and 13 to 15 percent rated it as fair or poor. Similarly, the last two questions show almost no differences concerning overall satisfaction with the hospital experience and lengths of hospital stays. The main differences—which are, by and large, still relatively small—involve physician care. American and British respondents were slightly less favorable about their overall physician care than Australians and Canadians. More revealing are the data concerning length of visits. U.K. residents report considerably more short visits, and Americans far more long visits. But Americans are also much more likely than others to say that the time the doctor spent with them was too short. A clear difference in expectations is evident; this topic was discussed at some length in Chapter 2.

Another survey by some of the same authors, conducted in 2000, asked physicians (about 400 general practitioners and primary care physicians, and about 100 cardiologists, gastroenterologists, and oncologists per country) about their perceptions of care in these same countries (Blendon et al. 2001). Table 6.13 shows that physicians are far more likely than consumers to show cross-national differences in their views. The top half of the table examines physician perceptions that community resources are inadequate in six areas: medical and diagnostic equipment, hospital beds, general practitioners, specialists/consultants, home care, and long-term care and rehabilitation facilities. In all six areas, physicians from other countries perceive more inadequacy of resources than do U.S. physicians. In the case of hospital beds, only 12 percent of U.S. physicians find the supply inadequate, compared to 67 percent to 79 percent in the other countries. Among the other three countries, Canadian and U.K. physicians are more likely than Australians to note insufficient resources for several of the measures.

The second half of the table focuses on physicians' own practices. U.S. physicians are much less likely to express concerns about long waits for specialists or for surgical or hospital referrals. The largest difference is

Table 6.13: Generalist and Medical Specialist Physicians' Views on Problems in Health Services, 1998 (%)

	Australia	Canada	United Kingdom	United States
Inadequate Community Resources				
Latest medical and diagnostic equipment	13*	63*	47*	8
Hospital beds	67*	72*	79*	12
General practitioners	17	55*	44*	19
Medical specialists or consultants	30*	61*	62*	13
Home care	55*	60*	66*	24
Long-term care and rehabilitation facilities	74*	74*	81*	35
"Major Problem" for Their Own Medical Practices				
Limitations on hospital care	34	35	51*	38
Limits/long waits for specialist referrals	54*	66*	84*	27
Long waits for surgical or hospital care	66*	64*	77*	7
Limits in ordering diagnostic tests/procedures	9*	37*	30*	21
Patients can't afford necessary drugs	10*	17*	10*	48
Limitations on drugs one can prescribe	12*	17*	8*	41
External review of clinical decisions to control costs	21*	13*	19*	37
Not having enough time with patients	37	42	62*	42

*Statistically significant difference from the United States value at the 95 percent confidence level.
Source: Blendon, R. J., et al. 2001. "Physicians' Views on Quality of Care: A Five-Country Comparison." *Health Affairs* 20 (3): 233–43. Used with permission.

surgical or hospital care, where only 7 percent of U.S. physicians find this to be a major problem, compared to 64 percent to 77 percent of those in the other countries. In contrast, U.S. physicians are far more likely than others to cite as a major problem patient inability to afford necessary drugs, limitations on drugs they can prescribe, and external review of clinical decisions to control costs.

Finally, we move to more systematic reviews of objective quality across countries. Unfortunately, little information of this type has been published. The two studies noted below simply compare Canada and the United States.

Perhaps the most notable studies to date have been conducted by Roos et al. (1990), who have examined postsurgical mortality in the New England states versus Manitoba. The researchers divided procedures according to low, moderate, and high mortality, and looked at mortality rates 30 days, one year, and three years after surgery. After adjusting the best they could for case-mix differences, they found mortality rates to be lower in Manitoba for both low-risk and moderate-risk procedures, over all three time intervals. Thirty-day mortality rates were lower in New England for high-mortality procedures, but these differences subsided over time (Roos et al. 1992).

The second study examined cancer survival rates in the United States and in Ontario (U.S. GAO 1994). Specifically, it examined survival of a large sample of patients over the period between 1978 and 1990 for four types of cancer: breast, lung, colon, and Hodgkin's disease. In general, the study found similar survival rates for three of the cancers, but higher survival rates in the United States for breast cancer patients. Ten years after diagnosis, 65 percent of U.S. breast cancer patients were still alive, compared to 60 percent of Canadians. The study, however, was not able to determine whether the better survival rates in the United States were due to better outcomes or simply earlier detection, concluding that, "Until the effect on survival of differences in detection practices can be determined, the implications of these results for assessing quality of care in the two locations are unclear" (p. 5). In general, though, most experts believe that early detection does increase the chances of survival.

6.3.5 Equity of Financing System

Each of the cross-national outcomes measures shown above concerns the delivery of care—who has access to it, how much they use, how much it costs, and resulting effects on quality and satisfaction. Here we examine a different issue: the equity of the system used to finance this care. Fortunately, a set of studies addresses just this topic and covers seven of the ten countries considered in this chapter—all except Australia, Canada, and Japan (Wagstaff et al. 1999; van Doorslaer et al. 1999).

The authors first examine the sources for financing health services, dividing them into five types, the first three of which are public and the last two, private: direct taxes, indirect taxes, social insurance, private insurance, and direct payments. Direct taxes are those that are paid directly by the taxpayer (e.g., income, sales, or property taxes). Indirect taxes are those that are borne, but not paid directly, by the consumer (e.g., value-added or excise taxes). Social insurance is direct contribution to welfare or health programs (e.g., payroll taxes for the U.S. Medicare program). Private insurance is premium payments by enrollees, while direct payments are out-of-pocket costs when services are used.

Table 6.14 shows the distribution of financing sources by country, and indicates a large amount of cross-national variation. Only two of the countries, Switzerland and the United States, rely mostly on private funding sources. Both have relatively high portions paid directly by consumers of health services, although the figure for France is also high. The other five countries rely on public funding sources, predominantly taxes (Sweden and the United Kingdom) or social insurance payments (France, Germany, and the Netherlands).

The authors then sought to compare this information on the incidence of the financial burden of health services with income data from the countries to see whether these payments are regressive or progressive. If a system is progressive, then wealthier people will pay more than their share, and poorer people, less. They find that Switzerland and the United States have the most regressive systems, and the United Kingdom, the most progressive. France is mildly progressive, Sweden moderately regressive, and Germany and the Netherlands, somewhat more regressive (Wagstaff et al. 1999). One of the main reasons that Switzerland and the United States are so regressive is their reliance on private insurance and out-of-pocket costs—in effect, systems in which people pay their own way, with little in the form of cross-subsidization. Tax-based systems such as that in the United Kingdom tend to be more progressive because income tax rates are higher for wealthier people. The mixed findings for the countries relying mainly on social insurance are explained largely by the fact that in France (a progressive country) all workers participate in

Table 6.14: Sources of Funds for Health Sector Financing* (%)

	Direct Taxes	Indirect Taxes	Social Insurance	Private Insurance	Direct Payments
France	0	0	74	6	20
Germany	11	7	65	7	10
Netherlands	6	5	65	16	8
Sweden	64	8	18	0	10
Switzerland	24	5	7	41	24
United Kingdom	29	35	20	7	9
United States	28	7	13	29	22

*Data are from the most recent year available between 1987 to 1993, which varies by country.
Source: Reprinted from Wagstaff, A., et al. 1999. "Equity in the Finance of Health Care: Some Further Internatinal Comparisions." *Journal of Health Economics* 18 (3): 263–90. Copyright 1999, with permission from Elsevier Science.

the system, whereas in Germany and the Netherlands (regressive countries) many wealthier individuals opt out of the public system.

6.3.6 Summary of Evidence

The differences shown in the tables and discussion presented above cannot be easily summarized. Among ten countries, 45 comparisons of sets of two countries are possible. Some of the main findings (emphasizing differences between the United States and other countries) are:

- Access is both higher and lower in the United States, depending on how it is defined. On the negative side, more Americans say that they are prevented from obtaining needed medical services, in large measure because of costs. In contrast, access is better in the United States if one defines it in terms of waiting times for obtaining care.
- Overall hospital and physician usage rates are somewhat lower in the United States than in other countries, but rates are much higher for "high-tech" medical procedures. Similarly, the United States has far higher expenditures than other countries.

- Countries that rely on private insurance and out-of-pocket costs, such as the United States and Switzerland, have less equitable financing systems than others.
- Less information is available on quality and satisfaction across countries. With respect to quality, what little research is available indicates similar statistics in the United States and Canada. Consumer satisfaction rates are also relatively comparable among the four countries examined. Physicians in other countries, however, appear to be less satisfied with the adequacy of resources in their medical care systems than U.S. physicians, presumably because these countries do indeed have fewer financial resources devoted to their systems.

6.4 TEN "LESSONS" ON THE ROLE OF GOVERNMENT IN HEALTH SYSTEMS

Fair comparisons between market and nonmarket alternatives are extremely difficult to make. Because there is no generally applicable formula for choosing between them, the results of such comparisons often depend more on the predispositions of the evaluators than on their analyses.

   Charles Wolf, Jr. (1993, p. 117)

Being objective is indeed difficult when drawing conclusions about whether one country's health system is superior to another's. As discussed in Chapter 1, answers about which system is best inevitably are a matter of (informed, one would hope) opinion. Moreover—and as illustrated in Section 6.3 when attempting to compare system outcomes in different countries—good data are severely lacking. As a result, finding evidence that is convincing enough to dislodge a person from his or her preconceived viewpoints is challenging. Finally, and perhaps most important of all, different countries may not want the same things from their health systems. Some may want to emphasize access, others cost control, others efficiency over equity, and still others the opposite.

Because of these challenges, the ten lessons presented in this section should be considered most cautiously. They are based on the author's reading of cross-national literature; only a small amount of this literature could be presented in this chapter. Although many will disagree with the lessons, others may find them to be fairly noncontroversial and not particularly bold. If so, this is because the author believes that generalizing too much is dangerous: strategies that work in some countries often will not be successful if applied to others. Furthermore, each country's system has its strengths. The United States, for example, generally gets high marks for organizational innovation but does poorly with respect to equity, whereas the United Kingdom traditionally has had the opposite reputation. Nevertheless, the advantage of these inquiries is that countries have the potential to learn something from each other (Hsiao 1992). The United Kingdom experimented with a system of internal markets, in part to improve organizational innovation (although undoubtedly part of a larger drive by the Thatcher government to privatize more of the economy), while the United States is gradually trying to enfranchise the uninsured through such initiatives as the State Children's Health Insurance Program.

Unfortunately, some of the characteristics that make for a successful health system are not terribly transferable because of a number of impediments. To give one example, some (but certainly not all) analysts have concluded that parliamentary-style governments are less susceptible to regulatory capture than the presidential system used in the United States. In the former, individual legislators tend to have less influence because they need to "toe the party line," thus, efforts of special interests to influence a few selected legislators will tend to be less effective (Weaver and Rockman 1993; Reinhardt 1994). In contrast, U.S. legislators have more freedom to deviate from their parties and therefore may be more sought after by special interests. Another example is that regulatory capture is probably less likely when a cadre of dedicated, upper-management civil servants retain their positions after a change in government occurs— something that is truer in most other developed countries than in the United States. In both of these examples, there is little chance that the systems of one country could be imported to others; countries are entrenched either constitutionally or by long historic tradition. Little would be gained by turning these observations into lessons.

Finally, in several instances the literature shows little in the way of strong evidence to favor one health system choice over another. This ambivalence may be largely the result of a relatively immature set of reliable cross-national data, but also because, as noted above, different countries legitimately look for different things from their health systems. Even ignoring these problems for a moment, each of the following choices has convincing advantages and disadvantages: the advisability of a having government provide coverage directly versus overseeing its provision by private organizations (e.g., sickness funds); choosing whether to focus health system administration at the national versus local level; whether patients should be able to self-refer to specialists; whether primary care physicians should have hospital privileges; and what services should be covered under a universal coverage program.

Lesson 1: Health Services Coverage Should Be Universal

Section 6.2.1 listed the advantages and disadvantages of universal health services coverage. Six major advantages were noted, ranging from improving the health of the population to avoiding risk selection to reducing costs. The only disadvantage was that comprehensive coverage could result in the overuse of services, particularly those of marginal value.

However, many methods can address the problem of overuse and its resulting effect on expenditures within a framework of universal coverage. Much of Section 6.2 was devoted to various ways in which different countries have attempted to keep costs manageable. These techniques include coordinating provider reimbursements across payers to avoid cost shifting, moving away from fee-for-service toward capitated payments, instituting patient cost-sharing requirements, establishing global budgets and controls on the diffusion of expensive medical technologies, and controlling the supply of hospitals and physicians.

No one template is correct; different policies are used in different countries. The point is that all other developed countries have managed to provide universal coverage while at the same time keeping their expenditures far lower than those in the United States—a country in which more than 15 percent of the under-65 population is uninsured.

Lesson 2: Coverage Should Be Financed Primarily from Public Sources or Government-Ensured Social Insurance Using Progressive Revenue Sources

The equity of a country's health system is enhanced when revenues are generated from progressive sources. Although less progressive, some degree of equity is also maintained when everyone contributes a percentage of earnings to insurance pools. But equity is reduced when people must pay out-of-pocket for care, because this constitutes a larger proportion of income for poorer persons. Equity is also reduced when private, "actuarially fair" insurance exists—that is, when people pay their own way, reducing the amount of cross-subsidization from the wealthy to the less wealthy. Countries relying on private insurance and out-of-pocket costs, and those allowing wealthier people to opt out of government-ensured coverage programs, have less equitable financing systems.

Why should we care about the equity of a health financing system? The answer is somewhat philosophical and certainly open to debate: poorer people, who on average also tend to be in poorer health, should not be doubly disadvantaged by paying more if they need health services. Although individuals, no doubt, have some control over their health through their actions and behaviors, much illness is the result of random events, or of circumstances over which individuals have little control. Those who do incur illnesses and who cannot afford care should have care subsidized by those who are better off. Requiring the already financially disadvantaged to pay more of their scarce incomes when they get sick is, in the view of many, unfair. As noted by Robert Evans and colleagues:

> [P]eople pay taxes in rough proportion to their incomes, and use health care in rough proportion to their health status or need for care. The relationships are not exact, but in general sicker people use more health care, and richer people pay more taxes. It follows that when health care is paid for from taxes, people with higher incomes pay a larger share of the total cost; when it is paid for by the users, sick people pay a larger share. . . . Whether one is a gainer or loser, then, depends upon where one is located in the distribution of both income . . . and health. . . . In general, a shift to more user fee financing redistributes net income . . . from lower to higher income people, and from sicker to healthier people. The wealthy and healthy gain, the poor and sick lose. (Evans, Barer, and Stoddart 1993, p. 4)

A remedy is having revenues progressively based and largely unrelated to the actual usage of services.

Lesson 3: The Delivery of Services Can Be Carried Out Privately Under the Oversight of Government, Which Acts as a Purchaser of Services

Universal coverage does not mean public ownership or even control of a country's health system. Although certain countries—the United Kingdom is the most well-known example—rely more on the public owner-ship of health resources, this is not a necessary precondition. For instance, Canadian researchers often point out that almost all health resources in that country are privately owned. Thus, government can choose to purchase services rather than provide them directly.

This is sometimes called a "make-or-buy" decision (Preker, Harding, and Travis 2000). Although much of the attention on this topic has been from the literature on developing countries, the concept can be applied to developed countries as well. In most instances, government can purchase services from the private market, taking advantage of competition among producers of these inputs. This can result in fewer inefficiencies because of competition among the producers of these inputs (Preker, Harding, and Travis 2000; Wolf 1993; Vining and Weimer 1990).

How does government decide whether to produce health-related goods and services itself or purchase them in the marketplace? One determinant is the "contestability" of the private market that would produce the input—that is, the potential for competition among suppliers (Vining and Weimer 1990; Preker, Harding, and Travis 2000). If competition is likely, then government purchase of a good or service has advantages over government production. A second determinant is the "trustworthiness" of private suppliers, which is determined, in part, by the degree to which potential suppliers can act opportunistically. When would opportunism likely be a major problem? The answer to this question leads to a third determinant of whether government should produce or purchase— "measurability" (Preker, Harding, and Travis 2000). If the quality of the outputs produced by private suppliers can be measured more easily, then there is less room for opportunism and more for reliance on "buying" rather than "making." If, in contrast, the quality or quantity of inputs is hard to determine, then a stronger case for government control of the production process exists.

Thus, even if government has a strong role in a health system, competition can be used as a method of enhancing efficiency. Separating the purchaser from the providers encourages competition among the latter— as long as an adequate number of providers compete so as to avoid monopolization. Many developed countries are relying more on purchasing and less on producing health services. The United Kingdom, a country whose reputation has been one of strong national control, offers a good example. As noted above, as part of the "internal markets" reform movement, hospital services were purchased by district health authorities, and specialty services were purchased by primary care physician "fundholders." As the United Kingdom now moves away from the internal markets system, regional groups of primary care physicians are taking on expanded roles, purchasing specialty and other services for area residents (Enthoven 2000; Bindman and Weiner 2000).

Donald Light (2001b), who has written critically on the subject of more market domination in health systems, argues that enhancing government's role as purchaser holds several advantages. Government as purchaser can result in a greater focus on purchasing the types of services that enhance a population's health as well as greater accountability on part of providers. He writes,

> [W]e are in a transitional period of dislocation as we pass from providing medical services to purchasing for health gain. Thus, the enduring contribution of the managed competition policy movement is likely to be not so much competition per se but the transformation of state control from service administrator to strong purchaser or commissioner for evidence-based quality and health gain. That, it turns out, is what we have been wanting all along. (p. 1164)

Lesson 4: Emphasis Should Be Placed on Containing Costs Through Supply-Side Methods

Most countries focus their cost-containment efforts on suppliers of services rather than consumers. A number of supply-side cost-containment methods have been discussed in this chapter. These include global budgets, control of the diffusion of medical technologies, limits on the number of hospital beds and physicians, hospital and physician payment incentives, practice guidelines, and utilization review.

Supply-side methods have two main advantages over those aimed at the demand side. First, with respect to efficiency, informational problems often make demand-side policies less effective. For example, as noted in Chapter 3, consumers often do not respond to information about health plan quality by choosing more cost-effective plans. Second, unlike demand-side policies such as increased patient cost-sharing, those aimed at suppliers are not, by their nature, regressive (Ellis and McGuire 1993).

Supply-side approaches do have their problems, however. Several of the methods just noted, especially limits on technologies and hospital beds and funding, may result in long waits for services. Conversely, reliance on price—the key market mechanism—tends to result in shorter waits because services are rationed on ability to pay. If waits are too long, prices will increase, removing some from the waiting lists and thereby shortening queues.

Some countries, notably the United States, Germany, and France, report little in the way of waits for services (White 1995). In contrast, the systems of the United Kingdom and Canada have been criticized for long waits, particularly for elective surgery and diagnostic testing, and the data show evidence of waiting lists for care in Australia (Willcox 2001), Japan (White 1995), the Netherlands (Laeven 2001), and Sweden (Hanning 2001) (also see Table 6.7, above). Much research is currently being conducted in various countries on the extent of waits and ways in which they can be reduced. As yet, no consensus has been reached on how best to deal with the problem.

The problem of patients waiting to receive services is largely one of equating supply and demand, so health systems that do not rely on price rationing often (but not always) have longer waits. Nevertheless, waiting can be lessened under such systems by:

- Having a centralized information system that records waits throughout the system, allowing patients to be treated at more remote facilities when space is available
- Using such a system to alert payers and policymakers of bottlenecks, thus allowing additional capacity to be targeted to problem areas
- Providing financial inducements to hospitals and other facilities, as well as physician specialists, that are able to keep waiting time down
- Making reasonable waits, however defined, an explicit policy goal, and perhaps even a right of citizens

Lesson 5: Patient Cost-Sharing Requirements Should Be Kept Reasonably Low

Various parts of this book have stressed problems inherent in relying on patient cost-sharing. It has been argued, for example, that high patient cost-sharing dissuades patients from using useful as well as less useful services; discourages preventive care; may not be successful if providers respond by inducing demand; and is particularly difficult on lower-income persons, who, as it turns out, also tend to have more health problems.

Not surprisingly, some countries rely on user charges more than others. Table 6.14 showed that France, the United States, and Switzerland relied on them far more than Germany, the Netherlands, Sweden, and the United Kingdom. User charges also were relatively low in Canada, but appear to be higher in Australia and Japan (Yoshikawa and Bhattacharya 2002; White 1995). In addition, user charges for prescription drugs are common (except for the poor) in almost all countries as a way of stemming unnecessary prescribing and utilization. On the whole, those countries that rely more on user charges tend to have less progressive financing systems than others (Wagstaff et al. 1999).[19]

When cost-sharing is used, efforts should be made to insulate those who are least able to afford such payments. Fortunately, this is indeed the case in most countries. In the United States, for example, Medicaid beneficiaries are exempted from these requirements. In France, among those exempted from substantial cost-sharing requirements are those with low incomes, the unemployed, and the disabled (Costich 2002).

Lesson 6: To the Extent Possible, Payments to Providers Should Be Coordinated Among Payers

When multiple (as opposed to a single) payers for services contribute, a number of advantages can be achieved by coordinating payments—that is, having each payer provide the same amount. (This is a decidedly non-market approach; it is the antithesis of markets to explicitly coordinate payment.) These advantages include horizontal equity—all patients are worth the same to providers so they are more likely to be treated equally well; better potential to control costs; and related to this, the inability of providers to shift costs from one payer to another. As noted above, the main disadvantage is that all-payer rates do not allow higher-quality providers to distinguish themselves. Because of this, if a country wishes to provide financial incentives to enhance quality, it needs to find other ways to reward providers. All together, however, little evidence indicates that providers in all-payer and single-payer countries provide poorer care than those in other countries.

According to Abel-Smith (1992), all-payer systems have been quite successful. He writes:

---

19. The one exception is France, which Wagstaff et al. (1999) found to be mildly progressive. In their study, progressivity was determined not only by out-of-pocket costs but by whether premiums were collected from all workers (as is the case in France) or alternatively, whether individuals can opt out of the system (as is the case in Germany and the Netherlands).

> The key to Europe's success [in controlling costs] is the use of monop-
> sony power whereby one purchaser dominates the market, and not
> just the hospital market. Where there are many purchasers, as in Ger-
> many, they are forced to act together. Because the insurers are not
> allowed more revenue, either from tax or contributions, and because
> what they can charge the insured in copayments is centrally deter-
> mined, they are forced either to confront providers or to ration their
> allowable resources. In most countries this does not lead to lines of
> patients waiting for treatment. (p. 414)

Another advantage is that pricing regulations tend to be less intrusive
than those aimed at controlling quantities.

Some countries, notably Australia, Germany, and the Netherlands, do
allow wealthier individuals to opt out of the public system by purchasing private coverage. As a result, these patients tend to be worth more to
providers and are likely to get favorable treatment. One key to preserving
support of the public system is to keep the proportion of the population
opting out of the public plan reasonably low. If too many people opt
out of the public system, there will be more inequality of treatment by
providers, as well as less cross-subsidization since people tend to pay their
own way when they have private insurance. The question, according to
James Morone (2000) is, "Will people continue to see themselves as citizens, as members of a shared community? Or will they turn into shoppers
looking for their own best deal?" (p. 967). Answers to these questions are
key to whether developed countries can keep their systems of solidarity
intact.

Lesson 7: Countries Should Proceed with Caution in Providing Consumers a Choice of Insurer

As part of the "consumer revolution" in the health services area, choice
has become a key buzzword. Economists usually consider more choice to
be highly desirable, but consumers can be given many types of choices.
Examples include whether to have universal coverage or allow individuals to choose whether or not to purchase coverage, whether to assign
an insurer or permit consumers to choose among them; whether patients
can go to any provider they like; and the extent to which patients are able
choose to obtain whichever medical services they like (Rice 2001).

From this list, perhaps the choice that has received the most attention
of late is whether consumers should have a choice among health insurers.

Until recently, most countries did not allow such a choice. Consumers received coverage through their national or regional public plan, or through a particular sickness fund to which they were assigned. The United States has been an exception; most working-age consumers have had a choice of health plans for many years.

As noted above, some European countries have begun to offer a choice of health plans as well. In general, these countries have found that it is necessary to proceed slowly. Some of the adverse consequences experienced have included:

- Insurers competing for healthier patients, in large measure because of difficulties involved in risk adjusting health insurance premiums (van Doorslaer and Schut 2000; Zweifel 2000)
- Consumer difficulties in obtaining and using comparative information on plan performance (van Doorslaer and Schut 2000)
- Greater monopolization in the hospital and physician markets (Light 2001b)
- Political difficulties as the perception grows that government is moving away from a system of solidarity (Morone 2000; Pfaff and Wassener 2000)

This is not to say that the movement toward providing a choice of insurers is necessarily undesirable. Rather, countries should proceed cautiously because the potential for experiencing these problems—and probably others—is increased when a choice of health plans is offered to consumers.

Lesson 8: Fee-for-Service Payment Should Be Re-evaluated

Another trend among developed countries is the gradual movement away from fee-for-service medicine. Fee-for-service does have one major advantage—in most cases it gives providers an incentive to provide a sufficient quantity and intensity of services. The other side of the coin, however, is that too many services may be provided, potentially compromising quality and making it more difficult to control expenditures.

This trend is perhaps most obvious in Europe. Even in Canada, a country known for its total reliance on fee-for-service for physician payment, a movement away from the practice may be afoot. In an interview conducted in 2000, Canada's Minister of Health, Allan Rock, stated that:

If we're going to keep Canada's public health care system, primary health care reform—moving away from fee-for-service as the standard form of remuneration—has to occur. I'm encouraged by movement in that direction. . . . [T]here is now growing support for a rostered approach to primary care, delivered to a defined population by a team of family doctors. . . . This includes . . . a method of payment for a physician that is other than fee-for-service. . . . More and more of the provinces seem to be moving toward negotiating for this type of care approach as they sit down with their medical associations to work out compensation arrangements for the coming years. (Iglehart 2000b, pp. 136–37)

This movement away from fee-for-service is not isolated, but is part of a larger one related to the establishment of regional budgets for the health services provided to a population (particularly in Europe). These budgets are capitated, in that regions receive a fixed amount of medical resources per service. This should not be construed as implying that providers are paid on a capitation basis; in some places they are, and in others, they are not. Within that context, Nigel Rice and Peter Smith (2001) write:

Capitation is, without doubt, here to stay. There is a remarkable degree of agreement that—whatever the structure of the health care system—a policy of cost containment and devolved responsibility for health care requires setting prospective budgets on the basis of capitation payments. The question is therefore not *whether* to set capitations, but *how* to do so. (p. 107)

Interestingly, this trend appears to exist both in countries that are moving toward markets as well as those that are not.

Lesson 9: Government Should Fund Impartial Research and Analysis on Health System Performance

No country's health system is ideal; reforms have the potential for improving efficiency and equity. Moreover, because of changes in medical technology, demographics, the economic environment, and even people's tastes, a static system will tend to be unresponsive.

In most areas of the economy, markets tend to be relatively efficient in terms of the distribution of information regarding prices and quality.

However, as discussed throughout this book, researchers have found that information problems are often severe in the health services area. Individuals have trouble determining such things as the most appropriate health plan when they have a choice of insurer, the best provider given their needs and associated costs, and even whether to seek care in the first place. Therefore, compelling reasons exist as to why the government should play a strong role in monitoring population health and the quality, financing, access, and outcomes of the health services system.

Most countries already invest resources into areas where private companies have either less incentive to conduct research (as in the case of monitoring the prevalence of disease in the population), or where the payoffs are uncertain (as in the case of basic medical research). Nevertheless, these activities are essential. Moreover, the quality of policymaking is improved when sophisticated, impartial analyses of alternative policy options are available and rigorous research of the state of the system is available. Research generated by private for-profit organizations (e.g., prescription drug companies), although oftentimes useful, is obviously of concern because of the potential of bias. Even if objective researchers carry out the work, concern remains that only projects likely to result in benefits to the funding organization will be carried out in the first place. Government should therefore play a major role in the funding of such research.

In this respect, the United States seems to perform very well compared to other countries. In addition to funding basic clinical medical research that results in new pharmaceutical and technological breakthroughs, a number of government agencies fund universities and research firms to conduct a great deal of health services research. To give a single example, because government has invested heavily in research, we know the true number of the uninsured in the United States. Especially notable is the Agency for Healthcare Research and Quality, which funds research concerning quality and efficiency in the health sector. But other agencies, such as the Centers for Medicare & Medicaid Studies (formerly, Health Care Financing Administration), as well as the Centers for Disease Control and Prevention; the National Library of Medicine; the Veterans Administration; and the National Institutes of Mental Health, Drug Abuse, and Alcohol Abuse and Alcoholism also provide critical data and analyses of these issues. In 2000 these agencies received almost $3 billion (U.S.) in federal funding (Association for Health Services Research 2000). Not all of it went to health services research, but it is safe to say that almost $1 billion did.[20]

One problem, of course, is that most of this research is focused on the U.S. setting, although often the results of publicly funded U.S. health services research are applied to other national settings, as in the case of the lessons of the RAND Health Insurance Experiment. Other countries should invest in their own research to solve problems particular to their citizens and systems. While investing domestically in research, countries should also share information through institutions such as the OECD, the World Bank, and the WHO to facilitate reliable cross-national comparisons of health systems.

Research and analysis of health systems is not necessarily easy, since some of the major barriers to good research and analysis are political and financial. Health services research is costly and requires a longer-term commitment to establishing systems and organizations of data collection and analysis, without an immediate payoff. Research may not be in the political interest of governments. Government might *claim* that it wants impartial information on the inputs and outputs of a national health system, but the actual process of scrutiny often reveals flaws that are embarrassing to a country's health leadership or even an entire government. A further problem is that the ruling parties in certain countries are reluctant to fund studies that might reach conclusions that are inconsistent with their philosophies and party platforms. This is unfortunate because it makes the development of appropriate reform policies a "data-free" exercise.

Adequate funding of health services research through independent or depoliticized government agencies is essential for improving the efficiency and equity of health systems.

---

20. The U.S. Congress requires that 15 percent of funds from the National Institutes of Health be spent on health services research. The four institutes noted had budgets of $2.17 billion, so a minimum of $325 million was devoted to health services research. Adding that to the budgets for the Agency for Healthcare Quality and Research ($204 million), the Centers for Disease Control's National Center for Health Statistics ($110 million), and the research budget of the Centers for Medicare & Medicaid Studies ($62 million) results in $700 million. This does not count the health services research conducted by the Veterans Administration, whose research budget exceeded $300 million.

Lesson 10: Government Failure Is Not Necessarily a Greater Problem than Market Failure in the Health Services Sector

The first section of this chapter focused on government failure in general, and regulatory capture in particular. This was appropriate because the previous chapters of the book concentrated on problems with markets. Government involvement in the health system is subject to its own set of problems.

The issue, of course, is not whether countries should use markets *or* government to organize, deliver, and finance health services, but rather, how to determine the roles played by each and the balance between them. This chapter has discussed the various choices that countries must make concerning this balance and presented some evidence that indicates— albeit quite inexactly—the relative success that ten countries have had.

Can this evidence presented earlier indicate what is the most successful balance between markets and government? Unfortunately, the answer is "no." At least four reasons contribute to this.

1. Different countries may not want the same things from their health systems. Some may want to emphasize access, others cost control, others efficiency over equity, and still others the opposite. More-over, historical and cultural factors are critical determinants of how different countries' health services systems have developed, making it risky to suggest that any one country's system be replicated by others.

2. Creating an agreed-on set of weights among the different outcomes would probably be impossible. How does one weigh, for example, the short waits (a characteristic of the U.S. system) against the eq-uity of health system financing (a characteristic of the U.K. system)?

3. Characterizing countries according to the reliance of each on markets versus government is difficult. Germany offers a good ex-ample. Although government involvement in health services financ-ing (which is largely left up to the sickness funds) is not explicit, a great deal of government oversight and direction occurs, particularly on the supply side. Further complicating matters is that countries' health systems change, sometimes fairly rapidly. Both the United Kingdom and the Netherlands, for example, went from fairly non-marketlike systems to ones relying much more on competition, after which each stepped back from the market somewhat.

4. Although cross-national measures of access and costs are reasonably good, little is known about the quality of care provided in different countries.

The first part of the first point is perhaps most important: different countries emphasize different objectives. This makes it almost impossible to say that one country has a better system than another. With that in mind, it is probably safe to say that developed countries with near universal coverage do a better job than the United States in ensuring that mainstream medical care can be accessed when a person has a medical need for it. Although much attention has focused on waiting times in some of these countries, long waits are almost always for elective procedures. Regarding efficiency, the United States provides excellent care to most of those with health insurance, but also at a cost far higher than any other country. As a result, generalizing about efficiency is difficult since this efficiency is properly viewed as the system's outputs in relation to the inputs expended. In conclusion then, to the extent that the U.S. system is most subject to market failure and other countries' systems, to government failure, little can be concluded about the relative susceptibility of health systems to market versus government failure.

Chapter 7

Conclusion

THE THEME OF this book has been much different from that of other health economics texts. Other texts generally accept that, without strong evidence to the contrary, relying on market competition will result in the best outcomes—at least with regard to efficiency. For example, one book that this author regards highly notes:

> The use of our economic tools may lead to predictions that turn out to be different than what we observe. . . . When predictions differ from what we observe . . . , it does not mean that the theory is wrong or not useful. Instead, it is an indication that one or more of the assumptions underlying the theory have been violated. . . . When the underlying assumptions are different from what is expected, there is a possible role for public policy. (Feldstein 1988, pp. 593–94)

This statement would appear—at least to most economists—to be eminently reasonable. Since economic theory shows that market competition will lead to Pareto-optimal outcomes, why not allow market forces to operate unencumbered by government interference, unless we have solid evidence that such intervention will result in better outcomes?

This book has taken (and justified, we hope) an entirely different approach. To understand this approach, it is necessary to give close consideration to the above quotation. Feldstein indeed allows for a role for government but *only* if we observe that the predictions of economic theory differ from our observations. In particular:

• The onus is on those who would contend that market forces will not result in the best outcomes.

• To justify government involvement, it is necessary to demonstrate that reality differs from the predictions of the theory.

One of the main themes of this book is that the viewpoint expressed by Feldstein, which pervades economic thought, is not the right way to approach the study of health economics and the formulation of health policy. There is no reason for supposing that a competitive marketplace will result in superior outcomes in the health area, so it is not necessary to demonstrate that market outcomes from the operation of a hypothetical competitive market will be different from what theory would predict.

Why is there no reason to believe that a competitive marketplace will result in the best outcomes? Because such a conclusion is based on many strong assumptions being met. This book examined over a dozen of the assumptions that need to be fulfilled to ensure that a free market results in the best outcomes for society; none of them were even close to being met in the health services. If these assumptions are not met, economic theory provides no basis for assuming the superiority of competitive approaches. Thus, the burden of proof should not fall on those who profess the superiority of alternative approaches.

To clarify this point, suppose a country is confronting a very important health policy decision: whether to enact limits on how much it will spend each year on health-related goods and services. The above quotation implies that such a policy should be considered only if costs under a truly competitive marketplace are higher than would be predicted by theory. But even if true, this would be very difficult to demonstrate because it involves trying to answer a "counterfactual"[1] question: how much would a perfectly competitive market spend on health services? Because an answer to this question is hardly obvious and would be the subject of much dispute, the above mindset makes it nearly impossible to justify most government involvement in health.

A better approach to policymaking does not put the burden of proof on those believing that government intervention is justified. Rather, all alternative policies being considered would start on an equal basis. Then, empirical evidence would be gathered to determine the likely effect of each alternative. In the global budget example, one would need to predict the effect of enacting (versus not enacting) such a policy on costs, quality

---

1. See Section 3.2.2 for a further discussion of counterfactual questions.

and outcomes, people's waiting time, and so on, and then weigh these various effects together to determine which policy is likely to be superior. Such an analysis might find that global budgets are not a good idea—but such a conclusion would be reached after, not before, conducting the research. Competitive (i.e., noninterventionist) approaches would not be *presumed* superior.

This distinction in approach may seem niggling to some, but it turns out to be fundamental. Viewing competition as just one possible policy alternative, instead of the presumed superior policy, opens up any number of possible policies that could indeed show themselves to be superior. Many such examples were given throughout the book; they are discussed in Section 4.3, which provides a number of possible supply-side interventions. Furthermore, one of the main conclusions of Chapter 6 was that when the empirical evidence is considered, one *cannot* draw the conclusion that a market-based system (to which the United States comes closest) actually performs better than those in other countries when resource expenditures are considered—not only from an equity standpoint, but with respect to efficiency as well.

In the conventional model, very few levers are actually available to policymakers who are interested in health services. Because such a model is driven by consumer demand, the primary tools involve influencing demand, either by changing out-of-pocket price, or by providing additional information to consumers. Influencing supply is not an option because the model presumes that suppliers will simply produce those things that are demanded.

What we see in health policy throughout the world, however, is the reliance instead on supply-side policies. These include such policy tools as capitation, DRGs, utilization review, practice guidelines, technology controls, and global budgets—just to name a few. None of these policies arise from the competitive model, nor would any be shown by economic theory to result in superior outcomes. Nevertheless, most countries rely on them, and many analysts would argue that these supply-side policies have resulted in superior outcomes in the health services marketplace.

Determining which policies are indeed superior, however that may be defined, is a challenging task. The answers, of course, will vary depending on the particular circumstances (e.g., the disease, the population group, the country). Health services and health policy researchers throughout the world are key participants in this undertaking and provide critically important information. But to prescribe the best possible set of policy options, these researchers must employ tools that expand rather than narrow this set of options.

The challenges facing health policymakers—to ensure that costs are kept manageable and quality remains acceptable in a world of limited budgets but expanding technological capabilities—are daunting. New and innovative ideas are essential. If analysts misinterpret economic theory as applied to health—by assuming that market forces are necessarily superior to alternative policies—then they will blind themselves to policy options that might actually be better at enhancing social welfare.

Appendix: Overview of the Health Services Systems in Ten Developed Countries

Miriam J. Laugesen[1] and Thomas Rice

AUSTRALIA

All Australian citizens and permanent residents are covered by Australia's national health insurance program, called Medicare. The Medicare program provides comprehensive coverage, including primary care, hospital care, and pharmaceuticals. Responsibility for the health service is shared between federal and six state governments.

In 1998 Australia spent $2,085 (U.S.) per person on health, which was 8.6 percent of its GDP. Seventy percent of this expenditure was financed by the public sector, 7.9 percent by private insurers, and 16.2 percent by individuals' out-of-pocket expenditures (OECD 2001).

The Federal (Commonwealth) Government finances 47 percent of total health expenditure and exerts considerable influence over the health sector through its financial grants to states and territories, regulation of private insurers, direct financial grants to organizations providing health services, and national priorities and programs (Hall 1999). The federal government also finances and regulates pharmaceuticals and long-term care, and makes grants to various organizations for major capital

---

1. Miriam J. Laugesen was, at the time of writing, a RAND-UCLA postdoctoral trainee in the Department of Health Services at the UCLA School of Public Health. She received training in health policy at Harvard University and she received her Ph.D. in political science from the University of Melbourne, Australia, in December 2000. Her dissertation examined successive episodes of health system reform in New Zealand. Dr. Laugesen's research is focused on the political actors and institutions that shape the organization and financing of health services, as applied to physician payment policy and health sector reform processes.

equipment, rural health services, Aboriginal health, and mental health services.

Australia's six state governments spend around 20 percent of national health expenditures. The states' major responsibility in health is for acute and psychiatric services, although they also regulate health professionals. The federal government and the states negotiate five-year funding contracts that establish the obligations of the federal government and state governments.

Historically, private and government roles in the Australian health system have oscillated between systems of public and private insurance and between systems of free and fee-based and means-tested hospital care (Gray 1996). Private health insurers operate as an additional option to Medicare rather than as an alternative payer for health services (Commonwealth Department of Health and Aged Care 1999a). Private insurance accounted for just 7.9 percent of health expenditure in 1998 (OECD 2001), although around 30 percent of Australians are enrolled in private health insurance. The role of private insurance is essentially to provide patients the choice of their physician in a hospital, faster access to hospital treatment, and greater privacy and comfort while in hospital. Various policies introduced between 1999 and 2001 suggest that the federal government may increase its role in financing health services while also encouraging increased enrollment in private insurance.

Private health insurance enrollment declined in the 1990s. As a result, in the late 1990s the government introduced policies—especially premium rebates—to encourage enrollment in private health insurance. Individuals receive a 30 percent rebate for premiums paid for private health insurance. Early statistics released in 1999 suggested the rebate was encouraging enrollment (Commonwealth Department of Health and Aged Care 1999b), although Hall (1999) suggests it was also allowing insurers to increase premiums.

The federal government uses its regulatory influence to correct various market failures in the insurance market, including regulating the prices of premiums and the benefits that insurers can offer. Insurers are required to have financial reserves and to fund a consumer-complaints bureau. Controls have been placed on contracting between private health insurers and hospitals (Commonwealth Department of Health and Aged Care 1999a). Private health insurers are prohibited from charging fees based on risk, and are required to provide community rating, or uniform insurance premiums, to all enrollees. A reinsurance system transfers funds from insurers with a low proportion of claims relating to aged and chronically ill members to insurers with a high proportion of such claims (Commonwealth Department of Health and Aged Care 1999a).

In 2000 the Australian government introduced a policy to encourage enrollees to remain insured over their lifetime. The government was concerned that individuals were buying insurance when they needed hospital care and then canceling it after they received treatment. The young and healthy have few incentives to buy insurance. The new policy, called Lifetime Cover, allows insurers to charge a late-entry fee for people who buy insurance for the first time over 30. The late-entry fee is 2 percent of the premium and applies for each year a member is aged above 30 when he or she first buys hospital coverage. Individuals who purchased hospital coverage before age 31 after July 2000, and who remain enrolled, pay less than first-time enrollees over the age of 30 after July 2000. Individuals can switch between insurers, but if they are without insurance for a defined period they lose their lifetime coverage status. A 50 year old will pay 40 percent over the base rate premium, up to a maximum loading of 70 percent, which applies to those aged over 65.

Hospital care perhaps best demonstrates the Australian mix of public-private roles. Australia has a free public hospital system managed by the states, while Medicare also subsidizes physician fees in private hospitals. Public hospitals provide quality care at no cost to the patient, but the public hospital system does not provide immediate access for nonurgent surgery or treatment, or choice of physician. In 1999, 17 percent of Australians surveyed said they had to wait more than four months for nonemergency surgery (see Table 6.7 in Chapter 6). Nevertheless, Australians are split on how serious the waiting times are, with only 25 percent "very worried" about waiting too long and 28 percent suggesting they are "somewhat worried." Almost half of respondents surveyed said they were "not too worried" about waiting for nonemergency care (see Table 6.6).

Individuals can receive "private" hospital treatment in public hospitals (as well as in private hospitals) and receive faster treatment and can choose their physician. Medicare covers 75 percent of the physician fee schedule amount for private hospital treatment. Private insurers or individuals pay the remaining 25 percent of the fee schedule amount. Often, patients treated privately pay high out-of-pocket charges for hospital treatment because no price regulation of physician fees above the fee schedule exists. Physicians can charge any fee in excess of the schedule fee. The federal government has recently introduced a policy called "Closing the Gap" to allow some insurers to offer policies that will cover the gap between the Medicare fee schedule benefit and the actual physician charge. Insurers can only offer "gap cover schemes" by agreement with Medicare.

In the nonhospital sector, private insurance has a lesser role and Medicare a more significant role, partly because of regulations limiting private insurance coverage for outpatient physician services. Medicare covers physicians, optometrists, and some dental surgery services in full or in part. Medicare pays for specialist treatment referred through a gatekeeper physician. Physicians are paid on a fee-for-service basis and patients can choose their own physician. As in the U.S. Medicare system, Australia uses a fee schedule to pay its providers, which lists fee amounts and benefits for medical services. Unlike the U.S. Medicare fee schedule, Medicare payments in Australia are sometimes less than 100 percent of the fee schedule. For example, an outpatient physician consultation is paid at 85 percent of the fee schedule. Around 80 percent of medical services are billed at or below the official fee schedule (Commonwealth Department of Health and Aged Care 2000).

Primary care services are largely free for patients as a result of government incentives for limiting out-of-pocket charges to patients. Primary care physicians are encouraged to bill Medicare directly for services (through a system known as "bulk billing") rather than billing patients. Bulk billing offers advantages for physicians, who are ensured payment for their services, while the system also reduces out-of-pocket costs for patients. A provider who is billing Medicare directly cannot charge patients additional fees. Around 70 percent of services for which Medicare benefits are paid are bulk billed and are therefore free to the patient (Commonwealth Department of Health and Aged Care 2000). Patients receiving care from providers who are not bulk billing are likely to pay higher out-of-pocket costs, because Commonwealth law does not restrict the fee physicians charge. Private insurers cannot offer coverage for the difference between the schedule and the fee paid.

Cost-sharing for health services in Australia accounted for around 16 percent of national health expenditure throughout the 1990s (OECD 2001). Cost-sharing is generally limited to copayments on prescribed medicines, private hospital care, and some noncovered services out of hospital. Welfare beneficiaries, the elderly, veterans, and low-income patients are eligible for reduced copayments, and an annual safety-net deductible limits the total amount of out-of-pocket charges. After the deductible amount is met, patients pay reduced copayments or no co-payments, depending on their eligibility status.

Medicare is funded by general tax revenue and a compulsory 1.5 percent levy on taxable income for taxpayers above defined income thresholds. The Medicare levy contributes just over a third of the revenue for Medicare. Higher income earners pay an additional 1 percent levy. Higher earning taxpayers are exempt from the additional 1 percent levy if they purchase private insurance (Commonwealth Department of Health and Aged Care 2000).

CANADA

Canada provides universal coverage for all medically necessary hospital and physician services. Because of its proximity to the United States, Canada's healthcare system is frequently compared and contrasted with the United States. Total per person health expenditure was $2,360 (U.S.) in 1998, a little more than half of the United States per person expenditure. Measured as a proportion of GDP, Canada's total health expenditure was 9.3 percent of GDP, compared with the U.S. level of 12.9 percent. The majority of health expenditures are financed from the public sector (70.1 percent), 11 percent by private heath insurance, and 16.6 percent from individuals' out-of-pocket payments.

As in most federal systems, financing and responsibility for health services is divided between provinces and territories (13 total, referred to as provinces below) and the federal government. Each province administers its own system, but these provincial systems comply with national standards set out in the country's main governing legislation, the Canada Health Act. The federal government can influence the provincial systems because it helps fund them and withholds a portion of funds from provinces that do not comply with the standards. Federal contributions have fallen in recent years, however, and constitute just 23 percent of total provincial expenditures, down from 45 percent in 1980 (Iglehart 2000a).

The Act stipulates that five standards must be met for each province to receive the maximum federal contribution (Canada Health Act Overview 2001):

1. Public administration—the system must be "administered and operated on a nonprofit basis by a public authority";
2. Comprehensiveness—the system must cover all necessary hospital and physician services;

3. Universality—all residents must be covered;
4. Portability—seamless coverage is provided when a person moves between provinces, and urgent care is covered when traveling outside of the country; and
5. Accessibility—there can be no unreasonable impediments to obtaining covered services such as user charges or extra billing by physicians.

The Canadian provinces have the reputation of having "single-payer systems," and this is true for services governed by the Canada Health Act. The provinces finance 92 percent of hospital payments and 98.5 percent of physician reimbursements. This prevents providers from "shifting" costs or charges between payers and gives provinces a great deal of leverage in negotiations with providers.

A number of services are not included in the Canada Health Act. Provinces cover these services only at their discretion, including outpatient prescription drugs (inpatient drugs are covered by hospital budgets), dental care, and home care services. Provinces provide coverage for outpatient prescription drugs for selected population groups, generally those on social assistance (the poor) and the elderly, usually with some patient cost-sharing required. Some provinces also provide drug coverage to the general population, but there tend to be substantial cost-sharing requirements. Dental coverage is provided mainly for poor persons (Goldsmith 2002).

Unlike in many other countries, private health insurance coverage for services that are covered by the provinces is either explicitly prohibited or restricted so heavily as to make it not economically viable to offer. Consequently, private insurance for hospital and physician services is not available. Such coverage is prevalent, however, for other care (e.g., drugs, dentistry, optometrist services), with about two-thirds of the population having some form of supplemental private insurance (Smee 1997). Premiums are sometimes subsidized by employers as part of a fringe benefit package, or are paid out-of-pocket by consumers.

Almost all hospitals are nonprofit. They are paid a global budget for their operating expenses. Historically, hospitals negotiated their budgets with provincial governments, but increasingly, regional health authorities in provinces such as British Columbia, Saskatchewan, and Alberta are responsible for determining the budgets for hospitals in their area. Global budgets have given hospitals strong incentives to keep down operating expenses, most of which are labor related. In that regard, one study for the 1980s found that the United States employed twice as many hospital employees per filled hospital bed compared to Ontario (Newhouse, Anderson, and Roos 1988). Data from 1998 indicate that total hospital employment per 1,000 population is 42 percent higher in the United States than Canada. In contrast, provinces fund most capital expenditure, including expensive medical equipment. In general, provinces need to approve such expenditures by hospitals, irrespective of the source of funding, or they will not be covered under the global budget. In most provinces, this has resulted in less diffusion of such equipment compared to many other countries (see Table 6.2).

Most physicians work outside of hospitals and do not have hospital privileges (White 1995). In general, they are also responsible for specialist referrals (Goldsmith 2002; White 1995). Physicians tend to practice privately and are paid on a fee-for-service basis. Little managed care exists in Canada, although some government officials would like to see a movement in that direction (Iglehart 2000b). Relative fee levels are established by the medical profession, with conversion factors (i.e., actual payment levels) determined mainly by the provinces.

Canadian provincial governments were able to use their monopsonistic power as purchasers to influence physician reimbursement rates during the 1990s. Constrained by low economic growth rates over a 20-year period, physician fees in Canada fell about 60 percent relative to those in the United States (White 1995). However, because fees were low and provinces were the only payers, physicians had a built-in financial incentive to "induce demand." As a result of this, as well as economic pressures faced by provinces, most provinces enacted systems of expenditure caps. As of the mid 1990s eight of the ten provinces had established "hard" caps in which fees are reduced in proportion to the degree to which the caps are exceeded. In addition, five of the ten had, as of the mid 1990s, adopted some form of individual income cap as well. Typically, this entailed reducing unit fees after a physician exceeded a certain income threshold (Lomas et al. 1996). Provinces also tried to control the supply of physicians by controlling medical school enrollment and, in some instances, restricting immigration of physicians from other provinces into areas that already have a high density of physicians (Goldsmith 2002).

The policies of the 1990s to restrict payments and to limit the number of physicians who were trained have been modified. Many provinces revised the expenditure cap policies substantially because of the political difficulties of imposing the expenditure caps on physicians. Restrictions on physician training were relaxed.

Health services are financed by a variety of sources. These include federal, provincial, and municipal taxes paid by individuals and corporations; employer payroll taxes and/or direct premiums paid by consumers in selected provinces; other government taxes; premiums paid by employers and individuals for services not covered by the provinces; and out-of-pocket costs for these services. The proportion of total expenditures paid from public sources declined in recent years because the cost of non–publicly covered services has increased faster than other costs, in part because of budget cutting by provinces (Goldsmith 2002; Evans 2000). However, since 1997 the proportion of total health expenditure financed by the public has increased relative to the private sector share.

FRANCE

The French population is almost universally covered by health insurance (Assurance-maladie), which is largely organized on the basis of professional sectors in the labor market. The national health insurance program is funded by employers and employees through a payroll tax. A second form of comprehensive universal coverage known as CMU (Couverture médicale universelle), which has been operating since 2000, covers the poor, those without stable employment, and legal migrants without coverage (Imai, Jacobzone, and Lenain 2000). Previously, 300,000 persons were without insurance in 1999 (Poullier and Sandier 2000; Lancry and Sandier 1999). The scheme enables beneficiaries to avoid high coinsurance costs and avoid paying point-of-service charges, since payments are made directly by this fund (Costich 2002). Illegal immigrants do not have access to health insurance (WHO 1997).

The French health system aims to balance freedom of choice with principles of social solidarity. Some analysts have described it as a hybrid Bismarckian-Beveridge system (Poullier and Sandier 2000). Total per person health expenditure was $2,043 (U.S.) in 1998 and healthcare expenditure was 9.4 percent of GDP. Almost 78 percent (77.7 percent) of health expenditure was financed by the public sector, including the 73.7 percent of health expenditure that was financed by social insurance schemes in 1998. The OECD regards social insurance expenditure in all countries as public expenditure. Private insurance financed 12.5 percent of health expenditure and individuals financed 10.2 percent of health expenditure in 1998.

The national government regulates the expenditure and distribution of hospital services and the price of pharmaceuticals and medical fees, and determines the level of financing for public hospitals (Poullier and Sandier 2000). In recent years, central government has sought more control over health expenditure through a national global budget target. Under the 1996 Juppé Plan, the French parliament adopted an annual national health expenditure target for physician, prescription, public hospital, and private clinical expenditures (Imai, Jacobzone, and Lenain 2000). The effectiveness of this measure is questionable, since total reimbursements are not capped. Increasing emphasis is also placed on national health priorities through such mechanisms as the National Health Congress (Conférence nationale de santé), which is a representative body that develops annual health policy priorities (High Committee on Public Health 1998). The government is also making efforts to assess the effectiveness of reimbursed services (Blanchard 2001).

Regional levels of the health system gained new responsibilities in the 1990s and devolution is increasing (High Committee on Public Health 1998). Regional hospitalization agencies (agences regionales hospitalieres) distribute global budgets and coordinate regional health services (Costich 2002) and work with the regional sickness funds. In principle, these agencies are behaving like regional health purchasers (Imai, Jacobzone, and Lenain 2000). These authorities are managed by directors who are appointed by the cabinet (WHO 1997). There are also 16 regional branches of the National Health Insurance Agency (Caisses régionales d'assurance maladie or CRAM), which are responsible for insurance enrollment and allocation of equipment for public and private hospitals on a non–profit-making basis (Daligand et al. 1998).

The National Health Insurance Agency for Salaried Workers (CNAMTS) is the main national health insurance fund and covers 80 percent of the population. Various other funds cover smaller, professionally based groups. Representatives of employers and employees govern insurance funds. Levels of insurance coverage vary according to the type of service, from full coverage of major surgery to around 75 percent coverage for physician consultations.

Private supplementary insurance covers almost 90 percent of the population. Individuals can obtain supplementary insurance to cover compulsory copayments such as per diem hospital charges. Supplementary insurance can also pay the difference between the insurance benefit and the fee schedule or fee charged by physicians. However, not every insurance fund reimburses patients for the difference between the fee schedule amount and the amount the patient paid (Costich 2002). Private insurers act as secondary payers, but they do not usually cover services excluded by the public insurers (Couffinhal and Paris 2001). Many employees receive or purchase private insurance through their employers.

Most physicians in France work in private practice (56 percent) on a fee-for-service basis. One-quarter of physicians (25 percent) are salaried employees of public hospitals, 11 percent work in other types of public institutions, and 8 percent are unclassified or not practicing (Couffinhal and Paris 2001). Payments for physicians in private practice are based on a fee schedule, which will, over time, have similarities with the resource-based relative value scale (RBRVS) used by the U.S. Medicare program. Patients can visit specialists without referrals.

The fee schedule is based on an agreement between physicians' unions and public insurance funds. The relationship between physicians and insurance funds has always been strained (Couffinhal and Paris 2001). Reductions to the fee schedule resulted in physician strikes in 2002 (Dorozynski 2002). Physicians can, however, increase their fees above the reimbursement level of the insurance funds, because these fees are met by supplementary insurance or out-of-pocket payments (Imai, Jacobzone, and Lenain 2000).

Hospitals are managed by the state (45 percent), nonprofit organizations (15 percent), and the private sector (35 percent). Hospitals receive global budgets, and local hospital managers and boards are responsible for the management and staffing decisions within the hospitals. Central government determines hospital allocations, but the sickness funds distribute the funds. Historic costs as well as estimates of future operating costs determine individual hospital allocations. Since 1996 hospitals have reported to regional hospitalization agencies (WHO 1997).

Regional planning has a long tradition in France through a map called the Carte Sanitaire, which is used to measure and plan the distribution of hospital services. The Schéma Régional d'Organisation Sanitaire (SROS) is used to plan the regional distribution of equipment and services. The Carte Sanitaire has limited expansion in the number of hospital beds, but it has not addressed the other costs that contribute to increased hospital expenditure (Lancry and Sandier 1999).

Despite these efforts at planning, significant restructuring of the supply of hospital services has been difficult. Local mayors are usually also presidents of hospital boards, and local political pressures to keep hospitals running are strong (WHO 1997; Freeman 2000). A decree passed in 1997 allowed for the closure of hospitals with occupancy rates below 60 percent; however, local communities have opposed hospital closures. As of 1999, the 1997 decree had not led to widespread closure of wards or hospitals (Lancry and Sandier 1999).

GERMANY

Germany has a national health insurance system that covers around 88 percent of the population through 453 nonprofit statutory health insurance funds (European Observatory on Health Care Systems 2000a). Membership in these funds is compulsory for middle-income and lower-income salary and wage earners (75 percent of the population) and voluntary for self-employed people, government employees, and higher-income earners (14 percent). Nine percent of the population is enrolled with private insurers. Two percent of the population is assisted by a separate scheme for the police and military. Less than 1 percent of the population is uninsured.

Germany spent about the same on health per person as Canada, or $2,361 (U.S.) per person in 1998. Measured as a proportion of GDP, Germany's expenditure on health was 10.3 percent, which is comparable with Switzerland. Three-quarters (75.8 percent) of health expenditure was from the public sector, including social insurance, which funded 70 percent of total health expenditures in 1998 (OECD 2001). Just under 13 percent (12.9 percent) of health expenditures were financed by out-of-pocket payments, and 7.1 percent from private insurance.

A key feature of the German health system is the dispersal of decision making among different tiers of government (federal and state) and nongovernmental organizations (see Wilhelm-Schwartz and Busse 1997) in a corporatist decision-making structure. In other words, physician associations and sickness funds essentially administer the health insurance system on behalf of the government by implementing federal policy through their negotiated collective agreements. As a result, the past history of German health policy has tended toward stability because of the multiple actors and veto power of interest groups in the health system (Giaimo and Manow 1997).

The federal government regulates long-term care, health professionals, and health insurance funds, including compulsory health insurance benefit packages, the organizational structure of the health insurance funds, the scope of negotiations between the sickness funds and providers of health services, and the financing of health services (Busse 1999). The 16 states (Länder) implement federal laws and are responsible for regional hospital planning, regulating the professions, public health, and emergency services.

Reforms designed to increase competition in the insurance sector were a feature of German health policy in the mid 1990s. In 1997, Germany allowed individuals to choose their statutory insurer. The transition to full-scale competition, such as allowing funds to offer different benefit packages and selective contracting with providers, was never made, partly because greater differentiation across insurers would result in the erosion of solidarity (Brown and Amelung 1999). By the year 2000, various policy changes had been introduced that increased the level of government health funding and reduced patient copayments (Federal Ministry of Health 2001).

The private insurance market in Germany is relatively small. Seven percent of health expenditure was funded from private insurance in 1998 (OECD 2001). All individuals are eligible to purchase supplementary private insurance regardless of their employment status or income. Comprehensive private coverage is restricted to the self-employed, higher-income earners, and government employees. Around 9 percent of the population receives comprehensive coverage from private insurance plans (European Observatory on Health Care Systems 2000a). In general, both comprehensive and supplementary private health insurance plans offered in Germany are not highly regulated, and premium prices and cost-sharing tend to be higher, since providers treating private patients have more discretion in setting their own fees.

Hospitals have traditionally received capital budgets from the federal and state governments that are funded from general taxation. Individual hospitals negotiate their annual operating budgets with health insurance funds. Just over half of all hospitals in Germany are in the public sector, 37 percent are nonprofit, and around 7 percent are in the private sector (European Observatory on Health Care Systems 2000a). The hospital sector in Germany is likely to undergo considerable change in the next decade because of a shift from global budgets to a DRG payment system (Altenstetter 2001).

Physician payments are based on relative values for different services established at the national level. However, actual payment rates, along with volume and expenditure caps, are determined by negotiations between physicians and the sickness funds in each state. Physicians are required to join physician associations in each Länder. Physician associations distribute payments from health insurance funds to their members. Federal reforms of 1999 introduced physician payment reductions that were unpopular with physician groups (Cooper-Makhorn 1999). Cuts to physician payment rates since 1996 and strikes in 1999 raised the question of whether corporatist negotiations would continue to structure physician-fund relations.

Health insurance is financed by payroll taxes shared between employees and employers. In 2000 the average contribution rate was 13.5 percent of pretax wages, split between employers and employees (European Observatory on Health Care Systems 2000a). Funds charge different prices (although the differences are not dramatic), so not all individuals pay the same amount. Contributions depend on income, and are limited by a contribution ceiling. Maximum contribution rates are determined annually. People who contribute to the health insurance funds receive coverage for dependent family members, within certain income limits. A reinsurance system compensates funds for the differences between funds in enrollment characteristics such as age, income, and number of dependents covered. People who are without wage earnings such as the retired, also make contributions, but the "employer role" is assumed by the retirement or unemployment fund in which they are enrolled (European Observatory on Health Care Systems 2000a).

JAPAN

Japan's universal compulsory health insurance system covers the entire population.

Individuals are assigned to one of 5,000 insurance funds based on their employment status, and the size or nature of the firm for which they work (Yoshikawa and Bhattacharya 2002). Three major types of insurance funds exist. Municipal government insurance funds, called Citizens' Health Insurance, are the largest, and cover 45.45 million subscribers. Municipal funds provide insurance to self-employed people, farmers, the unemployed, retirees and their dependents, and anyone else who does not otherwise qualify for health insurance (Yoshikawa and Bhattacharya 2002). The second largest type of insurance scheme is for employees of large companies. These individuals (32.58 million subscribers) receive their insurance from one of the 1,800 "Health Insurance

Society" schemes. Finally, the government-managed health insurance plan, a single fund at the national level, covers employees of small-sized to medium-sized companies. Insurance plans also exist for specific groups such as seamen, national public service employees, local public service employees, and teachers and staff employees of private schools (Health Insurance Bureau 2002).

In 1998 Japan spent 7.4 percent of its GDP on health, or $1,795 (U.S.) per person, which is slightly more than Sweden spends per person. Seventy-eight percent of health expenditure is funded from public sources, including social insurance, which funds the majority of health expenditure (69.9 percent). Seventeen percent of health expenditures were financed from out-of-pocket sources in 1998 (OECD 2001). Out-of-pocket payments are likely to increase relative to other financing sources in the future, because of proposals to raise copayments.

In a number of ways Japan's health system resembles those of many European countries, although government tax subsidies play a much more important role. The system features an employer/municipality-based insurance system, private provision, close involvement of interest groups in decision making, government regulation of the insurance industry, and a global health budget. Benefits are standardized, and risk selection is regulated. Premium prices are not regulated outside of the government-managed health insurance plan; however, the maximum premium is limited to a percentage of income. A compensation scheme for the higher health service costs of the elderly, called the *Roken* system, is managed by municipalities and financed through transfers from all insurers and the government (Yoshikawa and Bhattacharya 2002). The government uses supply-side regulation of number of medical students and hospital beds to restrict costs (Imai 2002).

The most important feature of the Japanese health system is the national medical fee schedule for physician services. The medical fee schedule and delivery of health services are inseparable, since "each shapes the other" (White 1995). The fee schedule is reviewed every two years by a council of 20 members representing professionals, business, government, labor, and expert labor (Ikegami 1991). In practice, the Japan Medical Association is the major player in the fee schedule negotiations (Ikegami and Campbell 1999).

Japan has a relatively successful record in restraining costs over the last two decades. This may explain why Japan did not follow other countries in experimenting with managed competition reforms in the 1990s.

However, while cost containment was successful, cost restraints did not compensate for diminishing resources. Slow economic growth toward the end of the 1990s meant that health costs were increasing faster than firms' revenues and employees' wages.

Some analysts suggest that despite the need for systemic changes, reforms have been limited because the decision-making process relies heavily on consensus between the service providers (mainly the Japan Medical Association, representing doctors in private practice), insurers, and the government (Imai 2002). However, others disagree that major changes are needed. Ikegami and Campbell (1999) argue that the principal problem facing Japan's health system is the economic recession, rather than the structure of the system itself.

Future reforms are likely to change hospital payment methods, such as the further extension of DRG payment methods. Eighty-one percent of hospitals are privately owned and 19 percent of hospitals are publicly owned. The hospital system in Japan comprises private, university, prefectural, and municipal hospitals. In Japan, a hospital is defined as any institution with 20 or more beds. Most private hospitals are owned by physicians, since for-profit investor-owned hospitals are prohibited (Campbell and Ikegami 1998).

Large public or university-run institutions provide the majority of acute and high-technology care. The Department of National Hospitals owns and subsidizes 218 hospitals and sanatoriums. The department pays for services that would otherwise be less attractive for private physicians to perform, such as organ transplants and positron radiation therapy for cancer. Sanatoriums provide services for conditions such as muscular dystrophy and mental health care. By 2004 the government is planning to reorganize the public hospital sector into independent administrative corporations (Department of National Hospitals 2002).

Physicians mainly work in private practice and are reimbursed through the fee schedule. Nearly all physicians are in solo practice because of the legal restrictions on sharing equipment and staff (Campbell and Ikegami 1998). Outpatient primary care, including pharmacy services, is reimbursed at the same rate as hospital treatment. Revenue from pharmaceuticals allows physicians to offset fee schedule reductions (Ikegami and Campbell 1999). As a result, pharmaceutical consumption is extremely high as a proportion of total expenditures. In addition, the number of consultations per person, per year is more than twice the OECD average. However, inpatient admission rates to general beds are well below the OECD average (Imai 2002). General practice medicine is not clearly established as a separate discipline, so specialist doctors are not differentiated from general practitioners. Doctors in private clinics try to treat all problems of their patients (Imai 2002).

The financing structure of the Japanese health system is complex and is not uniform across all insurance funds. It has been described as a hybrid of social insurance and a tax-based system (Ikegami and Campbell 1999). Funds receive varying levels of tax subsidies from the government. For example, the municipal insurance funds for the self-employed and pensioners receive 50 percent of total benefits from tax revenues, while the government-managed health insurance scheme that covers small firms receives 14 percent of its revenues from taxes.

THE NETHERLANDS

All Dutch residents are covered by a scheme called exceptional medical expenses (Algemene Wet Bijzondere Ziektekosten, AWBZ), which covers hospital care that lasts longer than 365 days, some outpatient treatment for physical and mental disorders, and preventive health services for the entire population. Around two-thirds of the Dutch population has compulsory health insurance, provided through 30 health insurance funds under the "Sickness Fund Insurance Act" (Ziekenfondswet, ZFW). This insurance covers all general practitioner, hospital, and some dental services, for employees and self-employed persons with lower incomes, certain groups of retired persons, and unemployed or welfare recipients (Ministry of Health, Welfare and Sport 2000). Finally, as in Germany, people with an income over a certain level can purchase comprehensive private insurance. Around one-third of the population qualify for the private insurance. Five percent of the population who work for regional governments are covered by a government health insurance scheme (WHO 1997). Although the system of health insurance has its roots in the Bismarckian welfare state, in recent years the eligibility for health insurance has become increasingly based on income rather than employment status (Okma 2001).

The Netherlands spent 8.7 percent of GDP on health in 1998, or $2,150 (U.S.) per person. Compared to other countries surveyed, per person expenditure is slightly more than Australia but less than Canada and Germany. Sixty-eight percent of health expenditure in The Netherlands was financed from public sources in 1998, including 64.5 percent from social insurance. Private expenditures financed around one-quarter of total health expenditure, including 17.5 percent from private insurance and 8 percent from out-of-pocket payments.

Analysts of the Dutch health system have stressed the unique mix of public and private financing by health insurance funds and private insurance, the corporatist nature of decision making (Schut 1995; Ministry of Health, Welfare and Sport 2000), as well as the government's centralized budgetary control over the health insurance system. Each year, the cabinet agrees on the level of total health expenditure, which is known as the macro health budget. The Minister of Health, Welare and Sport then determines how the expenditure will be divided (Okma 2001). The College of Health Insurance develops a set of policy rules that the Minister approves. Health insurance funds receive risk-adjusted capitated payments.

Traditionally, insurers and providers have been well-represented within the health policy decision-making structure. In the postwar period, the Health Insurance Board, which comprised 45 members and represented a wide range of interest groups and insurers, played an important role in Dutch health policy. After 1999, this structure was replaced by a board of individuals without direct ties to any of these groups, who are appointed by the Minister of Health, Welfare and Sport. Further changes were introduced in 2001 that increased the independence of this board.

Managed competition–style reforms were proposed in the early 1990s. Opposition to the reform plans was widespread (Okma 1997), and many of these policies were not implemented. Lieverdink (2001) argues that the government and health insurance funds had opposing interests that stymied change. However, others suggest that a number of managed or regulated competition reforms were introduced and continue to be implemented (Schut 2002). Whereas health insurance funds were previously paid on the basis of their costs, they now receive prospective risk-adjusted payments. Health insurance funds are now responsible for 40 percent of the medical expenses of their enrollees. Other policies that were introduced included freedom of choice of insurer in the annual open enrollment period, the introduction of price competition among sickness funds, and the abolition of any-willing-provider laws (selective contracting) (Schut 2002). In 2001, the cabinet released a paper that advocated less regulation of insurance companies and health service providers by central government.

Health insurance funds have directed considerable attention to expanding their market share in the private supplemental insurance sector

(Lieverdink 2001). All individuals may buy private supplemental insurance for other health services not covered by exceptional medical expenses or sickness fund insurance, such as nonpreventive dental care. As mentioned above, approximately one-third of the population (5 million) with an income above EURO 25,000 has the option of buying private health insurance. Insurers are required under the Medical Insurance Act to offer a standard insurance package with statutory regulations partly governing acceptance, the extent of the risk insured, and the maximum premium price (WHO 1997).

All hospitals in The Netherlands are nonprofit and funded by a mix of global operating budgets and capital budgets. Historically, hospital operating budgets were based on prior budgets, which penalized efficient institutions (WHO 1997). Today, hospitals receive a separate budget for capital costs and then negotiate with insurers about the volume and price of their services. As in many countries the waiting times for treatment are an important issue, and in 2001 the government pledged additional funding to reduce the number of patients on the lists. Starting in 2003, global budgets will be replaced with a financing system based on DRGs.

General practitioners receive capitated payments for their patients from sickness funds and are usually paid on a fee-for-service basis by their privately insured clients (Okma 2001). Dentists are paid on a fee-for-service basis. Members of the insurance funds choose their general practitioners and register with them, and thereafter patients may only receive services from that physician. Patients can switch or be referred to other physicians. Capitation amounts are based on the average number of physician visits made within the fund.

Employee, employer, and government contributions finance the social insurance schemes. Contributions to the social insurance funds are calculated as a percentage of income. In 2000 this share totaled 8.1 percent of income. All contributions are paid to the College of Health Insurance. In turn, this College pays the individual insurance funds based on the risk profile of each insurer. The funding is designed to cover 90 percent of the fund expenses. The remaining 10 percent of expenses are financed through a system of nominal, standard premiums for each member (Rice and Smith 1999). Funds are permitted to charge their enrollees a community-rated premium. Since they are free to determine the level of these premiums, they can compete on price, and in 2002 the cheapest sickness fund charged a 50 percent lower premium than the most expensive fund (Schut 2002).

SWEDEN

Sweden has a national health service that provides services to all residents, including foreigners. Sweden's national health expenditure was $1,732 (U.S.) per person in 1998, or 7.9 percent of GDP. Eighty-three percent of health expenditure in Sweden is financed publicly (OECD 2001). Around 15 percent is from out-of-pocket sources (Diderichsen 2000). Private insurance finances less than 1 percent of health expenditure.

Health services are a local responsibility in Sweden and are financed from central and local sources. Central government distributes funds to Sweden's 20 county councils and one local authority. The National Social Insurance Board collects employer contributions and provides capitated funds to county councils, but these funds were only 14 percent of total health expenditure in 1998 (European Observatory on Health Care Systems 2001). The National Social Insurance Board has a wide range of responsibilities, such as financing the costs of employee illness.

Central government institutions are involved in evaluating new technologies, public health, professional licensing and regulation, and oversight of the health sector. The Ministry of Health and Social Affairs (Socialdepartementet) and the National Board of Health and Social Welfare (Socialstyrelsen) supervise the county councils by developing national-level health legislation and evaluating the services provided by county councils (European Observatory on Health Care Systems 2001). The Swedish Federation of County Councils represents county councils at the national level. Drug benefits are financed centrally through the National Social Insurance Board.

County councils are elected every four years and the system of elections means voters can hold local politicians accountable for the delivery of health services (Calltorp 1999). County councils collect local taxes to finance health services and manage local hospitals and health centers. In general, county facilities operate as monopolies within each county, although more counties allowed patients to choose their own hospital in the 1990s (Anell 1996). Almost all services are provided at the county level, but more complicated and rare services are treated at regional centers (Swedish Federation of County Councils 2001).

The county councils are usually divided into health districts, and these are divided into primary care districts. The districts are controlled by elected board members. Some districts act as purchasers for their populations. Districts were traditionally organized around providers, such as a hospital and a primary care center, and within each district a primary health district often follows the geographical contours of the municipality. In 2000, Sweden had about 370 primary health districts (European Observatory on Health Care Systems 2001). Interspersed within the subregional level are Sweden's 289 municipalities, which are responsible for long-term care and nursing home care.

Sweden followed other countries in introducing elements of competition within their national health service in the 1990s. However, competition was pursued within the traditional Swedish framework of widespread county variation, and maintaining existing provider structures. Some of the policies included allowing choice of doctor and hospitals for patients. Until 1993 patients were assigned local doctors and they could not choose their primary care physician (Freeman 2000). Some counties created organizations at the district level to purchase health services for their populations, and in some counties a distinction was created between purchasing and providing activities (Anell 1996).

Most of the new purchasers that were established during this period tended to simply reflect previous geographical areas and council structures. The separation of providers and purchasers was weak compared to the separation in the United Kingdom (Anell 1996). Compared to the reforms in many other European countries, Swedish reforms were relatively minor, since purchasers continued to have a monopoly in each district. Purchasers also had very few opportunities to control costs. For example, free choice of hospital by patients meant that purchasers were required to pay the fee charged by the hospital (Andersen, Smedby, and Vågerö 2001). Other procompetitive policies appeared to be ineffective. For a brief period between 1994 and 1995, patients were required to sign up with one primary care provider to encourage continuity of care, and to encourage physicians to compete by providing higher-quality, more patient-oriented care. No significant differences in physician behavior were observed, and this policy was abandoned (Andersen, Smedby, and Vågerö 2001).

The Swedish hospital system is organized around 70 district hospitals and nine regional hospitals that provide more specialized care. Approximately 95 percent of general hospital beds are in the public sector. Hospitals often are managed by a combination of elected public officials and hospital managers, who are civil servants (European Observatory on Health Care Systems 2001). County council hospitals are responsible for acute care, but municipalities are responsible for longer-term care.

Sixteen out of 21 health authorities (counties) use the DRG system to pay hospitals. The DRG payment system was introduced in some counties in the 1990s to address waiting times for hospital treatment and the perceived lack of incentives for hospitals to increase their output. The Stockholm County Council found that hospital productivity increased under the DRG system, but costs also increased under this payment system (Andersen, Smedby, and Vågerö 2001). Some hospitals introduced volume caps to balance these incentives for increased output (Anell 1996), while other counties returned to fixed or global budgets (Diderichsen 2000). Regional hospitals are commonly reimbursed through retrospective fee-for-service payments (European Observatory on Health Care Systems 2001).

Sweden has one of the world's highest physician ratios, with one practitioner for every 350 inhabitants; however, practicing specialists in general or family medicine constitute less than one-fifth of all practicing specialists (Minister of Health 2001). Physician care is mainly provided through 900 health centers financed by the county councils, as well as by private practitioners. Most physicians are employed on salaries, but they also receive some payments depending on the number of patients they treat. Around 8 percent of physicians work on a fee-for-service basis in private practice. Private practitioners account for 26 percent of all physician visits (specialists and general practice) (Swedish Federation of County Councils 2001). Private providers are paid through councils. The National Social Insurance Board pays councils for care from private sector providers and the board also regulates the private sector payment rates.

The county councils' total health services budget is determined by income tax revenues, state grants, patient fees, and reimbursements from other sources for treatment of patients from outside the county council (European Observatory on Health Care Systems 2001). Taxes, employee and employer contributions, and specific transfer payments from central government also finance health services. The National Social Insurance Board collects payroll taxes. Both private and public employers pay a contribution per employee to the health insurance system, which in 2000 was 8.5 percent of the employee's salary (European Observatory on Health Care Systems 2001).

SWITZERLAND

Switzerland has only required compulsory health insurance since 1996, but a system of voluntary insurance combined with premium subsidies dates to 1911. Switzerland's health system is notable for the absence of a government-controlled social insurance fund, and for its high levels of per person health expenditure compared to other European countries. In 1998 Switzerland spent $2,853 (U.S.) per person.

Nevertheless, Switzerland's share of health services paid for by public expenditure, according to the OECD, is comparable to many other European countries (73.2 percent), and as a proportion of GDP, Switzerland's expenditure is relatively similar to Germany's (10.3 percent). Private insurance financed 9.8 percent of total health expenditure in 1998 (OECD 2001). Other estimates (European Observatory on Health Care Systems 2000b) suggest that public spending is lower than other European countries, and that for 1997, out-of-pocket payments financed 27.6 percent of total health expenditure.

Switzerland is composed of 23 "cantons," which operate like states, within Switzerland's federal system of government. At the national level, the Swiss national Confederation (representing cantons) has a role in financing premium subsidies, public health, research, safety, and professional accreditation. The 23 cantons are responsible for regulating and training health professionals, for public health, and for implementing federal laws (European Observatory on Health Care Systems 2000b). Both the Confederation and the cantons in Switzerland have a less important role in financing or controlling global health budgets and costs than the governments in Germany and The Netherlands. Subsidies for premiums remain the dominant mechanism for federal and cantonal governments to finance health services, along with canton subsidies for hospitals.

Compulsory health insurance is individually purchased and provided by nonprofit health insurance funds that are regulated in a number of ways by the federal government. Insurers must accept all individuals who apply for coverage, and they must charge uniform premiums to all subscribers, although different insurers can charge different amounts. All insurers are required to offer the same package of benefits. The benefits package encompasses all services received by a doctor, medical treatment in general hospital wards, and prescribed generic pharmaceuticals from a drug specialty list (Colombo 2001). Individuals can also choose policies that have a higher deductible with lower premiums, bonuses for no claims, and managed care plans (WHO 2001).

Government subsidizes the cost of health insurance for people in some cantons whose premiums exceed 8 percent to 10 percent of their incomes. About one-third of the population has this assistance (Bundesamt für

Sozialversicherung, cited in WHO 2001). Each canton fixes the allowable proportion, and the federal government matches these contributions (Zweifel 2000). A risk-adjustment scheme redistributes funds to insurers with higher-cost enrollees (Colombo 2001); however, Zweifel (2000) argues that the payments do not fully compensate for risk differences.

Supplementary insurance policies cover hotel costs and other benefits not provided by compulsory insurance. Only 20 percent of the population carried supplementary insurance in 1998 (Erdmann and Wilson 2001). Although private insurers can offer basic insurance plans as of 2001, no private insurance companies had registered to provide this type of coverage. Health insurance funds providing compulsory insurance plans can offer complementary private health insurance plans to their enrollees (Colombo 2001).

Hospitals receive subsidies from cantons as well as payments from health insurance funds and private insurance. Many of the cantons operate their own hospitals. The average length of stay in Switzerland hospitals is among the highest in Europe. Most payments are usually per day, but in some cantons global budgets are also standard. The federal health insurance law requires cantons to plan hospital provision and to limit the range of providers who will be reimbursed by compulsory insurance programs (European Observatory on Health Care Systems 2000b). This is essentially a control on the supply of hospitals.

Swiss physicians have traditionally operated under a corporatist model of fee negotiation similar to that found in other European countries. Switzerland has a national fee schedule that establishes relative values for each service. The national fee schedule is modified in each canton by negotiations between health insurers and physician associations (European Observatory on Health Care Systems 2000b). Physicians working in hospitals are mostly salaried. After the 1996 insurance reforms, there have been more instances of insurers creating modified physician payment arrangements such as preferred provider networks and health maintenance organizations.

Individuals pay premiums directly to insurance companies rather than to a centralized health insurance fund in Switzerland. They also pay taxes, which contribute to the health services and premium subsidies financed by cantons and the federal government.

UNITED KINGDOM

All residents of the United Kingdom receive care through the National Health Service (NHS). The United Kingdom consists of four countries:

England, Scotland, Northern Ireland, and Wales. Scotland and Wales have achieved greater independence from England in recent years. Health sector arrangements in these areas have been relatively similar to the NHS in England with some variation in the organization and number of purchasing organizations. England is responsible for 80 percent of health expenditures within the United Kingdom.

Of the ten countries surveyed here, the United Kingdom spent the least, either measured per person ($1,510 [U.S.]) or as a percentage of GDP (6.8 percent) in 1998. Eighty-three percent of health expenditure was financed from public sources, 3.5 percent by private insurance, and 11.1 percent by out-of-pocket payments in 1998 (OECD 2001).

The English NHS is comprised of organizations at the national, regional, district, and local levels. The national Department of Health is responsible for public health and health policy and for overseeing the NHS. The Department of Health determines the allocation of funding to 28 strategic health authorities. Strategic health authorities are required to develop plans for health services in their areas and are also responsible for monitoring the performance of local primary care trusts (PCTs) and NHS trusts. The 200 or so PCTs are the major commissioners of services for the populations they serve. NHS trusts are the main providers of secondary and tertiary services and include all major public hospitals (Department of Health 2002).

The NHS has a reputation for providing a good standard of care at a relatively low cost. It serves a population about one-fifth the size of that in the United States and spends "about one-fifteenth of the money while covering nearly everybody for nearly all medical services" (Light 1997). However, some analysts contend the low cost of the NHS might have been at the expense of quality of care. Since the mid 1980s the health service has been the target of repeated reforms. England developed an internal market for NHS health services in 1991. These reforms established regional and district purchasing organizations to buy health services from primary care providers and hospitals. General practitioners were also given the option of acting as purchasers for their patients. In theory, "American-style competition had replaced Soviet-style command and control" (Le Grand 1999).

Purchasers and providers, however, did not function in the internal market as anticipated. Rather than negotiating highly specific contracts with the lowest-cost provider, purchasers and providers had incentives to form stable relationships that reduced the need for specificity in contracts and reduced information and transaction costs (Tuohy 1999). Smee (2000) argues that the internal market was not effective because it was difficult to develop purchasers powerful enough to counter the information advantage of providers. Hospitals had a long history as local monopolists, and little information was available on either the cost or quality of care. Staff working in the government bureaucracy did not know enough about how markets worked.

Finally, optimal market processes tend to create winners and losers, but the NHS was accountable ultimately to Parliament. Voters did not support the reforms, and this provided few incentives for politicians to let the internal market operate as it was designed. Smee (2000) argues that politicians, who were accustomed to being responsible for the health service, did not allow purchasers sufficient autonomy. As a result, decisions such as hospital closures were too difficult to carry out, and little competition was allowed in order to avoid political embarrassment and preserve equity (Light 1997).

After almost a decade of attempting a provider-purchaser split and competition among providers, the new 1997 Labour government maintained the split but opted to encourage cooperation rather than competition. Since 1997, Labour introduced a number of reform plans that de-emphasized competition and stressed a commitment to increasing quality in the NHS, as well as higher levels of funding. Reform plans have focused on addressing the absence of national standards or clear incentives to improve performance, overcentralization, and poor responsiveness to patients (Secretary of State for Health 2000).

A reform plan announced in 2000 promised more ambitious improvements to the NHS, compared to previous reform plans. Supported by the largest sustained increase in funding ever planned for the NHS, the Secretary of State for Health promised major changes to the NHS, such as an increase in health funding, and in the number of hospitals, physicians, and nurses. Reduced waiting times for hospital and doctor appointments, cleaner wards, better food and facilities in hospitals, and improved health services for older people were also promised (Secretary of State for Health 2000).

In spite of these problems, the level of loyalty to the NHS has been relatively high. Private insurance has not played a major role in financing health services in England, especially compared to countries such as Australia, although many analysts suggest this could change. Around 10 percent of the population, or 6.8 million people, had private insurance coverage in 1998. The majority (around 5 million) of the privately insured are covered through their employers, while 1.8 million purchase private insurance (Koen 2000). Most insurance policies cover hospital inpatient, outpatient, and day treatment in a private hospital or a private ward in an NHS hospital; drugs; and x-rays. Policies do not generally cover the treatment of chronic or long-term illnesses that cannot be cured, such as asthma, diabetes, or multiple sclerosis. Private insurance does not cover pre-existing symptoms for two years and requires patients to be symptom free, nor does it cover dental or primary care services, treatment for HIV/AIDS, or pregnancy (Association of British Insurers 2002).

Hospitals in England are largely publicly owned, and care is provided free of charge, excluding small charges for amenities. Public hospitals were restructured into NHS trusts in the late 1990s. Regional centers provide more specialized care. Unless a patient needs emergency treatment, hospital treatment requires a referral from a primary care provider. For nonemergency care, waiting times traditionally have been long in the NHS, even for services such as heart surgery (Dobson 2000).

Prior to 1991 hospitals received an annual grant that depended on the size and characteristics of the population in their catchment area. This payment method did not provide strong incentives for increased volume or productivity. Under the internal market (1991 to 1997), a contracting system developed that strengthened incentives for efficiency as the contracts became more sophisticated. Since 1997 block contracts largely replaced cost and volume contracts and, arguably, the incentives for efficiency weakened.

Physician payment methods differ for physicians in primary care or hospital-based settings. Specialists are employed on salaries within public hospitals. However, publicly employed hospital specialists can—and often do—have limited part-time private fee-for-service practices. Physicians outside of hospitals are mainly self-employed. Most primary care physicians are paid according to an annual national contract that is an agreement between the government and the British Medical Association. The national contract specifies a mix of fixed allowances for practice expenses, capitation fees (which provide around half of physicians' income), and fee-for-service payments (European Observatory on Health Care Systems 1999). Since 1999, health authorities have also been able to develop individual contracts that are negotiated separately from this national contract on a pilot basis with groups of primary care providers.

Primary care is the first point of access for nonemergency care in the NHS. Around 90 percent of patient contacts with the NHS are with primary care physicians (European Observatory on Health Care Systems 1999). Primary care is provided free of charge to patients who register with a general practitioner. Most primary care physicians work in individual or group practices.

Reform of the primary care sector is gradually transforming and increasing the role of primary care physicians. In April 1999 the Labour Government introduced a new system of funding primary physician care through primary care groups, which later evolved into primary care trusts (PCTs). PCTs are responsible for all primary and hospital care (except some forms of tertiary and long-term care) for their enrolled patients. PCTs encompass groups of primary care practices in geographical areas covering 50,000 to 250,000 people (European Observatory on Health Care Systems 1999). Physicians working as part of primary care groups remain self-employed (European Observatory on Health Care Systems 1999). PCTs receive a fixed payment per patient and are allowed to retain budget surpluses, which can be spent on services or facilities of benefit to patients (Koen 2000). PCTs are rapidly taking responsibility for the mix and volume of health services supplied to their populations, and this trend is likely to continue (European Observatory on Health Care Systems 1999).

Health services are mainly financed by general government revenue, although around 12 percent of expenditure is financed by an earmarked tax called the national health insurance contribution. The amount of funding available for health services is determined by the cabinet and distributed by the treasury to the Department of Health and to the NHS.

UNITED STATES OF AMERICA

Unlike the other countries discussed in this book, the United States does not provide universal coverage for health services. Government has, however, an important role as insurer of the elderly, the disabled, and the poor. Around 98 percent of Americans aged 65 and over have some coverage through the Medicare program, and about 40 percent of those below the poverty level have Medicaid coverage. Among the under-65 population, just less than two-thirds of Americans (63 percent) had employer-provided health coverage in 1999, and 24 percent were covered by government insurance policies. Nevertheless, about 15 percent of those under age 65 are uninsured at any one point in time. Over a two-year period, it has been estimated that nearly one-third of the under-65 population is uninsured some of the time (Stone 2000).

In spite of these major gaps in coverage, the United States spent 12.9 percent of its GDP on health services in 1998; that is $4,165 per person, a figure that far exceeds all other countries in the world. The U.S. system is financed from a variety of sources. One-third of payments come from private insurance, another third from the federal government, 18 percent are out of pocket, about 10 percent are from state and local government, and the remaining 5 percent are from other sources (U.S. DHHS 2001).

Since 1965 the federal Medicare program has insured elderly Americans. Almost all U.S. citizens over age 65, as well as disabled individuals, are eligible for the Medicare program. All Americans who need a kidney transplant or renal dialysis because of chronic kidney disease are also entitled to benefits under Part A, regardless of their age. Medicare provides hospital, physician, and some nursing home and home health services, but does not cover outpatient prescription drugs. The program is divided into two parts. Part A mainly covers hospital (and some nursing home) care, and is akin to social insurance in that it is financed primarily through payroll deductions of 2.9 percent. The deduction is split between the employer and employee, and self-employed individuals pay both the employee and employer contribution. Part B mainly covers physician services both in and out of the hospital, medical equipment such as wheelchairs, home health care, and other outpatient services. Three-quarters of its costs come from general (federal) revenues, with the remaining 25 percent paid through beneficiary premiums. In 2001 the premium was $50 per month per person.

Medicare, however, has a number of gaps in coverage. The coinsurance and copayment requirements are substantial, including 20 percent of all Part B costs, as well as various uncovered services including most long-term care and outpatient prescription drugs. As a result, about 90 percent of Medicare beneficiaries have supplemental insurance coverage—36 percent through former employers, 27 percent through individual "Medigap" insurance policies, 17 percent through HMOs, and 11 percent through the Medicaid program (Rice and Bernstein 1999). More than one-third of seniors, however, have no coverage whatsoever for prescription drugs.

Medicaid coverage is more comprehensive but, unlike Medicare, the program is run by the states (and financed jointly with the federal government). As a result, eligibility requirements and benefits are not standardized. Eligibility tends to be "categorical"—that is, to be covered, individuals must meet certain requirements that vary among states. Most beneficiaries have low incomes and are dependent children, pregnant woman, seniors, or disabled. Whereas some states cover nearly all poor persons, others cover only a fraction of the poor. Nationally, about 37 percent of those below the poverty line have Medicaid coverage (U.S. DHHS 2001), although many others do have private insurance coverage through their own or a family member's employer. Some of the benefits are mandatory in all states (e.g., inpatient, outpatient, and physician services), but others are optional (e.g., prescription drugs, dental care). A significant portion—more than 20 percent of Medicaid spending—finances long-term care of low-income seniors. Because these individuals often spend most of their incomes and assets on nursing home care, once they become poor they often are eligible for Medicaid coverage.

Insurance coverage for the under-65 population is provided by employers. Coverage is usually extended to an employee's dependents and spouse, and most employers offer employees a choice of insurance plans. Employers purchase insurance on behalf of their employees through contracts that are usually negotiated annually with insurance carriers or managed care companies. Individually purchased coverage represents only 8 percent of the total (U.S. DHHS 2001). The reasons for this are many:

- Historically, coverage provided through the workplace has benefited from substantial tax advantages. Most importantly, employer contributions to employee health insurance are not considered income taxable to the employee.
- Employers can often elicit discounts from insurers as a result of economies of scale.
- Workers tend to be healthier (and therefore, less risky) than those not in the workforce.
- Coverage through the workplace helps ensure against adverse selection, in particular, people obtaining coverage specifically because they expect to incur substantial health service costs.

One of the main problems with this patchwork system is that many people remain uninsured, either because they are not employed, they are employed by a firm that does not offer coverage, their firm offers coverage but they are not eligible for it, or they are eligible for coverage but cannot afford it. Although each of these reasons is important, the latter appears to be most responsible for the upward trend in uninsurance. The number of uninsured in the United States rose from 33 million in 1989 to 39 million in 1998 (U.S. DHHS 2001).

In addition to their role in insuring the most vulnerable members of the population, the federal government and some state governments regulate insurers. For example, federal legislation known as COBRA (Consolidated Omnibus Budget Reconciliation Act) requires employers to offer employees the option of continuing their insurance coverage if they leave their job and have no coverage, either because insurance is not provided at their new place of employment or because they are not working. Some states require all health insurers to cover certain services, although most large employers are exempt from this because they self-insure and by law are not subject to state health insurance regulation. Both state and federal regulatory mechanisms are relatively weak, however, and pale in comparison to the types of regulations, or protections, insurers operate under in Australia, for example, or Europe. Although COBRA coverage may provide a safety net for people between jobs, the price of premiums is not regulated under this legislation, and employees therefore must pay much more out-of-pocket for premiums.

Most hospitals in the United States are nonprofit, although there is a trend toward more proprietary facilities. Seventy-one percent of beds in community hospitals are in nonprofit facilities, 13 percent are in for-profit facilities, and 16 percent are under the jurisdiction of state or local government. By international standards, occupancy rates are low, averaging 66 percent in 1999 (U.S. DHHS 2001). The Medicare program pays hospitals on the basis of DRGs—that is, a fixed amount per admission based on the patient's diagnosis. Other payers, however, use a variety of methods, including DRGs, per diems, and discounted usual charges.

The United States has a greater proportion of specialist physicians than most other countries. As discussed in Chapter 4 and shown in Table 4.1, U.S. physicians are paid in many different ways. The majority of Medicare beneficiaries receive their care from physicians who are paid on a fee-for-service basis based on a resource-based relative value scale (RBRVS). About 15 percent are in HMOs and therefore not part of the Medicare fee-for-service system. In private insurance, physicians can be paid by salary, capitation, and fee-for-service, and within these, can receive bonuses or "withholds" for meeting or not meeting certain productivity or cost-containment goals. Most HMOs pay their primary providers using capitation, but an even larger majority base specialist payment on fee-for-service. More than 40 percent of plans use bonuses or withholds for primary care physicians, and about 30 percent, for specialists (Medicare Payment Advisory Commission 2000).

As noted, the source of federal payments is a combination of payroll taxes and general revenues. Private insurance is paid largely through premiums paid by employers and employees.

Although many calls have been made for fundamental reform of the U.S. system and the introduction of a national health insurance program, most changes have been incremental in scope. The major significant development in recent years was the establishment of the State Children's Health Insurance Program in 1997, aimed at covering a large proportion of the country's uninsured children. A great deal of attention has been paid to adding prescription drug coverage to the Medicare program, but at time of writing no proposal has garnered the support of either house of Congress.

References

Aaron, H. J. 1994. "Public Policy, Values, and Consciousness." *Journal of Economic Perspectives* 8 (2): 3–21.

Aaron, H. J., and R. D. Reischauer. 1995. "The Medicare Debate: What Is the Next Step?" *Health Affairs* 14 (4): 8–30.

Abel-Smith, B. 1992. "Cost Containment and New Priorities in the European Community." *Milbank Quarterly* 70 (3): 393–422.

Aday, L. A., R. Andersen, and G. V. Fleming. 1980. *Health Care in the U.S.: Equitable to Whom?* Beverly Hills, CA: Sage Publications.

Ahern, M. M., M. S. Hendryx, and K. Siddharthan. 1996. "The Importance of Sense of Community in People's Perceptions of Their Health-Care Experiences." *Medical Care* 34 (9): 911–23.

Akerlof, G. A., and W. T. Dickens. 1992. "The Economic Consequences of Cognitive Dissonance." *American Economic Review* 72 (3): 307–19.

Altenstetter, C. 2001. "Health Care Reform in Germany in Comparative Perspective, with Special Attention to Funding and Reimbursement Issues of Medical and Hospital Services." Paper presented at the 29th European Consortium for Political Research Joint Sessions of Workshops, April 6–11, Grenoble.

Andersen, R. M., B. Smedby, and D. Vågerö. 2001. "Cost Containment, Solidarity and Cautious Experimentation: Swedish Dilemmas." *Social Science and Medicine* 52: 1195–204.

Anderson, G., C. Black, E. Dunn, et al. 1997. "Willingness to Pay to Shorten Waiting Time for Cataract Surgery." *Health Affairs* 16 (5): 181–90.

Anell, A. 1996. "The Monopolistic Integrated Model and Health Care Reform: The Swedish Experience." *Health Policy* 37: 19–33.

Aronson, E. 1972. *The Social Animal.* San Francisco: W. H. Freeman & Co.

Arrow, K. J. 1963a. *Social Choice and Individual Values.* New York: John Wiley.

———. 1963b. "Uncertainty and the Welfare Economics of Medical Care." *American Economic Review* 53 (5): 940–73.

———. 1983. "Some Ordinalist-Utilitarian Notes of Rawls's Theory of Justice." In *Social Choice and Justice: Collected Papers of Kenneth J. Arrow*, pp. 96–117. Cambridge, MA: Belknap Press of Harvard University Press.

Association of British Insurers. 2002. "Fact Sheet on Private Medical Insurance. [Online article.] http://www.abi.org.uk.

Association for Health Services Research. 2000. "HSR Reports." [Newsletter.] Washington, DC: AHSR, April.

Bamezai, A., J. Zwanziger, G. A. Melnick, and J. M. Mann. 1999. "Price Competition and Hospital Cost Growth in the United States (1989–1994)." *Health Economics* 8: 233–43.

Barer, M. L., R. G. Evans, and R. J. Labelle. 1988. "Fee Controls as Cost Controls: Tales from the Frozen North." *Milbank Quarterly* 66 (1): 1–64.

Barer, M. L., J. Lomas, and C. Sanmartin. 1996. "Re-Minding Our Ps and Qs: Medical Cost Controls in Canada." *Health Affairs* 15 (2): 216–34.

Barr, M. D. 2001. "Medical Savings Accounts in Singapore: A Critical Inquiry." *Journal of Health Politics, Policy and Law* 26 (4): 709–26.

Bator, F. M. 1958. "The Anatomy of Market Failure." *Quarterly Journal of Economics* 52 (3): 351–79.

Becker, G. S. 1979. "Economic Analysis and Human Behavior." In *Sociological Economics*, edited by L. Levy-Garboua. Beverly Hills, CA: Sage Publications.

Becker, G. S., and K. M. Murphy. 1988. "A Theory of Rational Addiction." *Journal of Political Economy* 96 (4): 675–700.

Bentham, J. 1791. *Principles of Morals and Legislation*. London: Doubleday.

———. 1968. "An Introduction to the Principles of Morals and Legislation." In *Utility Theory: A Book of Readings*, edited by A. N. Page, pp. 3–29. New York: John Wiley.

Berk, M. L., and A. C. Monheit. 2001. "The Concentration of Health Expenditures, Revisited." *Health Affairs* 20 (2): 9–18.

Bindman, A. B., and J. P. Weiner. 2000. "The Modern NHS: An Underfunded Model of Efficiency and Integration." *Health Affairs* 19 (3): 120–23.

Blackorby, C., and D. Donaldson. 1990. "A Review Article: The Case Against the Use of the Sum of Compensating Variations in Cost-Benefit Analysis." *Canadian Journal of Economics* 23 (3): 471–94.

Blanchard, S. 2001. "Pourquoi Rembourser les Médicaments Inutiles?" *Le Monde* 21 Juillet.

Blendon, R. J., and J. M. Benson. 2001. "Americans' Views on Health Policy: A Fifty-Year Historical Perspective." *Health Affairs* 20 (2): 33–46.

Blendon, R. J., J. Marttila, J. M. Benson, M. C. Shelter, F. J. Connolly, and T. Kiley. 1994. "The Beliefs and Values Shaping Today's Health Reform Debate." *Health Affairs* 13 (1): 274–84.

Blendon, R. J., D. E. Altman, J. Benson, M. Brodie, M. James, and G. Chervinsky. 1995a. "The Public and the Welfare Reform Debate." *Archives of Pediatric and Adolescent Medicine* 149 (10): 1065–69.

Blendon, R. J., J. Benson, K. Donelan, et al. 1995b. "Who Has the Best Health Care System? A Second Look." *Health Affairs* 14 (4): 220–30.

Blendon, R. J., C. Schoen, K. Donelan, et al. 2001. "Physicians' Views on Quality of Care: A Five-Country Comparison." *Health Affairs* 20 (3): 233–43.

Boulding, K. E. 1969. "Economics as a Moral Science." *American Economic Review* 59 (1): 1–12.

Brenner, G., and D. Rublee. 2002. "Germany." In *World Health Systems: Challenges and Perspectives,* edited by B. J. Fried and L. M. Gaydos, pp. 121–36. Chicago: Health Administration Press.

Brook, R. H., J. E. Ware, Jr., W. H. Rogers, et al. 1983. "Does Free Care Improve Adults' Health?" *The New England Journal of Medicine* 309 (23): 1426–34.

Brown, L. D., and V. E. Amelung. 1999. "Manacled Competition: Market Reforms in German Health Care" *Health Affairs* 18 (3): 76–91.

Buchanan, J. M. 1977. "Political Equality and Private Property: The Distributional Paradox." In *Markets and Morals,* edited by G. Dworkin, G. Bermant, and P. G. Brow. Washington, DC: Hemisphere Publishing Corp.

Buchmueller, T. C. 1998. "Does a Fixed-Dollar Premium Contribution Lower Spending?" *Health Affairs* 17 (6): 228–35.

Bundesamt für Sozialversicherung. 2000. *Analyse des Effects de la LAMal dans le Financement du Système de Santé et d'Autres Régimes de Protection de Sociale.* Neuchâtel, Budesamt für Statistik (Cited in WHO 2001).

Bunker, J., and B. Brown. 1974. "The Physician-Patient as an Informed Consumer of Surgical Services." *The New England Journal of Medicine* 290 (19): 1051–55.

Busse, R. 1999. "Priority-Setting and Rationing in German Health Care." *Health Policy* 50 1 (2): 71–90.

Calltorp, J. 1999. "Priority Setting in Health Policy in Sweden and a Comparison with Norway." *Health Policy* 50: 1–22.

Campbell, J. C., and N. Ikegami. 1998. *Art of Balance in Health Policy: Maintaining Japan's Low-Cost, Egalitarian System.* Cambridge, UK: Cambridge University Press.

Canada Health Act Overview. 2001. [Online article.] http://www.hc-sc.gc.ca/medicare/chaover.htm.

Cantril, H. 1965. *The Pattern of Human Concerns.* New Brunswick, NJ: Rutgers University Press.

Carlsen, F., and J. Grytten. 1998. "More Physicians: Improved Availability or Induced Demand?" *Health Economics* 7: 495–508.

Chernew, M., and D. P. Scanlon. 1998. "Health Plan Report Cards and Insurance Choice." *Inquiry* 35: 9–22.

Christianson, J., B. Dowd, J. Kralewski, S. Hayes, and C. Wisner. 1995. "Managed Care in the Twin Cities: What Can We Learn?" *Health Affairs* 14 (2): 114–30.

Christianson, J. B., C. S. Lessor, L. E. Felland, et al. 2000. "Increased Consolidation Raises Concerns." Community Report No. 02. Washington, DC: Center for Studying Health Systems Change, Fall.

Coburn, D. 2000. "Income Inequality, Social Cohesion and the Health Status of Populations: The Role of Neo-Liberalism." *Social Science and Medicine* 51: 135–46.

Collard, D. 1978. *Altruism and Economy: A Study in Non-Selfish Economics.* Oxford: Martin Robertson & Co.

Colombo, F. 2001. "Towards More Choice in Social Protection? Individual Choice of Insurer in Basic Mandatory Health Insurance in Switzerland." OECD *Labour Market and Social Policy Occasional Papers* No. 53. Paris: OECD.

Commonwealth Department of Health and Aged Care. 1999a. "Public and Private—In Partnership for Australia's Health." *Occasional Papers*: *Health Financing Series.* Canberra: Commonwealth Department of Health and Aged Care.

———. 1999b. "Private Health Insurance." *Occasional Papers*: *New Series* No. 4. Canberra: Commonwealth Department of Health and Aged Care.

———. 2000. "The Australian Health Care System: An Outline." [Online article.] Financing and Analysis Branch, Commonwealth Department of Health and Aged Care, Canberra. http://www.health.gov.au/haf/ozhealth/.

Congressional Budget Office. 1994. *Effects of Managed Care: An Update.* Washington, DC: CBO.

Cooper-Makhorn, D. 1999. "German Doctors Strike Against Health Budget Cuts." *British Medical Journal* 318: 76.

Costich, J. F. 2002. "France." In *World Health Systems: Challenges and Perspectives,* edited by B. J., Fried and L. M. Gyados, pp. 153–72. Chicago: Health Administration Press.

Couffinhal, A., and V. Paris. 2001. "Utilization Fees Imposed to Public Health Care System Users in France." Paper presented at the Workshop Organized by the Commission on the Future of Health Care in Canada, November 29.

Coulam, R. F., and G. L. Gaumer. 1991. "Medicare's Prospective Payment System: A Critical Appraisal." *Health Care Financing Review* 13 (Annual Supplement): 45–77.

Council for Affordable Health Insurance. 1997. *Mandated Health Insurance Benefits.* Alexandria, VA: Council for Affordable Health Insurance, August 4.

Cromwell, J., and J. Mitchell. 1986. "Physician-Induced Demand for Surgery." *Journal of Health Economics* 5 (3): 293–313.

Culyer, A. J. 1982. "The Quest for Efficiency in the Public Sector: Economists Versus Dr. Pangloss." In *Public Finance and the Quest for Efficiency, Proceedings of the 38th Congress of the International Institute of Public Finance,* edited by H. Hanusch, pp. 39–48. Copenhagen.

———. 1989. "The Normative Economics of Health Care Finance and Provision." *Oxford Review of Economic Policy* 5 (1): 34–58.

———. 1993. "Health, Health Expenditures, and Equity." In *Equity in the Finance and Delivery of Health Care: An International Perspective,* edited by E. van Doorslaer, A. Wagstaff, and F. Rutten, pp. 299–319. Oxford, UK: Oxford Medical Publications.

———. 2001. "Equity—Some Theory and Its Policy Implications." *Journal of Medical Ethics* 27: 275–83.

Cunningham, P. J., C. Denk, and M. Sinclair. 2001. "Do Consumers Know How Their Health Plan Works?" *Health Affairs* 20 (2): 159–66.

Cutler, D. M., and S. J. Reber. 1998. "Paying for Health Insurance: The Trade-off Between Competition and Adverse Selection." *Quarterly Journal of Economics* 113 (2): 433–66.

Daligand, L., M. C. Jacques, S. Marvalin, et al. 1998. *Sécurité Sociale.* 4th edition. Paris: Masson.

Daly, G., and F. Giertz. 1972. "Welfare Economics and Welfare Reform." *American Economic Review* 62 (1): 131–38.

Daly, M. C., G. J. Duncan, G. A. Kaplan, and J. W. Lynch. 1998. "Macro-to-Micro Links in the Relation Between Income Inequality and Mortality." *Milbank Quarterly* 76 (3): 315–39.

Daniels, N. 1985. "Health Care Needs and Distributive Justice." In *In Search of Equity: Health Needs and the Health Care System,* edited by R. Bayer, A. O. Caplan, and N. Daniels. New York: Plenum Press.

Daniels, N., B. Kennedy, and I. Kawachi. 2000. *Is Inequality Bad for Our Health?* Boston: Beacon Press.

Deaton, A. 2001. "Health, Inequality, and Economic Development." NBER Working Paper No. W8318. Cambridge, MA: National Bureau of Economic Research.

Deber, R. B. 2000. "Getting What We Pay For: Myths and Realities About Financing Canada's Health Care System." Toronto: Department of Health Administration, University of Toronto.

Department of Health, England. 2002. "NHS Performance Indicators: February 2002." [Online article.] http://www.doh.gov.uk/nhsperformanceindicators/2002/ha_intro.html.

Department of National Hospitals, Japan. 2002. "Department of National Hospitals, Ministry of Health, Labour and Welfare." [Online article.] http://www.mhlw.go.jp/english/org/policy/p12.html.

Devers, K., J. B. Christianson, L. E. Felland, S. Felt-Lisk, L. Rudell, and J. L. Hargraves. 2001. "Highly Consolidated Market Poses Cost Control Challenges." Community Report No. 06. Washington, DC: Center for Studying Health Systems Change, Winter.

Diderichsen, F. 2000. "Sweden." In: "Reconsidering the Role of Competition in Health Care Markets." *Journal of Health Politics, Policy and Law* 25 (5): 931–35.

Dobson, R. 2000. "Blair Tackled on Heart Deaths." *British Medical Journal* 320: 670.

Donelan, K., R. J. Blendon, C. Schoen, K. Davis, and K. Binns. 1999. "The Cost of Health System Change: Public Discontent in Five Nations." *Health Affairs* 18 (3): 206–16.

Dorozynski, A. 2002. "French Healthcare System Beset by Strikes." *British Medical Journal* 324: 258.

Dowd, B. 1999. "An Unusual View of Health Economics." *Health Affairs* 18 (1): 266–69.

Dranove, D. 1995. "A Problem with Consumer Surplus Measures of the Cost of Practice Variations." *Journal of Health Economics* 14 (2): 243–51.

Duan, N., W. G. Manning, C. N. Morris, and J. P. Newhouse. 1984. "Choosing Between the Sample-Selection Model and the Multi-Part Model." *Journal of Business and Economic Statistics* 2 (3): 283–89.

Duesenberry, J. S. 1952. *Income, Saving and the Theory of Consumer Behavior.* Cambridge, MA: Harvard University Press.

Dworkin, R. 1981. "What Is Equality? Part 2: Equality of Resources." *Philosophy & Public Affairs* 10 (4): 283–345.

Easterlin, R. 1974. "Does Economic Growth Improve the Human Lot? Some Empirical Evidence." In *Nations and Households in Economic Growth: Essays in Honor of Moses Abramovitz,* edited by P. A. David and M. W. Reder, pp. 89–125. New York: Academic Press.

Economist. 2001. "The New Rich May Worry About Envy, but Everyone Should Worry About Poverty." June 14.

Ellis, R. P., and T. G. McGuire. 1993. "Supply-Side and Demand-Side Cost Sharing in Health Care." *Journal of Economic Perspectives* 7 (4): 135–51.

Elster, J. 1992. *Local Justice: How Institutions Allocate Scarce Goods and Necessary Burdens.* New York: Russell Sage Foundation.

Enthoven, A. 1978a. "Consumer Choice Health Plan." *The New England Journal of Medicine* 298 (12): 650–58.

———. 1978b. "Consumer Choice Health Plan." *The New England Journal of Medicine* 298 (13): 709–20.

———. 1980. *Health Plan: The Only Practical Solution to the Soaring Cost of Medical Care.* Reading, MA: Addison-Wesley.

———. 1988. *Theory and Practice of Managed Competition in Health Care Finance.* Amsterdam: North-Holland.

———. 2000. "In Pursuit of an Improving National Health Service." *Health Affairs* 19 (3): 102–19.

Enthoven, A., and R. Kronick. 1989a. "A Consumer-Choice Health Plan for the 1990s." *The New England Journal of Medicine* 320 (1): 29–37.

———. 1989b. "A Consumer-Choice Health Plan for the 1990s." *The New England Journal of Medicine* 320 (2): 94–101.

Erdmann, Y., and R. Wilson. 2001. "Managed Care: A View from Europe." *Annual Review of Public Health* 22: 273–91.

Escarce, J. J. 1992. "Explaining the Association Between Surgeon Supply and Utilization." *Inquiry* 29 (4): 403–15.

———. 1993a. "Effects of Lower Surgical Fees on the Use of Physician Services Under Medicare." *JAMA* 269 (19): 2513–18.

———. 1993b. "Medicare Patients' Use of Overpriced Procedures Before and After the Omnibus Budget Reconciliation Act of 1987." *American Journal of Public Health* 83 (3): 349–55.

European Observatory on Health Care Systems. 1999. *Health Care Systems in Transition: United Kingdom.* Copenhagen: WHO Regional Office for Europe.

———. 2000a. *Health Care Systems in Transition: Germany.* Copenhagen: WHO Regional Office for Europe.

———. 2000b. *Health Care Systems in Transition: Switzerland.* Copenhagen: WHO Regional Office for Europe.

———. 2001. *Health Care Systems in Transition: Sweden.* Copenhagen: WHO Regional Office for Europe.

Evans, R. G. 1983. "Health Care in Canada: Patterns of Funding and Regulation." *Journal of Health Politics, Policy and Law* 8 (1): 1–43.

———. 1984. *Strained Mercy.* Toronto, Ontario: Butterworth.

———. 1999. "What We Do—and Don't—Know About Social Inequalities in Health." In *Social Inequalities in Health: Keynote Addresses from the Annual Meeting on Health Philanthropy.* Washington, DC: Grantmakers in Health.

———. 2000. "Canada." In: "Reconsidering the Role of Competition in Health Care Markets." *Journal of Health Politics, Policy and Law* 25 (5): 889–97.

Evans, R. G., M. L. Barer, and G. L. Stoddart. 1993. "The Truth About

User Fees." In *Policy Option*. Montreal, Quebec: Institute for Research on Public Policy.

Evans, R. G., M. L. Barer, G. L. Stoddart, and V. Bhatia. 1983. *It's Not the Money, It's the Principle: Why User Changes for Some Services and Not Others?* Vancouver: Centre for Health Services and Policy Research, University of British Columbia.

Evans, R. G., E. M. A. Parish, and F. Sully. 1973. "Medical Productivity, Scale Effects, and Demand Generation." *Canadian Journal of Economics* 6 (3): 376–93.

Evans, R. G., and G. L. Stoddart. 1990. "Producing Health, Consuming Health Care." *Social Science and Medicine* 31 (12): 1347–63.

Fahs, M. C. 1992. "Physician Response to the United Mine Workers' Cost-Sharing Program: The Other Side of the Coin." *Health Services Research* 27 (1): 25–45.

Federal Ministry of Health, Germany. 2001. "Health Care in Germany Including the Health Care Reform 2000." [Online article.] http://www.bmgesundheit.de/engl/healthcare.htm.

Feldman, R., and B. Dowd. 1991. "A New Estimate of the Welfare Loss of Excess Health Insurance." *American Economic Review* 81 (1): 297–301.

———. 1993. "What Does the Demand Curve for Medical Care Measure?" *Journal of Health Economics* 12 (2): 192–200.

Feldman, R., and M. A. Morrisey. 1990. "Health Economics: A Report on the Field." *Journal of Health Politics, Policy and Law* 15 (3): 627–46.

Feldman, R., and F. Sloan. 1988. "Competition Among Physicians, Revisited." *Journal of Health Politics, Policy and Law* 13 (2): 239–61.

Feldstein, M. S. 1973. "The Welfare Loss of Excess Health Insurance." *Journal of Political Economy* 81 (2): 251–80.

Feldstein, P. J. 1988. *Health Care Economics*. New York: John Wiley.

———. 1996. *The Politics of Health Legislation: An Economic Perspective*. Chicago: Health Administration Press.

———. 1998. *Health Care Economics*. New York: John Wiley.

Fielding, J. E., and P. J. Lancry. 1993. "Lessons from France—'Viva la Difference.'" *JAMA* 270 (6): 748–56.

Fielding, J. E., and T. Rice. 1993. "Can Managed Care Competition Solve the Problems of Market Failure?" *Health Affairs* 12 (Supplement): 216–28.

Finkler, S. A. 1979. "Cost-Effectiveness of Regionalization: The Heart Surgery Example." *Inquiry* 16 (3): 264–70.

Fishlow, A. 1965. *American Railroads and the Transformation of the Antebellum Economy*. Cambridge, MA: Harvard University Press.

Fogel, R. A. 1964. *Railroads and American Economic Growth: Essays in Econometric History*. Baltimore: Johns Hopkins Press.

Fox, D. M., and H. M. Leichter. 1993. "The Ups and Downs of Oregon's Rationing Plan." *Health Affairs* 12 (2): 66–70.

Frank, R. H. 1985. *Choosing the Right Pond: Human Behavior and the Quest for Status.* New York: Oxford University Press.

———. 1999. *Luxury Fever.* New York: Free Press.

Frank, R., and T. McGuire. 2000. "Economics and Mental Health." In *Handbook of Health Economics,* vol. 1B, edited by A. J. Culyer and J. P. Newhouse, pp. 895–954. Amsterdam: Elsevier.

Freeman, R. 2000. *The Politics of Health Care in Europe.* New York: Manchester University Press and St. Martins Press.

Fried, B. J., and L. M. Gaydos. 2002. *World Health Systems: Challenges and Perspectives.* Chicago: Health Administration Press.

Friedman, M. 1962. *Price Theory.* Chicago: Aldine Press.

Fuchs, V. 1978. "The Supply of Surgeons and the Demand for Operations." *Journal of Human Resources* 12 (Supplement): 35–56.

———. 1983. *Who Shall Live?* New York: Basic Books.

———. 1996. "Economics, Values, and Health Care Reform." *American Economic Review* 86 (1): 1–23.

Fuchs, V. R., and J. S. Hahn. 1990. "How Does Canada Do It? A Comparison of Expenditures for Physicians' Services in the United States and Canada." *The New England Journal of Medicine* 323 (13): 884–90.

Gabel, J. R., and G. A. Jensen. 1989. "The Price of State Mandated Benefits." *Inquiry* 26 (3): 419–31.

Gabel, J. R., and T. H. Rice. 1985. "Reducing Public Expenditures for Physician Services: The Price of Paying Less." *Journal of Health Politics, Policy and Law* 9 (4): 595–609.

Gabel, J., S. DiCarlo, C. Sullivan, and T. Rice. 1990. "Employer-Sponsored Health Insurance, 1989." *Health Affairs* 9 (3): 161–75.

Gabel, J., D. Liston, G. Jensen, and J. Marsteller. 1994. "The Health Insurance Picture in 1993: Some Rare Good News." *Health Affairs* 13 (1): 327–36.

Gabel, J., L. Levitt, J. Pickreign, et al. 2001. "Job-Based Health Insurance in 2001: Inflation Hits Double Digits, Managed Care Retreats." *Health Affairs* 20 (5): 180–86.

Giaimo, S., and P. Manow. 1997. "Institutions and Ideas into Politics: Health Care Reform in Britain and Germany." In *Health Policy Reform, National Variations and Globalization,* edited by C. Altenstetter and J. Warner Björkman. New York: St. Martins Press.

Ginsburg, P. B., L. B. LeRoy, and G. T. Hammons. 1990. "Medicare Physician Payment Reform." *Health Affairs* 9 (1): 178–88.

Gintis, H. 1970. *Neo-Classical Welfare Economics and Individual Development.* Cambridge, MA: Union for Radical Political Economists.

Glaser, W. A. 1991. *Health Insurance in Practice: International Variations in Financing, Benefits, and Problems.* San Francisco: Jossey-Bass.

Gold, M. R., R. Hurley, T. Lake, T. Ensor, and R. Berenson. 1995. "A National Survey of the Arrangements Managed Care Plans Make with Physicians." *The New England Journal of Medicine* 333 (25): 1678–83.

Goldsmith, L. J. 2002. "Canada." In *World Health Systems: Challenges and Perspectives,* edited by B. J. Fried and L. M. Gaydos, pp. 227–48. Chicago: Health Administration Press.

Goldstein, E., and J. Fyock. 2001. "Reporting of CAHPS Quality Information to Medicare Beneficiaries." *Health Services Research* 36 (3): 477–88.

Gornick, M. E. 2000. *Vulnerable Populations and Medicare Services.* New York: Century Foundation Press.

Graaff, J. V. 1971. *Theoretical Warfare Economics.* London: Cambridge University Press.

Gravelle, H. 1998. "How Much of the Relation Between Population Mortality and Unequal Distribution of Income Is a Statistical Artifact?" *British Medical Journal* 316: 382–85.

Gray, G. 1996. "Reform and Reaction in Australian Health Policy." *Journal of Health Politics, Policy and Law* 21 (3): 587–615.

Green, D. P., and I. Shapiro. 1994. *Pathologies of Rational Choice Theory.* New Haven, CT: Yale University Press.

Green, R. M. 1976. "Health Care and Justice in Contract Theory Perspective." In *Ethics and Health Policy,* edited by R. M. Veatch and R. Branson. Cambridge, MA: Ballinger.

Greenfield, S., E. C. Nelson, M. Zubkoff, et al. 1992. "Variations in Resource Utilization Among Medical Specialties and Systems of Care: Results from the Medical Outcomes Study." *JAMA* 267 (12): 1624–30.

Grytten, J., and R. Sorensen. 2001. "Type of Contract and Supplier-Induced Demand for Primary Care Physicians in Norway." *Journal of Health Economics* 20: 379–93.

Hadley, J., J. Holahan, and W. Scanlon. 1979. "Can Fee-for-Service Reimbursement Coexist with Demand Creation?" *Inquiry* 16 (3): 247–58.

Hahnel, R., and M. Albert. 1990. *Quiet Revolution in Welfare Economics.* Princeton, NJ: Princeton University Press.

Hall, J. 1999. "Incremental Change in the Australian Health Care System." *Health Affairs* 18 (3): 95–113.

Hannan, E. L., H. Kilburn, Jr., H. Bernard, J. F. O'Donnell, G. Lukacik, and E. P. Shields. 1991. "Coronary Artery Bypass Surgery: The Relationship Between In-Hospital Mortality Rate and Surgical Volume after Controlling for Clinical Risk Factors." *Medical Care* 29 (11): 1094–107.

Hanning, M. 2001. "Waiting Lists Initiatives in Sweden." Paper presented at the session, "Incentives for Reduced Waiting Times in Health Systems: A Comparison of Experiences in Different Countries," International Health Economics Association Third International Conference. York, UK, July 23.

Hausman, D. M., and M. S. McPherson. 1993. "Taking Ethics Seriously: Economics and Contemporary Moral Philosophy." *Journal of Economic Literature* 31 (2): 671–731.

Hay, J., and M. J. Leahy. 1982. "Physician-Induced Demand: An Empirical Analysis of the Consumer Information Gap." *Journal of Health Economics* 1 (3): 231–44.

Hay, J. W., and R. J. Olsen. 1984. "Let Them Eat Cake: A Note on Comparing Alternative Models of the Demand for Medical Care." *Journal of Business and Economic Statistics* 2 (3): 279–82.

Hayek, F. A. 1945. "The Use of Knowledge by Society." *American Economic Review* 35 (4): 519–34.

Health Insurance Bureau, Japan. 2002. [Online article.] http://www.mhlw.go.jp/english/org/policy/p34-35.html.

Hellinger, F. J., and H. S. Wong. 2000. "Selection Bias in HMOs: A Review of the Evidence." *Medicare Care Research and Review* 57 (4): 405–39.

Hemenway, D., and D. Fallon. 1985. "Testing for Physician-Induced Demand with Hypothetical Cases." *Medical Care* 23 (4): 344–49.

Henderson, and Quandt. 1980. *Microeconomic Theory.* New York: McGraw-Hill.

Henke, K.-D., M. A. Murray, and C. Ade. 1994. "Global Budgeting in Germany: Lessons for the United States." *Health Affairs* 13 (4): 7–22.

Hertzman, C. 2001. "Population Health and Children Development: A View from Canada." In *Income, Socioeconomic Status, and Health: Exploring the Relationships*, edited by J. A. Auerbach and B. K. Krimgold. Washington, DC: National Policy Association.

Hester, J., and I. Leveson. 1974. "The Health Insurance Study: A Critical Appraisal." *Inquiry* 11 (1): 53–60.

Hibbard, J. H., and J. J. Jewett. 1996. "What Type of Quality Information Do Consumers Want in a Health Care Report Card?" *Medical Care Research and Review* 53 (1): 28–47.

———. 1997. "Will Quality Report Cards Help Consumers?" *Health Affairs* 16 (3): 218–28.

Hibbard, J. H., J. J. Jewett, S. Engelmann, and M. Tusler. 1998. "Can

Medicare Beneficiaries Make Informed Choices?" *Health Affairs* 17 (6): 181–93.

Hibbard, J. H., P. Slovic, E. Peters, M. L. Finucane, and M. Tusler. 2001. "Is the Informed-Choice Policy Approach Appropriate for Medicare Beneficiaries?" *Health Affairs* 20 (3): 199–203.

Hibbard, J. H., S. Sofaer, and J. J. Jewett. 1996. "Condition-Specific Performance Information: Assessing Salience, Comprehension, and Approaches for Communicating Quality." *Health Care Financing Review* 18 (1): 95–109.

Hibbard, J. H., and E. C. Weeks. 1989a. "The Dissemination of Physician Fee Information: Impact on Consumer Knowledge, Attitudes, and Behaviors." *Journal of Health & Social Policy* 1 (1): 75–87.

———. 1989b. "Does the Dissemination for Comparative Data on Physician Fees Affect Consumer Use of Services?" *Medical Care* 27 (12): 1167–74.

High Committee on Public Health. 1998. *Health in France.* Montrogue: Editions John Libbey Eurotext.

High, J. 1991. *Regulation: Economic Theory and History.* Ann Arbor, MI: University of Michigan Press.

Hillman, A. L., M. V. Pauly, and J. J. Kerstein. 1989. "How Do Financial Incentives Affect Physicians' Clinical Decisions and the Financial Performance of Health Maintenance Organizations?" *The New England Journal of Medicine* 321 (1): 86–92.

Hillman, A. L., W. P. Welch, and M. V. Pauly. 1992. "Contractual Arrangements Between HMOs and Primary Care Physicians: Three-Tiered HMOs and Risk Pools." *Medical Care* 30 (2): 136–48.

Hoerger, T. J., and L. Z. Howard. 1995. "Search Behavior and Choice of Physician in the Market for Prenatal Care." *Medical Care* 33 (4): 332–49.

Hoffman, C., and A. Schlobohm. 2000. *Uninsured in America: A Chart Book.* Washington, DC: Kaiser Family Foundation.

Holahan, J., and W. Scanlon. 1979. "Physician Pricing in California: Price Controls, Physician Fees, and Physician Incomes from Medicare and Medicaid." *Grants and Contracts Report, Pub. No. 03006.* Washington, DC: Health Care Financing Administration.

House, J. S., K. R. Landis, and D. Umberson. 1999. "Social Relationships and Health." In *Income Inequality and Health,* edited by I. Kawachi, B. P. Kennedy, and R. G. Wilkinson. New York: New Press.

Hsiao, W. C., P. Braun, D. Yntema, and E. R. Becker. 1988. "Estimating Physicians' Work for a Resource-Based Relative Value Scale." *The New England Journal of Medicine* 319 (13): 835–41.

Hsiao, W. C. 1992. "Comparing Health Care Systems: What Nations

Can Learn from One Another." *Journal of Health Politics, Policy and Law* 17 (4): 613–36.

Hurley, J., and R. Labelle. 1995. "Relative Fees and the Utilization of Physicians' Services in Canada." *Health Economics* 4 (6): 419–38.

Hurley, J., R. Labelle, and T. Rice. 1990. "The Relationship Between Physician Fees and the Utilization of Medical Services in Ontario." *Advances in Health Economics and Health Services Research* 11: 49–78.

Hurley, J. 2002. Personal communication.

Iglehart, J. K. 2000a. "Revisiting the Canadian Health Care System." *The New England Journal of Medicine* 342 (26): 2007–12.

———. 2000b. "Restoring the Status of an Icon: A Talk with Canada's Minister of Health." *Health Affairs* 19 (3): 132–40.

Ikegami, N. 1991. "Japanese Health Care: Low Cost Through Regulated Fees." *Health Affairs* 10 (3): 87–109.

Ikegami, N., and J. C. Campbell. 1999. "Health Care Reform in Japan: The Virtues of Muddling Through." *Health Affairs* 18 (3): 56–75.

Imai, Y. 2002. "Health Care Reform in Japan." OECD Economics Department *Working Papers* No. 321. Paris: OECD.

Imai, Y., S. Jacobzone, and P. Lenain. 2000. "The Changing Health System in France." OECD Economics Department *Working Papers* No. 269. Paris: OECD.

Institute of Medicine. 2001. *Coverage Matters: Insurance and Health Care.* Washington, DC: National Academy Press.

Isaacs, S. L. 1996. "Consumers' Information Needs: Results of a National Survey." *Health Affairs* 15 (4): 31–41.

Jamison, D. T., and M. E. Sandbu. 2001. "WHO Rankings of Health System Performance." *Science* 293: 1595–96.

Jensen, G. A., and M. A. Morrisey. 1999. "Employer-Sponsored Health Insurance and Mandated Benefit Laws." *Milbank Quarterly* 77 (4): 425–59.

Jensen, G. A., M. A. Morrisey, S. Gaffney, and D. K. Liston. 1997. "The New Dominance of Managed Care: Insurance Trends in the 1990s." *Health Affairs* 16 (1): 125–36.

Jewett, J. J., and J. H. Hibbard. 1996. "Comprehension of Quality Indicators: Differences Among Privately Insured, Publicly Insured, and Uninsured." *Health Care Financing Review* 18 (1): 75–94.

Jonsson, B. 1989. "What Can Americans Learn from Europeans?" *Health Care Financing Review* 11 (Supplement): 79–109.

Judge, K. 1995. "Income Distribution and Life Expectancy: A Critical Appraisal." *British Medical Journal* 311: 1285–87.

Kahn, K. L., E. B. Keeler, M. J. Sherwood, et al. 1990. "Comparing Outcomes of Care Before and After Implementation of the DRG-Based Prospective Payment System." *JAMA* 264 (15): 1984–88.

Kaiser Family Foundation and Health Research and Educational Trust. 2000. *Employer Health Benefits: 2000 Annual Survey.* Washington, DC: Kaiser Family Foundation.

Kaplan, G. A., E. R. Pamuk, J. W. Lynch, R. D. Cohen, and J. L. Balfour. 1996. "Inequality in Income and Mortality in the United States: Analysis of Mortality and Potential Pathways." *British Medical Journal* 312 (7037): 999–1003.

Kawachi, I. 2000. "Income Inequality and Health." In *Social Epidemiology*, edited by L. F. Berman and I. Kawachi. New York: Oxford University Press.

Kawachi, I., and B. P. Kennedy. 1999. "Health and Social Cohesion: Why Care About Income Inequality?" In *Income Inequality and Health,* edited by I. Kawachi, B. P. Kennedy, and R. G. Wilkinson. New York: New Press.

———. 2001. "How Income Inequality Affects Health: Evidence from Research in the United States." In *Income, Socioeconomic Status, and Health: Exploring the Relationships,* edited by J. A. Auerbach and B. K. Krimgold. Washington, DC: National Policy Association.

Kawachi, I., B. P. Kennedy, and R. G. Wilkinson. 1999. *Income Inequality and Health.* New York: New Press.

Keeler, E. B. 1987. "Effect of Cost Sharing on Physiological Health, Health Practices, and Worry." *Health Services Research* 22 (3): 279–306.

Kennedy, B. P., I. Kawachi, and D. Prothrow-Stith. 1996. "Income Distribution and Mortality: Cross-Sectional Ecological Study of the Robin Hood Index in the United States." *British Medical Journal* 312: 1004–07.

Kirkman-Liff, B. L. 1990. "Physician Payment and Cost-Containment Strategies in West Germany: Suggestions for Medicare Reform." *Journal of Health Politics, Policy and Law* 15 (1): 69–100.

Koen, V. 2000. "Public Expenditure Reform: The Health Care Sector in the United Kingdom." OECD Economics Department *Working Papers* No. 256. Paris: OECD.

Kosecoff, J., K. L. Kahn, W. H. Rogers, et al. 1990. "Prospective Payment System and Impairment at Discharge: The 'Quicker-and-Sicker' Story Revisited." *JAMA* 264 (15): 1980–83.

Krasnik, A., P. P. Groenewegen, P. A. Pedersen, et al. 1990. "Changing Remuneration Systems: Effects on Activity in General Practice." *British Medical Journal* 300 (6741): 1698–1701.

Kronick, R., D. C. Goodman, and J. Wennberg. 1993. "The Marketplace in Health Care Reform: The Demographic Limitations of Managed Competition." *The New England Journal of Medicine* 328 (2): 148–52.

Kuttner, R. 1984. *The Economic Illusion: False Choices Between Prosperity and Social Justice.* Boston: Houghton Mifflin.

————. 1997. *Everything for Sale: The Virtue and Limits of Markets.* New York: Alfred A. Knopf.

Labelle, R., G. Stoddart, and T. Rice. 1994. "A Re-Examination of the Meaning and Importance of Supplier-Induced Demand." *Journal of Health Economics* 13 (3): 347–68.

Laeven. 2001. "Incentives and Waiting Lists: Interventions on Waiting Lists and Their Impact on Demand." Paper presented at the session, "Incentives for Reduced Waiting Times in Health Systems: A Comparison of Experiences in Different Countries," International Health Economics Association Third International Conference. York, UK, July 23.

Lancry, P. J., and S. Sandier. 1999. "Rationing Health Care in France." *Health Policy* 50 (1): 23–38.

Leape, L. 1989. "Unnecessary Surgery." *Health Services Research* 24 (3): 351–407.

Le Grand, J. 1992. "The Theory of Government Failure." *British Journal of Political Science* 21 (4): 423–42.

————. 1999. "Competition, Cooperation, or Control? Tales from the British National Health Service." *Health Affairs* 18 (3): 27–39.

Leibenstein, H. 1966. "Allocative Efficiency vs. 'X-Efficiency.'" *American Economic Review* 392–415.

————. 1976. *Beyond Economic Man.* Cambridge, MA: Harvard University Press.

Levit, K. R., H. Lazenby, D. R. Waldo, and L. M. Davidoff. 1985. "National Health Expenditures, 1984." *Health Care Financing Review* 7 (1): 1–35.

Levit, K., C. Smith, C. Cowan, H. Lazenby, and A. Martin. 2002. "Inflation Spurs Health Spending in 2000." *Health Affairs* 21 (1): 172–81.

Lieverdink, H. 2001. "The Marginal Success of Regulated Competition Policy in The Netherlands." *Social Science and Medicine* 52: 1183–94.

Light, D. W. 1995. "*Homo Economicus*: Escaping the Traps of Managed Competition." *European Journal of Public Health* 5 (3): 145–54.

————. 1997. "From Managed Competition to Managed Cooperation: Theory and Lessons from the British Experience." *Milbank Quarterly* 75 (3): 297–342.

————. 2001a. "Managed Competition, Governmentality and Institutional Response in the United Kingdom." *Social Science and Medicine* 52 (8): 1167–81.

————. 2001b. "Comparative Institutional Response to Economic Policy, Managed Competition and Governmentality." *Social Science and Medicine* 52 (8): 1151–66.

Lindsey, P. A., and J. P. Newhouse. 1990. "The Cost and Value of Second Surgical Opinion Programs: A Critical Review of the Literature." *Journal of Health Politics, Policy and Law* 15 (3): 543–70.

Lipsey, R. G., and K. Lancaster. 1956–1957. "The General Theory of the Second Best." *Review of Economic Studies* 24 (1): 11–32.

Little, I. M. D. 1957. *A Critique of Welfare Economics*. London: Oxford at the Clarendon Press, Oxford University Press.

Lohr, K. N., R. H. Brook, C. J. Kamberg, et al. 1986. "Effect of Cost Sharing on Use of Medically Effective and Less Effective Care." *Medical Care* 24 (Supplement): S31–S38.

Luft, H. S. 1973. "The Impact of Poor Health on Earnings." *Health Care Policy Discussion Paper No. 10*. Boston: Harvard Center for Community Health and Medical Care, Program on Health Care Policy, Harvard University.

———. 1978. *Poverty and Health*. Cambridge, MA: Ballinger.

———. 1981. *Health Maintenance Organizations: Dimensions of Performance*. New York: John Wiley.

———. 1997. Personal communication.

Luft, H. S., J. P. Bunker, and A. C. Enthoven. 1979. "Should Operations Be Regionalized? The Empirical Relation Between Surgical Volume and Mortality." *The New England Journal of Medicine* 301 (25): 1364–69.

Macinko, J., and B. Starfield. 2001. "The Utility of Social Capita in Research on Health Determinants." *Milbank Quarterly* 79 (3): 387–427.

Manning, W. G., A. Leibowitz, G. A. Goldberg, W. H. Rogers, and J. P. Newhouse. 1984. "A Controlled Trial of the Effect of a Prepaid Group Practice on Use of Services." *The New England Journal of Medicine* 310 (23): 1505–10.

Manning, W. G., J. P. Newhouse, N. Duan, E. B. Keeler, A. Leibowitz, and M. S. Marquis. 1987. "Health Insurance and the Demand for Medical Care: Evidence from a Randomized Experiment." *American Economic Review* 77 (3): 251–77.

Manning, W. G., and M. S. Marquis. 2001. "Health Insurance: Tradeoffs Revisited." *Journal of Health Economics* 20: 289–93.

Margolis, H. 1982. *Selfishness, Altruism, and Rationality*. Cambridge, UK: Cambridge University Press.

Marmor, T. R., and A. Dunham. 1983. "Political Science and Health Services Administration." In *Political Analysis and American Medical Care: Essays*, edited by T. R. Marmor, pp. 3–44. London: Cambridge University Press.

Marmot, M. G., H. Bosma, H. Hemingway, E. Brunner, and S. Stansfeld. 1997. "Contribution of Job Control and Other Risk Factors to Social Variations in Coronary Heart Disease Incidence." *Lancet* (350): 235–39.

Marquis, M. S., and G. F. Kominski. 1994. "Alternative Volume Performance Standards for Medicare Physicians' Services." *Milbank Quarterly* 72 (2): 329–57.

Marshall, A. 1920. *Principles of Economics.* London: Macmillan and Co.

McCarthy, T. R. 1985. "The Competitive Nature of the Primary Care Physician Services Market." *Journal of Health Economics* 4 (2): 93–117.

McClellan, M., and D. Kessler for the TECH Investigators. 1999. "A Global Analysis of Technological Change in Health Care: The Case of Heart Attacks." *Health Affairs* 18 (3): 250–55.

McGuire, T. G., and M. Pauly. 1991. "Physician Response to Fee Changes with Multiple Payers." *Journal of Health Economics* 10 (4): 385–410.

Mechanic, D. 1979. *Future Issues in Health Care.* New York: The Free Press, Macmillan and Co.

———. 1990. "The Role of Sociology in Health Affairs." *Health Affairs* 9 (1): 85–97.

Medicare Payment Advisory Commission. 2000. "Health Plans' Selection and Payment of Health Care Providers, 1999." Washington, DC: Medicare Payment Advisory Commission.

Mellor, J. M., and J. Milyo. 2001. "Reexamining the Evidence of an Ecological Association Between Income Inequality and Health." *Journal of Health Politics, Policy and Law* 26 (3): 487–521.

Menke, T. J., and N. P. Wray. 1999. "Cost Implications of Regionalizing Open Heart Surgery Units." *Inquiry* 36: 57–67.

Mennemeyer, S. T., M. A. Morrisey, and L. Z. Howard. 1997. "Death and Reputation: How Consumers Acted upon HCFA Mortality Information." *Inquiry* 34: 117–28.

Milgram, S. 1963. "Behavioral Study of Obedience." *Journal of Abnormal and Social Psychology* 67 (4): 371–78.

Miller, D. 1992. "Distributive Justice." *Ethics* 102 (April): 555–93.

Miller, M. E., W. P. Welch, and E. Englert. 1995. "Physicians Practicing in Hospitals: Implications for a Medical Staff Policy." *Inquiry* 32 (2): 204–10.

Miller, R. H. 1996. "Competition in the Health System: Good News and Bad News." *Health Affairs* 15 (2): 107–20.

Miller, R. H., and H. S. Luft. 1997. "Does Managed Care Lead to Better or Worse Quality of Care?" *Health Affairs* 16 (5): 7–25.

Minister of Health, Sweden. 2001. "Challenges to the Health Care of the Future: Summary and Translation of 'National Action Plan for the Development of Health Care.'" Gov. bill 1999/2000:149. Stockholm: Printing Works of the Riksdag Riksdagens Tryckeriexpedition.

Ministry of Health, Welfare and Sport, The Netherlands. 2000. "Health Insurance in The Netherlands." *International Publication Series,*

Health Welfare and Sport 1. The Hague: Ministry of Health, Welfare and Sport.

Mishan, E. J. 1969a. *Welfare Economics: Ten Introductory Essays*. New York: Random House.

———. 1969b. *Welfare Economics: An Assessment*. Amsterdam: North-Holland.

Mitchell, J. B., and F. Bentley. 2000. "Impact of Oregon's Priority List on Medicaid Beneficiaries." *Medical Care Research and Review* 57 (2): 216–34.

Mitchell, J. B., G. Wedig, and J. Cromwell. 1989. "The Medicare Physician Fee Freeze: What Really Happened?" *Health Affairs* 8 (1): 21–33.

Mitchell, J. M., J. Hadley, and D. J. Gaskin. 2000. "Physicians' Response to Medicare Fee Schedule Reductions." *Medical Care* 38 (10): 1029–39.

Mooney, G. 1994. *Key Issues in Health Economics*. New York: Harvester Wheatsheaf.

———. 1996a. "And Now for Vertical Equity? Some Concerns Arising from Aboriginal Health in Australia." *Health Economics* 5 (2): 99–103.

———. 1996b. "A Communitarian Critique of Health (Care) Economics." Presented at the inaugural meetings of the International Health Economics Association, Vancouver, British Columbia.

———. 1997. Personal communication.

Mooney, G., J. Hall, C. Donaldson, and K. Gerard. 1991. "Utilisation as a Measure of Equity: Weighing Heat?" *Journal of Health Economics* 10 (4): 475–80.

Mooney, G., and V. Wiseman. 2000. "World Health Report: Challenging a World View." *Journal of Health Services Research and Policy* 5 (4): 198–99.

Moore, F. C. 1877. *Fires: Their Causes, Prevention, and Extinction*. New York: F. C. Moore.

Morone, J. A. 2000. "Citizens or Shoppers? Solidarity Under Siege." *Journal of Health Politics, Policy and Law* 25 (5): 959–68.

Mueller, D. C. 1989. *Public Choice II*. Cambridge, UK: Cambridge University Press.

Muller, A. 2002. "Education, Income Inequality, and Mortality: A Multiple Regression Analysis." *British Medical Journal* 324 (1): 23–25.

Nath, S. K. 1969. *A Reappraisal of Welfare Economics*. London: Routledge & Kegan Paul.

National Health Policy Forum. 1995. *Consolidation in the Health Care Marketplace and Antitrust Policy*. Washington, DC: George Washington University.

Newhouse, J. P. 1974. "The Health Insurance Study: Response to Hester and Leveson." *Inquiry* 11 (3): 236–41.

———. 1978. *The Economics of Medical Care.* Reading, MA: Addison-Wesley.

———. 1993. *Free for All? Lessons from the* RAND *Health Insurance Experiment.* Cambridge, MA: Harvard University Press.

———. 1993. "An Iconoclastic View of Health Cost Containment." *Health Affairs* 12 (Supplement): 152–71.

———. 1994. "Patients at Risk: Health Reform and Risk Adjustment." *Health Affairs* 13 (1): 132–46.

Newhouse, J. P., G. Anderson, and L. L. Roos. 1988. "Hospital Spending in the United States and Canada: A Comparison." *Health Affairs* 7 (3): 6–24.

Newhouse, J. P., W. G. Manning, N. Duan, et al. 1987. "Findings of the RAND Health Insurance Experiment—A Response to Welch et al." *Medical Care* 25 (2): 157–79.

Ng, Y.-K. 1979. *Welfare Economics.* London: Macmillan and Co.

Nozick, R. 1974. *Anarchy, State, and Utopia.* New York: Basic Books.

Nyman, J. A. 1999a. "The Economics of Moral Hazard Revisited." *Journal of Health Economics* 18: 811–24.

———. 1999b. "The Value of Health Insurance: The Access Motive." *Journal of Health Economics* 18: 141–52.

OECD. 2001. "OECD Health Data 2001: A Comparative Analysis of 30 Countries." [CD-ROM.] Paris: OECD.

Ogden, D., R. Carlson, and G. Bernstein. 1990. "The Effect of Primary Care Incentives." In *Proceedings from the 1990 Group Health Institute.* Washington, DC: Group Health Association of America.

Okma, K. G. H. 1997. *Studies on Dutch Health Politics, Policies and Law.* Ph.D. Thesis, University of Utrecht, Germany.

———. 2001. "Health Care, Health Policies and Health Care Reforms in The Netherlands." *International Publication Series, Health Welfare and Sport* 7. The Hague: Ministry of Health, Welfare and Sport.

Olson, M. 1965. *The Logic of Collective Action.* Cambridge, MA: Harvard University Press.

Osler, M., E. Prescott, M. Gronbaek, et al. 2002. "Income Inequality, Individual Income, and Mortality in Danish Adults: Analysis of Pooled Data from Two Cohort Studies." *British Medical Journal* 324 (1): 13–15.

Parkin, M. 1999. *Microeconomics.* Reading, MA: Addison-Wesley.

Paul-Shaheen, P., J. D. Clark, and D. Williams. 1987. "Small Area Analysis: A Review and Analysis of the North American Literature." *Journal of Health Politics, Policy and Law* 12 (4): 741–809.

Pauly, M. V. 1968. "The Economics of Moral Hazard: Comment." *American Economic Review* 58 (4): 531–37.

———. 1978. "Is Medical Care Different?" In *Competition in the Health Care Sector: Past, Present, and Future,* edited by W. Greenberg, pp.

19–48. Washington, DC: Bureau of Economics, Federal Trade Commission.

———. 1996. "The Fall and Rise of Health Care Reform: A Dialogue." In *Looking Back, Looking Forward: "Staying Power" in Issues in Health Care Reform*, pp. 7–38. Washington, DC: Institute of Medicine.

———. 1997. "Who Was That Straw Man Anyway? A Comment on Evans and Rice." *Journal of Health Politics, Policy and Law* 22 (2): 467–73.

Peter, L., and R. Hull. 1969. *The Peter Principle.* New York: William Morrow.

Pfaff, M., and D. Wassener. 2000. "Germany." In: "Reconsidering the Role of Competition in Health Care Markets." *Journal of Health Politics, Policy and Law* 25 (5): 907–13.

Phelps, C. E. 1995. "Welfare Loss from Variations: Further Considerations." *Journal of Health Economics* 14 (2): 253–60.

———. 1997. *Health Economics.* New York: HarperCollins.

Phelps, C. E., and C. Mooney. 1992. "Correction and Update on Priority Setting in Medical Technology Assessment in Medical Care." *Medical Care* 30 (8): 744–51.

Phelps, C. E., and S. T. Parente. 1990. "Priority Setting in Medical Technology and Medical Practice Assessment." *Medical Care* 29 (8): 703–23.

Physician Payment Review Commission. 1993. *Annual Report to Congress.* Washington, DC: PPRC.

Pigou, A. C. 1932. *The Economics of Welfare*, 4th ed. London: Macmillan and Co.

Pollack, R. A. 1978. "Endogenous Tastes in Demand and Welfare Analysis." *American Economic Review* 68 (2): 374–79.

Pollack, D. A., B. H. McFarland, R. A. George, and R. H. Angell. 1994. "Prioritization of Mental Health Services in Oregon." *Milbank Quarterly* 72 (3): 515–50.

Poullier, J. P., and S. Sandier. 2000. "France." *Journal of Health Politics, Policy and Law* 25 (5): 899–905.

Preker, A. S., A. Harding, and P. Travis. 2000. " 'Make or Buy' Decisions in the Production of Health Care Goods and Services: New Insights from Institutional Economics and Organizational Theory." *Bulletin of the World Health Organization* 78 (6): 779–90.

Rawls, J. 1971. *A Theory of Justice.* Cambridge, MA: Belknap Press of Harvard University.

Reinhardt, U. E. 1978. "Comment on Paper by Frank A. Sloan and Roger Feldman." In *Competition in the Health Care Sector: Past, Present, and Future*, edited by W. Greenberg, pp. 156–90. Washington, DC: Bureau of Economics, Federal Trade Commission.

———. 1985. "The Theory of Physician-Induced Demand: Reflections After a Decade." *Journal of Health Economics* 4 (2): 187–93.

———. 1989. "Economists in Health Care: Saviors, or Elephants in a Porcelain Shop?" *American Economic Review Papers and Proceedings* 79 (2): 337–42.

———. 1992. "Reflections on the Meaning of Efficiency: Can Efficiency Be Separated from Equity?" *Yale Law & Policy Review* 10: 302–15.

———. 1994. "Germany's Health Care System: It's Not the American Way." *Health Affairs* 13 (4): 22–24.

———. 1996. "Comment on Mark Pauly." In *Looking Back, Looking Forward: "Staying Power" in Issues in Health Care Reform*, pp. 7–38. Washington, DC: Institute of Medicine.

———. 1998. "Abstracting from Distributional Effects, this Policy Is Efficient." In *Health, Health Care and Health Economics: Perspectives on Distribution*, edited by M. L. Barer, T. E. Getzen, and G. L. Stoddart. New York: John Wiley.

———. 2001. "Can Efficiency in Health Care Be Left to the Market?" *Journal of Health Politics, Policy and Law* 26 (5): 967–92.

Rice, N., and P. Smith. 1999. *Approaches to Capitation and Risk Adjustment in Health Care: An International Survey.* York, UK: University of York, Center for Health Economics.

———. 2001. "Capitation and Risk Adjustment in Health Care Financing: An International Progress Report." *Milbank Quarterly* 79 (1): 81–113.

Rice, T. H. 1983. "The Impact of Changing Medicare Reimbursement Rates on Physician-Induced Demand." *Medical Care* 21 (8): 803–15.

———. 1984. "Physician-Induced Demand for Medical Care: New Evidence from the Medicare Program." *Advances in Health Economics and Health Services Research* 5: 129–60.

———. 1992a. "An Alternative Framework for Evaluating Welfare Losses in the Health Care Market." *Journal of Health Economics* 11 (1): 88–92.

———. 1992b. "Containing Health Care Costs in the United States." *Medical Care Review* 49 (1): 19–65.

———. 1998. "The Case for Universal Coverage." In *The Future of the U.S. Healthcare System: Who Will Care for the Poor and Uninsured?* edited by S. H. Altman, U. E. Reinhardt, and A. E. Shields, pp. 387–404. Chicago: Health Administration Press.

———. 2001. "Should Consumer Choice Be Encouraged in Health Care?" In *Social Economics and Health Care*, edited by J. B. Davis. London: Routledge.

Rice, T., and J. Bernstein. 1990. "Volume Performance Standards: Can They Control Growth in Medicare Services?" *Milbank Quarterly* 68: 295–319.

————. 1999. "Supplemental Health Insurance for Medicare Beneficiaries." Medicare Brief No. 6. Washington, DC: National Academy of Social Insurance, November.

Rice, T., E. R. Brown, and R. Wyn. 1993. "Holes in the Jackson Hole Approach to Health Care Reform." *JAMA* 270 (11): 1357–62.

Rice, T., and K. A. Desmond. 2002. "An Analysis of Reforming Medicare Through a 'Premium Support' Program." Washington, DC: Kaiser Family Foundation.

Rice, T., B. Biles, E. R. Brown, F. Diderichsen, and H. Kuehn. 2000. "Reconsidering the Role of Competition in Health Care Markets." *Journal of Health Politics, Policy and Law* 25 (5): 863–73.

Rice, T. H., and R. J. Labelle. 1989. "Do Physicians Induce Demand for Medical Services?" *Journal of Health Politics, Policy and Law* 14 (3): 587–600.

Rice, T., and K. R. Morrison. 1994. "Patient Cost Sharing for Medical Services: A Review of the Literature and Implications for Health Care Reform." *Medical Care Review* 51 (3): 235–87.

Rice, T., and K. E. Thorpe. 1993. "Income-Related Cost Sharing in Health Insurance." *Health Affairs* 12 (1): 21–39.

Rizzo, J. A., and D. Blumenthal. 1996. "Is the Target Income Hypothesis an Economic Heresy?" *Medical Care Research and Review* 53 (3): 243–66.

Robbins, A. 2001. "WHO Ranking of Health Systems." [Letter to the editor.] *Science* 294: 1832–33.

Robbins, L. 1984. "Economics and Political Economy." In *An Essay on the Nature and Significance of Economic Science*, 3rd ed., pp. xi–xxxiii. London, Macmillan Press.

Robert Wood Johnson Foundation. 1994. *Annual Report: Cost Containment.* Princeton, NJ: RWJF.

Robinson, J. 1962. *Economic Philosophy.* Chicago: Aldine Publishing Company.

Robinson, J. C. 2001. "Theory and Practice in the Design of Physician Payment Incentives." *Milbank Quarterly* 79 (2): 149–77.

Robinson, J. C., and L. P. Casalino. 2001. "Reevaluation of Capitation Contracting in New York and California." [Online article.] *Health Affairs* http://www.healthaffairs.org

Rodgers, G. B. 1979. "Income and Inequality as Determinants of Mortality: An International Cross-Section Analysis." *Population Studies* 33: 343–51.

Rodwin, M. A. 1993. *Medicine, Money, and Morals: Physicians' Conflicts of Interest.* New York: Oxford University Press.

————. 1996. "Consumer Protection and Managed Care: The Need for Organized Consumers." *Health Affairs* 15 (3): 110–21.

———. 2001. "Consumer Voice and Representation in Managed Health-care." *Journal of Health Law* 34 (2): 233–76.

Roemer, J. E. 1994. *Egalitarian Perspectives.* Cambridge, MA: Cambridge University Press.

———. 1995. "Equality and Responsibility." *Boston Review* 20 (2): 3–7.

Roemer, M. I. 1991. *National Health Systems of the World: Volume One, The Countries.* New York: Oxford University Press.

Roos, L. L., E. S. Fisher, R. Brazauskas, S. M. Sharp, and E. Shapiro. 1992. "Health and Surgical Outcomes in Canada and the United States." *Health Affairs* 11 (2): 56–72.

Roos, N. P., L. L. Roos, M. Cohen, et al. 1990. "Postsurgical Mortality in Manitoba and New England." *JAMA* 263 (18): 2453–58.

Ross, L. D. 1988. "Situational Perspectives on the Obedience Experiments." *Contemporary Psychology* 33 (2): 101–104.

Ross, L., and R. E. Nisbett. 1991. *The Person and the Situation: Perspectives of Social Psychology.* Philadelphia: Temple University Press.

Rowley, C. K., and A. T. Peacock. 1975. *Welfare Economics: A Liberal Restatement.* New York: John Wiley.

Rubin, H. R., B. Gandek, W. H. Rogers, M. Kosinski, C. A. McHorney, and J. E. Ware, Jr. 1993. "Patients' Ratings of Outpatient Visits in Different Practice Settings: Results from the Medical Outcomes Study." *JAMA* 270 (7): 835–40.

Safran, D. G., A. R. Tarlov, and W. H. Rogers. 1994. "Primary Care Performance in Fee-for-Service and Prepaid Health Care Systems: Results from the Medical Outcomes Study." *JAMA* 271 (20): 1579–86.

Sagoff, M. 1986. "Values and Preferences." *Ethics* 96 (January): 301–16.

Salkeld, G., M. Ryan, and L. Short. 2000. "The Veil of Experience: Do Consumers Prefer What They Know Best?" *Health Economics* 9: 267–70.

Saltman, R. B., and J. Figueras. 1998. "Analyzing the Evidence on European Health Care Reforms." *Health Affairs* 17 (2): 85–108.

Samuelson, P. A. 1938. "A Note on the Pure Theory of Consumer Behavior." *Economica* 5 (17): 61–71.

———. 1947. *Foundations of Economic Analysis.* New York: Atheneum.

Sapolsky, R. M., S. C. Alberts, and J. Altmann. 1997. "Hypercortisolism Associated with Social Subordinance or Social Isolation Among Wild Baboons." *Archives of General Psychiatry* 54 (12): 1137–43.

Scheffler, R. M., S. D. Sullivan, and T. H. Ko. 1991. "The Impact of Blue Cross and Blue Shield Plan Utilization Management Programs 1980–1988." *Inquiry* 28 (3): 263–75.

Schieber, G. J., J. P. Poullier, and L. M. Greenwald. 1994. "Health System Performance in OECD Countries, 1980–1992." *Health Affairs* 13 (4): 100–12.

Schor, J. 1993. *The Overworked American: The Unexpected Decline of Leisure*. New York: Basic Books.

Schroeder, S. A. 1984. "Western European Responses to Physician Oversupply: Lessons for the United States." *JAMA* 252: 373–84.

Schuster, M. A., E. A., McGlynn, and R. H. Brook. 1998. "How Good Is the Quality of Health Care in the United States?" *Milbank Quarterly* 76 (4): 517–63.

Schut, F. T. 1995. "Health Care Reform in The Netherlands: Balancing Corporatism, Etatism, and Market Mechanisms." *Journal of Health Politics, Policy and Law* 20 (3): 615–52.

———. 2002. Personal communication, March 13.

Schweitzer, M., J. C. Hershey, and D. A. Asch. 1996. "Individual Choice in Spending Accounts: Can We Rely on Employees to Choose Well?" *Medical Care* 34 (6): 583–93.

Scitovsky, T. 1976. *The Joyless Economy*. New York: Oxford University Press.

Secretary of State for Health, England. 2000. *The NHS Plan*. London: HMSO.

Sen, A. K. 1970. *Collective Choice and Social Welfare*. San Francisco: Holden-Day.

———. 1982. *Choice, Welfare, and Measurement*. Oxford, UK: Basil Blackwell.

———. 1987. *On Ethics and Economics*. Oxford, UK: Basil Blackwell.

———. 1992. *Inequality Revisited*. Cambridge, MA: Harvard University Press.

Shapiro, M. F., J. E. Ware, Jr., and C. D. Sherbourne. 1986. "Effects of Cost Sharing on Seeking Care for Serious and Minor Symptoms." *Annals of Internal Medicine* 104 (2): 246–51.

Shain, M., and M. I. Roemer. 1959. "Hospital Costs Relate to the Supply of Beds." *Modern Hospital* (April): 71–73, 168.

Shibuya, K., H. Hashimoto, and E. Yano. 2002. "Individual Income, Income Distribution, and Self Rated Health in Japan: Cross Sectional Analysis of Nationally Representative Sample." *British Medical Journal* 324 (1): 16–19.

Shively, C. A., and T. B. Clarkson. 1994. "Social Status and Coronary Artery Atherosclerosis in Female Monkeys." *Arteriosclerosis and Thrombosis* 14: 721–26.

Sidgwick, H. 1887. *Principles of Political Economy*. London: MacMillan.

Siu, A. L., F. A. Sonnenberg, W. G. Manning, et al. 1986. "Inappropriate Use of Hospitals in a Randomized Trial of Health Insurance Plans." *The New England Journal of Medicine* 315 (20): 1259–66.

Sloan, F. A., and R. Feldman. 1978. "Competition Among Physicians." In *Competition in the Health Care Sector: Past, Present, and Future*, edited by W. Greenberg. Washington, DC: Bureau of Economics, Federal Trade Commission.

Smee, C. H. 1997. "Bridging the Gap Between Public Expectations and Public Willingness to Pay." *Health Economics* 6 (1): 1–9.

Smee, C. 2000. "United Kingdom." In: "Reconsidering the Role of Competition in Health Care Markets." *Journal of Health Politics, Policy and Law* 25 (5): 945–51.

Smith, A. 1776. *Wealth of Nations: An Inquiry into the Nature and Causes.* New York: Modern Library (reprinted in 1994).

Stanbury, W. T. 1986. *Business-Government Relations in Canada.* Toronto: Methuen.

Stano, M. 1985. "An Analysis of the Evidence on Competition in the Physician Services Market." *Journal of Health Economics* 4 (3): 197–211.

Stearns, S., B. Wolfe, and D. Kindig. 1992. "Physician Responses to Fee-for-Service and Capitation Payment." *Inquiry* 29 (4): 416–25.

Stevens, B., and J. Mittler. 2000. "Understanding and Meeting the Information Needs of Beneficiaries at the Local Level." Washington, DC: Mathematica Policy Research, Inc., November.

Stigler, G. J. 1971. "The Theory of Economic Regulation." *Bell Journal of Economics and Management Science* 2: 3–21.

Stigler, G. J., and G. S. Becker. 1977. "*De Gustibus Non Est Disputandum.*" *American Economic Review* 67 (2): 76–90.

Stoddart, G. L., M. L. Barer, and R. G. Evans. 1993. *User Changes, Snares, and Delusions: Another Look at the Literature.* Hamilton, Ontario: Centre for Health Economics and Policy Analysis, McMaster University.

Stone, D. A. 1996. *Policy Paradox: The Art of Political Decision-Making.* New York: Norton.

———. 2000. "United States." In: "Reconsidering the Role of Competition in Health Care Markets." *Journal of Health Politics, Policy and Law* 25 (5): 953–58.

Sturm, R., and C. R. Gresenz. 2002. "Relations of Income Inequality and Family Income to Chronic Medical Conditions and Mental Health Disorders: National Survey." *British Medical Journal* 324 (1): 20–22.

Sugden, R. 1993. "Welfare, Resources, and Capabilities: A Review of Inequality Reeexamined by Amartya Sen." *Journal of Economic Literature* 31: 1947–62.

Swedish Federation of County Councils. 2001. *Publicly Financed Ambulatory Care 2000.* Offentligt Finansierad Privat Öppen vård 2000 2001-11-15. [Online article.] http://www.lf.se/sek/tankstatistik.htm.

Tai-Seale, M., T. H. Rice, and S. C. Stearns. 1998. "Volume Response to Medicare Payment Reductions with Multiple Payers: A Test of the McGuire-Pauly Model." *Health Economics* 7: 199–219.

Technological Change in Health Care (TECH) Research Network. 2001. "Technological Change Around the World: Evidence from Heart Attack Care." *Health Affairs* 20 (3): 25–42.

Thaler, R. H. 1992. *The Winner's Curse: Paradoxes and Anomalies of Economic Life.* New York: Free Press, Macmillan and Co.

Thorpe, K. E. 1997. "The Health System in Transition: Care, Cost, and Coverage." *Journal of Health Politics, Policy and Law* 22 (2): 339–61.

Thurow, L. C. 1977. "Government Expenditures: Cash or In-Kind Aid?" In *Markets and Morals,* edited by G. Dworkin, G. Bermant, and P. G. Brow. Washington, DC: Hemisphere Publishing Corp.

———. 1980. *The Zero-Sum Society.* New York: Penguin Books.

———. 1983. *Dangerous Currents: The State of Economics.* New York: Random House.

Trude, S., and P. B. Ginsburg. 2000. "Are Defined Contributions a New Direction for Employer-Sponsored Coverage?" Issue Brief no. 32. Washington, DC: Center for Health System Change, October.

Tu, J. V., C. L. Pashos, C. D. Naylor, et al. 1997. "Use of Cardiac Procedures and Outcomes in Elderly Patients with Myocardial Infarction in the United States and Canada." *The New England Journal of Medicine* 336 (21): 1500–05.

Tullock, G. 1979. "Objectives of Income Redistribution." In *Sociological Economics,* edited by L. Levy-Garboua. Beverly Hills, CA: Sage Publications.

Tuohy, C. H. 1999. *Accidental Logics: The Dynamics of Change in the Health Care Arena in the United States, Britain, and Canada.* New York: Oxford University Press.

Tussing, A. D., and M. A. Wojtowycz. 1986. "Physician-Induced Demand by Irish GPs." *Social Science and Medicine* 23 (9): 851–60.

Tversky, A., and D. Kahneman. 1981. "The Framing of Decisions and the Psychology of Choice." *Science* 211 (30 January): 453–58.

University of California. 2001. *Getting the Most from Your Benefits Plan.* [Online report.] http://www.ucop.edu/bencom/hw/ygip/ygip2001.pdf.

U.S. Census Bureau. 2000. *Statistical Abstract of the United States: 2000.* [Online report.] http://www.census.gov/prod/2001pubs/statab/sec14.pdf.

———. 2001. *Statistical Abstract of the United Staes: 2001.* [Online report.] http://www.census.gov/prod/2002pubs/01statab/stat-ab01.html.

U.S. Department of Health and Human Services. 1999. *Health, United States, 1999 with Health and Aging Chartbook.* [Online report.] http://www.cdc.gov/nchs/data/hus/hus99.pdf.

————. 2000. *Health, United States, 2000, with Adolescent Health Chartbook.* [Online report.] http://www.cdc.gov/nchs/data/hus00.pdf.

————. 2001. *Health, United States, 2001, with Urban and Rural Chartbook.* [Online report.] http://www.cdc.gov/nchs/products/pubs/pubd/hus/hus.htm.

U.S. Department of Labor, Bureau of Labor Statistics. 2000. "Occupational Outlook Handbook." [Online report.] http://stats.bls.gov/oco/ocos074.htm.

U.S. General Accounting Office. 1994. *Cancer Survival: An International Comparison of Outcomes.* Washington, DC: GAO.

Valdez, R. O. 1986. *The Effects of Cost Sharing on the Health of Children.* Santa Monica, CA: RAND Corp.

van Doorslaer, E., and F. T. Schut. 2000. "Belgium and The Netherlands Revisited." In: "Reconsidering the Role of Competition in Health Care Markets." *Journal of Health Politics, Policy and Law* 25 (5):875–87.

van Doorslaer, E., A. Wagstaff, and F. Rutten. 1993. *Equity in the Finance and Delivery of Health Care: An International Perspective.* Oxford, UK: Oxford Medical Publications.

van Doorslaer, E., A. Wagstaff, H. van der Burg, et al. 1999. "The Redistributive Effect of Health Care Finance in Twelve OECD Countries." *Journal of Health Economics* 18 (3): 291–313.

Verrilli, D. K., R. Berenson, and S. J. Katz. 1998. "A Comparison of Cardiovascular Procedure Use Between the United States and Canada." *Health Services Research* 33 (3, Part I): 467–87.

Vining, A. R., and D. L. Weimer. 1990. "Government Supply and Government Production Failure: A Framework Based on Contestability." *Journal of Public Policy* 10 (1): 1–22.

Vladeck, B. C. 1990. *Simple, Elegant, and Wrong.* New York: United Hospital Fund.

Voltaire, F.-M. A. 1759. *Candide.* Translated by L. Bair. New York: Bantam Books.

Wagstaff, A., E. van Doorslaer, S. Calonge, et al. 1992. "Equity in the Finance of Health Care: Some International Comparisons." *Journal of Health Economics* 11 (4): 361–87.

Wagstaff, A., and E. van Doorslaer. 1993. "Equity in Finance and Delivery of Health Care: Concepts and Definitions." In *Equity in the Finance and Delivery of Health Care: An International Perspective,* edited by E. van Doorslaer, A. Wagstaff, and F. Rutten, pp. 7–19. Oxford, UK: Oxford Medical Publications.

————. 2000. "Income Inequality and Health: What Does the Literature Tell Us?" *Annual Review of Public Health* 21: 543–67.

Wagstaff A, E. van Doorslaer, H. van der Burg, et al. 1999. "Equity in the

Finance of Health Care: Some Further International Comparisons." *Journal of Health Economics* 18 (3): 263–90.

Ware, J. E., Jr., R. H. Brook, W. H. Rogers, et al. 1986. "Comparison of Health Outcomes at a Health Maintenance Organization with Those of Fee-for-Service Care." *Lancet* 1 (8488): 1017–22.

Ware, J. E., Jr., M. S. Bayliss, W. H. Rogers, M. Kosinski, and A. R. Tarlov. 1996. "Differences in 4-Year Health Outcomes for Elderly and Poor, Chronically Ill Patients Treated in HMO and Fee-for-Service Systems: Results from the Medical Outcomes Study." *JAMA* 276 (13): 1039–47.

Weaver, R. K., and B. A. Rockman. 1993. "When and How Do Institutions Matter?" In *Do Institutions Matter?* edited by R. K. Weaver and B. A. Rockman. Washington, DC: Brookings Institution.

Wedig, G., J. B. Mitchell, and J. Cromwell. 1989. "Can Price Controls Induce Optimal Physician Behavior?" *Journal of Health Politics, Policy and Law* 14 (3): 601–20.

Weisbrod, B. A. 1978. "Comment on Paper by Mark Pauly." In: *Competition in the Health Care Sector: Past, Present, and Future*, edited by W. Greenberg, pp. 49–56. Washington, DC: Bureau of Economics, Federal Trade Commission.

Welch, B. L., J. W. Hay, D. S. Miller, R. J. Olsen, R. M. Rippey, and A. S. Welch. 1987. "The RAND Health Insurance Study: A Summary Critique." *Medical Care* 25 (2): 148–56.

Welch, W. P., A. L. Hillman, and M. V. Pauly. 1990. "Toward New Topologies for HMOs." *Milbank Quarterly* 68 (2): 221–43.

Wennberg, J., and A. Gittlesohn. 1982. "Variations in Medical Care Among Small Areas." *Scientific American* 246 (4): 120–34.

White, J. 1995. *Competing Solutions: American Health Care Proposals and International Experience.* Washington, DC: Brookings Institution.

Wickizer, T. M., and D. Lessler. 1998. "Effects of Utilization Management on Patterns of Hospital Care Among Privately Insured Adult Patients." *Medical Care* 36 (11): 1545–54.

Wickizer, T. M., R. C. Wheeler, and P. J. Feldstein. 1989. "Does Utilization Review Reduce Unnecessary Hospital Care and Contain Costs?" *Medical Care* 27 (6): 632–47.

Wilensky, G. R., and L. F. Rossiter. 1983. "The Relative Importance of Physician-Induced Demand in the Demand for Medical Care." *Milbank Memorial Fund Quarterly* 61 (2): 252–77.

Wiley, M. 2002. Personal communication. February.

Wilhelm-Schwartz, F., and R. Busse. 1997. "Germany." In *Health Care Reform: Learning From International Experience*, edited by C. Ham. Philadelphia: Open University Press.

Wilkinson, R. G. 1999. "Income Inequality, Social Cohesion, and Health: Clarifying the Theory—A Reply to Muntaner and Lynch." *International Journal of Health Services* 29 (3): 525–43.

Willcox, S. 2001. "Promoting Private Health Insurance in Australia." *Health Affairs* 20 (3): 152–61.

Williams, A. 1997. "Intergenerational Equity: An Exploration of the 'Fair Innings' Argument." *Health Economics* 6 (2): 117–32.

Williams, B. 1962. "The Idea of Equality." In *Philosophy, Politics, and Society,* 2nd ed., edited by P. Laslett and W. G. Runciman. Oxford, UK: Blackwell.

Wolf, C., Jr. 1979. "A Theory of Nonmarket Failure: Framework for Implementation Analysis." *Journal of Law and Economics* 22 (1): 107–39.

———. 1993. *Markets or Governments: Choosing Between Imperfect Alternatives.* Cambridge, MA: MIT Press.

Wolfe, P. R., and D. W. Moran. 1993. "Global Budgeting in the OECD Countries." *Health Care Financing Review* 14 (3): 55–76.

World Health Organization. 1997. *Highlights on Health in France.* European Commission, WHO Regional Office for Europe.

———. 2000. *Health Systems: Improving Performance.* Geneva: WHO.

———. 2001. *Highlights on Health in Switzerland.* Copenhagen: WHO Regional Office for Europe.

Yip, W. C. 1998. "Physician Response to Medicare Fee Reductions: Changes in the Volume of Coronary Artery Bypass Graft (CABG) Surgeries in the Medicare and Private Sectors." *Journal of Health Economics* 17 (6): 675–99.

Yip, W. C., and W. C. Hsiao. 1997. "Medical Savings Accounts: Lessons from China." *Health Affairs* 16 (6): 244–51.

Yoshikawa, A., and J. Bhattacharya. 2002. "Japan." In *World Health Systems: Challenges and Perspectives,* edited by B. J. Fried and L. M. Gaydos, pp. 249–66. Chicago: Health Administration Press.

Young, H. P. 1994. *Equity in Theory and Practice.* Princeton, NJ: Princeton University Press.

Zabinski, D., T. M. Selden, J. F. Moeller, and J. S. Banthin. 1999. "Medical Savings Accounts: Microsimulation Results from a Model with Adverse Selection." *Journal of Health Economics* 18 (2): 195–218.

Zwanziger, J., and G. A. Melnick. 1996. "Can Managed Care Plans Control Health Care Costs?" *Health Affairs* 15 (2): 185–99.

Zweifel, P. 2000. "Switzerland." In: "Reconsidering the Role of Competition in Health Care Markets." *Journal of Health Politics, Policy and Law* 25 (5): 937–44.

Index

About the Author

THOMAS RICE, PH.D., is professor and former chair of the Department of Health Services at the UCLA School of Public Health, and past editor of the journal, *Medical Care Research and Review*. Dr. Rice received his doctorate in economics at the University of California at Berkeley in 1982. He served on the faculty at the University of North Carolina School of Public Health from 1983 to 1991, when he joined UCLA. Dr. Rice has published widely on issues such as competition and regulation in health services, physicians' economic behavior, cost containment, health insurance, and the Medicare program. In 1988, he received the Association for Health Services Research (AHSR) Young Investigator Award, given to the outstanding health services researcher in the United States age 35 or under. In 1992, he received the Thompson Prize from the Association of University Programs in Health Administration, awarded annually to the outstanding health services researcher in the country age 40 or under. In 1998, he received the Article-of-the-Year Award from the Academy for Health Services Research and Health Policy for a piece published in the *Journal of Health Politics, Policy and Law*, which formed the basis of Chapters 2 and 3 of this book.